Pharmacologic Therapy

Editors

KIM M. O'CONNOR
DOUGLAS S. PAAUW

MEDICAL CLINICS
OF NORTH AMERICA

www.medical.theclinics.com

Consulting Editors
DOUGLAS S. PAAUW
EDWARD R. BOLLARD

July 2016 • Volume 100 • Number 4

ELSEVIER

1600 John F. Kennedy Boulevard • Suite 1800 • Philadelphia, Pennsylvania, 19103-2899

http://www.theclinics.com

MEDICAL CLINICS OF NORTH AMERICA Volume 100, Number 4
July 2016 ISSN 0025-7125, ISBN-13: 978-0-323-44848-2

Editor: Jessica McCool
Developmental Editor: Alison Swety

Medical Clinics of North America (ISSN 0025-7125) is published bimonthly by Elsevier Inc., 360 Park Avenue South, New York, New York 10010-1710. Months of publication are January, March, May, July, September, and November. Business and editorial offices: 1600 John F. Kennedy Boulevard, Suite 1800, Philadelphia, PA 19103-2899. Periodicals postage paid at New York, NY, and additional mailing offices. Subscription prices are USD $260.00 per year (US individuals), $531.00 per year (US institutions), $100.00 per year (US Students), $320.00 per year (Canadian individuals), $690.00 per year (Canadian institutions), $200.00 per year (Canadian and foreign students), $390.00 per year (foreign individuals), and $690.00 per year (foreign institutions). To receive student/resident rate, orders must be accompanied by name of affiliated institution, date of term, and the signature of program/residency coordinator on institution letterhead. Orders will be billed at individual rate until proof of status is received. Foreign air speed delivery is included in all Clinics' subscription prices. All prices are subject to change without notice. **POSTMASTER:** Send address changes to *Medical Clinics of North America*, Elsevier Health Sciences Division, Subscription Customer Service, 3251 Riverport Lane, Maryland Heights, MO 63043. **Customer Service: Telephone: 1-800-654-2452** (U.S. and Canada); **1-314-447-8871** (outside U.S. and Canada). **Fax: 314-447-8029. E-mail: journalscustomerserviceusa@elsevier.com** (for print support); **journalsonlinesupport-usa@elsevier.com** (for online support).

Reprints. For copies of 100 or more of articles in this publication, please contact the Commercial Reprints Department, Elsevier Inc., 360 Park Avenue South, New York, NY 10010-1710. Tel.: 212-633-3874; Fax: 212-633-3820; E-mail: reprints@elsevier.com.

Medical Clinics of North America is also published in Spanish by McGraw-Hill Interamericana Editores S. A., P.O. Box 5-237, 06500 Mexico, D.F., Mexico.

Medical Clinics of North America is covered in *MEDLINE/PubMed (Index Medicus), Current Contents, ASCA, Excerpta Medica, Science Citation Index, and ISI/BIOMED.*

PROGRAM OBJECTIVE

The goal of the *Medical Clinics of North America* is to keep practicing physicians up to date with current clinical practice by providing timely articles reviewing the state of the art in patient care.

TARGET AUDIENCE

All practicing physicians and other healthcare professionals.

LEARNING OBJECTIVES

Upon completion of this activity, participants will be able to:

1. Review pharmacologic options for musculoskeletal, rheumatologic, pulmonary, and cardiovascular disorders.
2. Discuss pharmacologic therapies for men's and women's health.
3. Recognize recently approved pharmacologic agents.

ACCREDITATION

The Elsevier Office of Continuing Medical Education (EOCME) is accredited by the Accreditation Council for Continuing Medical Education (ACCME) to provide continuing medical education for physicians.

The EOCME designates this enduring material for a maximum of 15 *AMA PRA Category 1 Credit*(s)™. Physicians should claim only the credit commensurate with the extent of their participation in the activity.

All other health care professionals requesting continuing education credit for this enduring material will be issued a certificate of participation.

DISCLOSURE OF CONFLICTS OF INTEREST

The EOCME assesses conflict of interest with its instructors, faculty, planners, and other individuals who are in a position to control the content of CME activities. All relevant conflicts of interest that are identified are thoroughly vetted by EOCME for fair balance, scientific objectivity, and patient care recommendations. EOCME is committed to providing its learners with CME activities that promote improvements or quality in healthcare and not a specific proprietary business or a commercial interest.

The planning committee, staff, authors and editors listed below have identified no financial relationships or relationships to products or devices they or their spouse/life partner have with commercial interest related to the content of this CME activity:

Caitlin Allen, MD; Matthew C. Altman, MD; John K. Amory, MD, MPH; Andrew G. Ayars, MD; Alison M. Bays, MD, MPH&TM; Kathryn E. Berkseth, MD; Edward R. Bollard, MD, DDS, FACP; Ginger Evans, MD; Joana Lima Ferreira, MD; Rena K. Fox, MD; Anjali Fortna; Adrielle L. Fry, MD; Gregory Gardner, MD, FACP; Andrew W. Hahn, MD; Rupali Jain, PharmD; Anthony Julius, MD; Aley G. Kalapila, MD, PhD; Jared Wilson Klein, MD, MPH; Katelan Longfellow, MD; Melinda S. Loveless, MD; Leonard A. Mankin, MD, FACP; Jeanne Marrazzo, MD, MPH; Jessica McCool; Thiruvengadam Muniraj, MD, PhD; Premkumar Nandhakumar; Kim M. O'Connor, MD, FACP; Douglas S. Paauw, MD, MACP; David H. Spach, MD; Megan Suermann; Eliza L. Sutton, MD; Arthi Thirumalai, MBBS; Tracy S. Tylee, MD; Joyce E. Wipf, MD; Jennifer J. Wright, MD.

UNAPPROVED/OFF-LABEL USE DISCLOSURE

The EOCME requires CME faculty to disclose to the participants:

1. When products or procedures being discussed are off-label, unlabelled, experimental, and/or investigational (not US Food and Drug Administration [FDA] approved); and
2. Any limitations on the information presented, such as data that are preliminary or that represent ongoing research, interim analyses, and/or unsupported opinions. Faculty may discuss information about pharmaceutical agents that is outside of FDA-approved labelling. This information is intended solely for CME and is not intended to promote off-label use of these medications. If you have any questions, contact the medical affairs department of the manufacturer for the most recent prescribing information.

TO ENROLL

To enroll in the *Medical Clinics of North America* Continuing Medical Education program, call customer service at 1-800-654-2452 or sign up online at http://www.theclinics.com/home/cme. The CME program is available to subscribers for an additional annual fee of USD $295.

METHOD OF PARTICIPATION

In order to claim credit, participants must complete the following:

1. Complete enrolment as indicated above.
2. Read the activity.
3. Complete the CME Test and Evaluation. Participants must achieve a score of 70% on the test. All CME Tests and Evaluations must be completed online.

CME INQUIRIES/SPECIAL NEEDS

For all CME inquiries or special needs, please contact elsevierCME@elsevier.com.

MEDICAL CLINICS OF NORTH AMERICA

THE CLINICS ARE AVAILABLE ONLINE!
Access your subscription at:
www.theclinics.com

Contributors

CONSULTING EDITORS

DOUGLAS S. PAAUW, MD, MACP
Professor of Medicine, Division of General Internal Medicine, Rathmann Family Foundation Endowed Chair for Patient-Centered Clinical Education; Medicine Student Programs, Professor of Medicine, University of Washington School of Medicine, Seattle, Washington

EDWARD R. BOLLARD, MD, DDS, FACP
Professor of Medicine, Associate Dean of Graduate Medical Education, Designated Institutional Official, Department of Medicine, Penn State-Hershey Medical Center, Penn State University College of Medicine, Hershey, Pennsylvania

EDITORS

KIM M. O'CONNOR, MD, FACP
Associate Professor, Division of General Internal Medicine, Department of Medicine, Roosevelt General Internal Medicine Clinic, University of Washington School of Medicine and Medical Center, Seattle, Washington

DOUGLAS S. PAAUW, MD, MACP
Professor of Medicine, Division of General Internal Medicine, Rathmann Family Foundation Endowed Chair for Patient-Centered Clinical Education; Medicine Student Programs, Professor of Medicine, University of Washington School of Medicine, Seattle, Washington

AUTHORS

CAITLIN ALLEN, MD
Resident Physician, Department of Medicine, University of Wisconsin School of Medicine and Public Health, Madison, Wisconsin

MATTHEW C. ALTMAN, MD
Division of Allergy and Infectious Diseases, University of Washington School of Medicine; Center for Allergy and Inflammation, UW Medicine at South Lake Union, Seattle, Washington

JOHN K. AMORY, MD, MPH
Professor, Department of Medicine, University of Washington, Seattle, Washington

ANDREW G. AYARS, MD
Division of Allergy and Infectious Diseases, University of Washington School of Medicine; Center for Allergy and Inflammation, UW Medicine at South Lake Union, Seattle, Washington

ALISON M. BAYS, MD, MPH&TM
Acting Instructor, Division of Rheumatology, Department of Internal Medicine, Harborview Medical Center, Seattle, Washington

KATHRYN E. BERKSETH, MD
Division of Metabolism, Endocrinology and Nutrition, Acting Instructor, Department of Medicine, University of Washington, Seattle, Washington

GINGER EVANS, MD
Acting Assistant Professor, Department of Medicine, VA Puget Sound Health Care System, University of Washington, Seattle, Washington

JOANA LIMA FERREIRA, MD
Clinical Instructor, Division of General Internal Medicine, Department of Medicine, University of Washington, Seattle, Washington

RENA K. FOX, MD
Professor of Medicine, Division of General Internal Medicine, Department of Medicine, University of California, San Francisco, San Francisco, California

ADRIELLE L. FRY, MD
Sports Medicine Fellow, Department of Rehabilitation Medicine, University of Washington, Seattle, Washington

GREGORY GARDNER, MD, FACP
Division of Rheumatology, Professor, Department of Internal Medicine, University of Washington, Seattle, Washington

ANDREW W. HAHN, MD
Infectious Diseases Fellow, Division of Infectious Diseases, University of Washington School of Medicine, Seattle, Washington

RUPALI JAIN, PharmD
Clinical Associate Professor, University of Washington School of Pharmacy, Seattle, Washington

ANTHONY JULIUS, MD
VA Puget Sound, University of Washington Medical Center, Seattle, Washington

ALEY G. KALAPILA, MD, PhD
Assistant Professor, Division of Infectious Diseases, Department of Medicine, Emory University School of Medicine, Atlanta, Georgia

JARED WILSON KLEIN, MD, MPH
Division of General Internal Medicine, Department of Medicine, Clinical Instructor, Harborview Medical Center, University of Washington, Seattle, Washington

KATELAN LONGFELLOW, MD
VA Puget Sound, University of Washington Medical Center, Bothell, Washington

MELINDA S. LOVELESS, MD
Clinical Assistant Professor, Department of Rehabilitation Medicine, University of Washington, Seattle, Washington

LEONARD A. MANKIN, MD, FACP
Associate Professor of Medicine, Oregon Health and Science University, Legacy Health, Portland, Oregon

JEANNE MARRAZZO, MD, MPH
Professor of Medicine; Director, Division of Infectious Diseases, University of Alabama at Birmingham, Birmingham, Alabama

THIRUVENGADAM MUNIRAJ, MD, PhD
Advanced Endoscopy Fellow, Division of Gastroenterology, Department of Medicine, Yale University School of Medicine, New Haven, Connecticut

KIM M. O'CONNOR, MD, FACP
Associate Professor, Division of General Internal Medicine, Department of Medicine, Roosevelt General Internal Medicine Clinic, University of Washington School of Medicine and Medical Center, Seattle, Washington

DAVID H. SPACH, MD
Professor of Medicine, Division of Infectious Diseases, University of Washington School of Medicine, Seattle, Washington

ELIZA L. SUTTON, MD
Associate Professor, Department of Medicine, Medical Director, Women's Health Care Center, University of Washington, Seattle, Washington

ARTHI THIRUMALAI, MBBS
Division of Metabolism, Endocrinology and Nutrition, Acting Instructor and Senior Fellow, Department of Medicine, University of Washington, Seattle, Washington

TRACY S. TYLEE, MD
Clinical Assistant Professor of Medicine, Department of Medicine, Division of Metabolism, Endocrinology and Nutrition, Endocrine and Diabetes Care Center, University of Washington, Seattle, Washington

JOYCE E. WIPF, MD
Section Chief of General Internal Medicine; Director, Center of Excellence in Primary Care Education, Seattle VA Puget Sound Health Care System, Professor of Medicine, University of Washington, Seattle, Washington

JENNIFER J. WRIGHT, MD
Assistant Professor, Department of Medicine, Division of General Internal Medicine, University of Washington, Seattle, Washington

Contents

alpha1-adrenergic antagonists, 5-alpha-reductase inhibitors, anticholinergic agents, and herbal therapies in the management of BPH.

As the population ages, the rates of osteoporotic fractures will increase, with postmenopausal women incurring most of these fractures. Diagnosis and treatment of osteoporosis are extremely important. Dual-energy x-ray absorptiometry scan screening is recommended in all women more than 65 years of age or in women aged 50 to 64 years with certain risk factors. Treatment should be considered if osteoporosis is present, there is a history of fragility fracture, or in the setting of osteopenia plus high risk for fracture.

Several key areas in gastroenterology pharmacotherapy are rapidly evolving, including the treatment of hepatitis C virus (HCV), irritable bowel syndrome, gastroesophageal reflux disease (GERD), and peptic ulcer disease. HCV treatment has radically changed in the past 2 years and now most patients are treatment candidates and have a high likelihood of permanent cure. Pharmacotherapy is now first-line treatment for patients with moderate to severe symptoms of irritable bowel syndrome. Proton pump inhibitors (PPIs) are the mainstay of therapy in gastric and duodenal ulcers and GERD, although long-term use carries the risk of several side effects that should be considered.

Conditions such as chronic rhinitis, urticaria, angioedema, and asthma are frequently seen in clinics and hospitals, and there are a core group of medications that are often used to treat these conditions. Knowing the indications, optimal dosing, and side-effect profile of these medications can improve outcomes. Chronic rhinitis due to various causes is one of the most common reasons for primary care physician visits. Knowing the indications for use, forms of administration, and side-effect profiles of these medications can help improve patient outcomes in these common conditions. This article focuses on the medications used to treat these conditions.

Musculoskeletal conditions are common, and there are many options for pharmacologic therapy. Unfortunately, there is not strong evidence for the use of many of these medications. Acetaminophen and nonsteroidal anti-inflammatory drugs (NSAIDs) are generally first-line medications for most musculoskeletal pain, but there is more evidence these medications are not as safe as once thought. Other analgesic and antispasmodic medications can be effective for acute pain but generally are not as effective for chronic pain. Antidepressants and anticonvulsants can be more effective for chronic or neuropathic pain. Topical formulations of NSAIDs can be effective for pain with fewer side effects.

This article reviews the current pharmacotherapy options available for the treatment of patients with substance use disorders. In the United States there are medications available to treat tobacco use disorders (nicotine replacement, bupropion, and varenicline), alcohol use disorders (naltrexone and acamprosate), and opioid use disorders (methadone and buprenorphine). These medications are likely underused and physicians should more readily prescribe for eligible patients.

Antimicrobial drug-resistance continues to force adaptation in our clinical practice. We explore new evidence regarding adjunctive antibiotic therapy for skin and soft tissue abscesses as well as duration of therapy for intra-abdominal abscesses. As new evidence refines optimal practice, it is essential to support clinicians in adopting practice patterns concordant with evidence-based guidelines. We review a simple approach that can 'nudge' clinicians towards concordant practices. Finally, the use of novel antimicrobials will play an increasingly important role in contemporary therapy. We review five new antimicrobials recently FDA-approved for use in drug-resistant infections: dalbavancin, oritavancin, ceftaroline, ceftolozane-tazobactam, and ceftazidime-avibactam.

Human immunodeficiency virus (HIV) infection is considered a chronic medical condition. Several new drugs are available, including fixed-dose combination tablets, that have greatly simplified combination antiretroviral therapy (ART) regimens to treat HIV, while increasing the life-expectancy of infected individuals. In the last decade, multiple well-regarded studies have established the benefits of using ART in high-risk, HIV-negative persons to prevent HIV acquisition. The primary care provider must not only understand commonly encountered issues pertaining to ART, such as toxicities and drug interactions, but also needs to be aware of using ART for HIV prevention.

Foreword

Pharmacologic Therapy

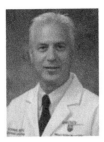

Edward R. Bollard, MD, DDS, FACP
Consulting Editor

Recent studies have continued to demonstrate that over two-thirds of Americans are currently taking prescription medications. Fifty percent of the population is taking at least two prescription drugs, and these numbers are considerably higher in our patients over the age of 65 years. The field of pharmacotherapeutics continues to expand, and the choice of medications to treat the variety of medical and psychiatric conditions is increasing in number while becoming more "personized" in their application. More than ever, it has become essential that the practicing clinician have an understanding of the pharmacology of these drugs, their indications for usage, and most importantly, the potential drug interactions and adverse side effects that they may pose.

In this issue of *Medical Clinics of North America*, Dr Kim M. O'Connor and Dr Douglas S. Paauw have assembled an extraordinary cohort of expert authors that provide the necessary overview of the pharmacotherapy that would apply to the patients seen by both primary care physicians and specialists in care. The topics range from the most recent updates in the management of hypertension and diabetes mellitus to the new oral anticoagulant agents and the advancing field of immunosuppressive therapy and immune-modulating agents.

Although development of the software for our electronic medical records continues to evolve in reference to the "alerts" we are provided when we prescribe medications, they will never replace the deeper understanding of what would be the "right medication for my particular patient." I believe you will find that the following articles in

Med Clin N Am 100 (2016) xv–xvi
http://dx.doi.org/10.1016/j.mcna.2016.04.003
0025-7125/16/$ – see front matter © 2016 Published by Elsevier Inc.

"Pharmacologic Therapy" provide the detailed understanding as well as the practical information necessary to make these decisions.

Edward R. Bollard, MD, DDS, FACP
Department of Medicine
Penn State–Hershey Medical Center
Penn State University College of Medicine
500 University Drive
PO Box 850 (Mail Code H039)
Hershey, PA 17033-0850, USA

E-mail address:
ebollard@hmc.psu.edu

Preface

Pharmacologic Therapies: Updates and Clinical Pearls

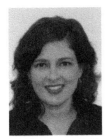 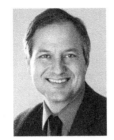

Kim M. O'Connor, MD, FACP   Douglas S. Paauw, MD, MACP
Editors

As health care providers, a large proportion of our clinical encounters focuses on the prescribing of pharmaceuticals. The evaluation and diagnosis of common clinical conditions have not changed significantly over time; however, novel pharmaceuticals and new uses for old drugs are developing at an alarming rate. In addition, since the institution of direct-to-consumer advertising in 1997, patients frequently request specific medications to treat their medical conditions. As a result, practicing providers are required to be up-to-date on new medications, their appropriate clinical uses, side effects, and drug interactions. For many care providers, the symptoms and illness that a patient presents with are manifestations of medication side effects. This issue focuses on common medical conditions encountered in a primary care practice or inpatient medicine service. The aim of this issue is not on diagnosis and evaluation but rather on the appropriate use and monitoring of medications. The issue focuses on a number of areas that have experienced rapid change and where the physician needs to have access to current, specific pharmacologic knowledge. A few examples of these are:

- Anticoagulant management of venous thromboembolism and nonvalvular atrial fibrillation has changed dramatically over the past few years with the introduction of numerous direct oral anticoagulants. Understanding the appropriate candidates for these medications, risks, and contraindications can be challenging.
- Hepatitis C is the leading cause of liver-related death, hepatocellular cancer, and liver transplant. In the past, treatments for hepatitis C were extremely toxic and poorly efficacious. The treatment of hepatitis C has dramatically changed since the development of direct-acting antivirals, with cure rates exceeding 90% and low risk for toxicities.
- The management of chronic pain is a common occurrence in most primary care practices with an estimated 20% of patients receiving an opioid prescription. As the rate of opioid prescriptions increased, so did the development of opioid use

Med Clin N Am 100 (2016) xvii–xviii
http://dx.doi.org/10.1016/j.mcna.2016.04.002
0025-7125/16/$ – see front matter © 2016 Published by Elsevier Inc.

disorders and opioid-related overdose deaths. In March 2016, the Centers for Disease Control and Prevention released guidelines for prescribing opioids for the management of chronic pain. Outside of treatment for patients with active cancer, palliative, or end-of-life care, the recommendation is to use nonopioid therapy when at all possible. This issue reviews nonopioid treatment options for common pain conditions as well as treatment options for substance use disorders.

- As life expectancy for patients living with HIV has caught up with the general population, many patients living with HIV will engage with primary care providers for routine health care maintenance and common medical conditions. Consequently, it is imperative that primary care providers are familiar with potential drug interactions and toxicities related to combination antiviral therapy. Robust data also support the use of pre-exposure prophylaxis with daily Tenofovir/Emtricitabine in patients at high risk for HIV acquisition. Providers will be called on to prescribe pre-exposure prophylaxis.

All the articles in this issue focus on an easy-to-use approach to equip the provider with information, prescribing pearls, and what to watch for in regard to drug interactions and side effects of different pharmacologic therapies. We are grateful to the educators and clinicians who contributed outstanding articles to this issue. We hope that this issue helps distill a large amount of rapidly changing information on pharmacologic therapy into a useful, clinically relevant text.

Kim M. O'Connor, MD, FACP
Division of General Internal Medicine
Department of Medicine
University of Washington School of Medicine
4245 Roosevelt Way NE
Box 354760
Seattle, WA 98105, USA

Douglas S. Paauw, MD, MACP
Division of General Internal Medicine
Department of Medicine
University of Washington School of Medicine
1959 NE Pacific Street
Seattle, WA 98195-6429, USA

E-mail addresses:
koconnor@uw.edu (K.M. O'Connor)
dpaauw@uw.edu (D.S. Paauw)

Pharmacologic Therapy of Type 2 Diabetes

Jennifer J. Wright, MD[a],*, Tracy S. Tylee, MD[b]

KEYWORDS

- Type 2 diabetes • Metformin • Sulfonylurea • Insulin • GLP-1 analog
- DPP-4 inhibitor • SGLT-2 inhibitor

KEY POINTS

- For glycemic control, metformin is the optimal first-line therapy for most patients.
- There are many issues to consider when deciding on additional therapies, including: effects on blood sugar lowering, weight, risk of hypoglycemia, costs, and route of administration.
- In patients with renal impairment, some medications have more pronounced adverse effects, and some are contraindicated.
- Elderly patients often need adjustment in their diabetes regimens due to less aggressive glucose lowering goals, and increased sensitivity to adverse effects of certain medications.
- Do not to overlook important therapies that reduce the risk of cardiovascular disease, independent of blood sugar lowering, including statins, antihypertensives and aspirin.

INTRODUCTION

Type 2 diabetes (T2DM) is a common condition, affecting 9.3% of the US population in 2014, 21 million people with the diagnosis and an estimated 8.1 million people who are undiagnosed.[1] Treatment of diabetes and related complications can be complex. In addition to lifestyle changes, medications play an important role in controlling patients' blood glucose levels and preventing complications from diabetes including kidney failure, blindness, amputations, and heart disease. From an individual and societal standpoint, it is also an expensive disease. Medical spending attributed to diabetes per individual is significant. For a patient diagnosed at age 50, it is estimated that he or she will have an excess of $91,200 in medical spending over his or her lifetime compared to a matched individual without diabetes, with 44% of this spent on prescription medications.[2] With appropriate therapy, patients can lead full, healthy lives

---

Disclosure Statement: The authors have nothing to disclose.
[a] Department of Medicine, Division of General Internal Medicine, University of Washington, 4245 Roosevelt Way Northeast, Seattle, WA 98105, USA; [b] Department of Medicine, Division of Metabolism, Endocrinology and Nutrition, Endocrine and Diabetes Care Center, University of Washington, 4245 Roosevelt Way Northeast, Seattle, WA 98105, USA
* Corresponding author.
E-mail address: sonic@uw.edu

Med Clin N Am 100 (2016) 647–663
http://dx.doi.org/10.1016/j.mcna.2016.03.014
0025-7125/16/$ – see front matter © 2016 Elsevier Inc. All rights reserved.

with the disease, so making informed decisions regarding pharmacotherapy for T2DM is clearly of great importance.

Treatment in Context

Prior to discussing the various pharmacologic agents that can be used to manage diabetes, one must put the medications into the context of the clinical benefits of treatment. Microvascular complications of diabetes include retinopathy, neuropathy, and nephropathy. The UKPDS (UK Prospective Diabetes Study) trial was a landmark study in treatment of T2DM, finding a reduction in microvascular complications with HbA1c lowering in patients with newly diagnosed T2DM. Patients randomized to pharmacologic treatment achieving HbA1c lowering to 7% versus 7.9% in the control arm showed a significant 25% reduction in aggregate microvascular endpoints–retinopathy requiring photocoagulation, vitreous hemorrhage, and/or fatal or non-fatal renal failure.[3] Observational UKPDS follow-up studies found evidence of a legacy effect, with persistent reduction in microvascular complications in the years following the study, despite no long-term difference in glucose control between the 2 groups.[4]

Macrovascular complications of diabetes include cardiovascular disease (CVD) and cerebrovascular accidents (CVAs). A benefit of glucose-lowering therapy in reducing the risk of these complications is less clear. A notable study, which did find benefit, is the UKPDS series of studies.[3–5] In the overweight subgroup of the original UKPDS study, patients who were treated with metformin had a statistically significant reduction in myocardial infarction (39%) in addition to all-cause death (36%).[5] In the posttrial observational follow-up study, this reduction in coronary events and all-cause death persisted (33% and 27% RRR [relative risk reduction] respectively). As well, a long-term benefit of early treatment with insulin and sulfonylureas was found (15% RRR for myocardial infarction, and 13% RRR for all-cause death).[4] However, several subsequent long-term studies failed to show benefit with intensive blood glucose lowering. In fact, the ACCORD (Action to Control Cardiovascular Risk in Diabetes) trial was ended early because of an excess risk of all-cause death in the intensive treatment arm (hazard ratio [HR] 1.22).[6] In contrast to the UKPDS, participants in these trials had long-standing diabetes, with established CVD or CVD risk factors, suggesting that intensive glucose control early in the course of T2DM may be important for reducing CVD risk. **Table 1** has a summary.

From the standpoint of preventing microvascular and macrovascular complications of diabetes through improved glycemic control, there are several factors to consider.

Table 1 Landmark clinical trials assessing for macrovascular benefits of glycemic control in type 2 diabetes	
Long-Standing Poorly Controlled Type 2 Diabetes, Aggressive HbA1c Lowering	**Newly Diagnosed Patients with Type 2 Diabetes**
ACCORD: increase in all-cause death, no benefit/harm in: CV outcomes ADVANCE: no benefit/harm in CV outcomes VADT: no benefit/harm in CV outcomes during the trial, observational follow-up trial with reduction in CV events, although not CV or all-cause death	UKPDS 10 y follow-up: reduction in CV events and all-cause death with metformin treatment > insulin or sulfonylurea treatment

Abbreviations: ADVANCE, Action in diabetes and vascular disease: PreterAx and diamicron MR controlled evaluation; VADT, Veterans affairs diabetes trial.
Data from Refs.[5–8]

Regarding specific drug choice, metformin has the best evidence for the reduction of macrovascular complications. Regarding intensity of therapy, there may be both short-term microvascular benefits and long-term macrovascular benefits to more aggressive blood glucose lowering therapies early in a patient's disease course, but in older patients with long-standing diabetes and other cardiovascular risk factors, the benefit of aggressive blood glucose-lowering therapy is less clear. Current guidelines recommend HbA1C target of 6.5% to 7.0% for most patients, and there are many options for achieving these goals.[9,10] This article aims to provide some guidance on how best to use medications to achieve these goals.

ORAL AGENTS
Metformin

There is near universal agreement that metformin is first-line therapy for most patients with T2DM, with initiation of treatment considered at the time of diagnosis. In addition to the established cardiovascular benefits previously discussed, metformin has several other favorable characteristics. This medication leads to a decrease in hepatic gluconeogenesis with an increase in insulin sensitivity and glucose uptake at the level of the tissue. By virtue of this mechanism of action, metformin does not increase insulin levels and therefore cannot cause hypoglycemia. In contrast to other agents used to treat diabetes, metformin does not cause weight gain and is frequently associated with modest weight loss. In the UKPDS study, patients on both insulin and sulfonylureas gained weight, while those on metformin did not.[11] In addition, it is inexpensive and thus should be available to all patients, regardless of insurance coverage or finances.

Unfortunately there are several conditions that limit the use of metformin. The most common concern is the risk of lactic acidosis in the setting of renal insufficiency, leading to the US Food and Drug Administration (FDA) labeling indicating metformin should not be prescribed to males with creatinine $\geq$ 1.5 or females with creatinine $\geq$ 1.4. But, though metformin is renally cleared, drug levels remain in the therapeutic range even as renal function declines towards an eGFR of 30 mL/min per 1.73 m^2, and there is no evidence for an increase in lactate levels with decreasing renal function in patients taking metformin.[12] In addition, a Cochrane Systematic Review did not find evidence of an increased risk of lactic acidosis in patients prescribed metformin compared with diabetic patients on other medications.[13] Based on these developments, one could consider taking the approach outlined in **Table 2** in prescribing metformin to patients with renal insufficiency.[12]

Table 2
Use of metformin in patients with renal insufficiency

Chronic Kidney Disease Stage	eGFR mL/min/1.73 m^2	Maximum Daily Dose (mg)	Other Comments
1	$\geq$90	2550	—
2	60–<90	2550	—
3A	45–<60	2000	—
3B	30–<45	1000	Do not initiate therapy, but acceptable to continue at this reduced maximum dose
4 and 5	<30	Do not use	—

Adapted from Inzucchi SE, Lipska KJ, Mayo H, et al. Metformin in patients with type 2 diabetes and kidney disease: a systematic review. JAMA 2014;312(24):2668–75.

In addition to renal insufficiency, there are other conditions and situations in which metformin is not recommended, including significant liver dysfunction and unstable congestive heart failure, although it is safe to use in patients with stable congestive heart failure. In addition, there is increasing evidence that metformin is safe to use in patients with significant liver dysfunction with an observational study of diabetic patients on metformin subsequently diagnosed with cirrhosis, where continuation of metformin was associated with a 57% RRR in all-cause death.[14] Advanced age is also frequently cited as a reason a patient is not prescribed metformin, but this is actually a preferred agent in elderly patients.[15] Situations in which it is reasonable to hold metformin include hospitalized patients, as they are likely at risk of both fluctuations in renal profusion and lactic acidosis by virtue of the illness leading to their hospitalization, and patients undergoing contrast-enhanced computed tomography (CT) studies, as these frequently lead to temporary fluctuations in renal function. Metformin can safely be restarted 48 hours after completion of the contrast study.

Adverse effects more commonly associated with metformin use are gastrointestinal adverse effects including diarrhea, abdominal bloating, and intestinal gas. It is estimated that 25% of patients may experience these adverse effects. Strategies to reduce these symptoms include starting metformin at a low dose (500 mg daily) and slowly increasing the dose (every 3–7 days) by 500 mg intervals to a typical target dose of 1000 mg twice a day. If patients are intolerant of the immediate-release formulation, there is also an extended-release formulation, metformin ER, which can be dosed once a day and may have less severe gastrointestinal adverse effects because of the slower release and decreased peak drug levels.

Once a patient is on metformin, this medication should be continued indefinitely unless the patient develops a contraindication. Prescribers should be aware that in the setting of long-term metformin use, there is a risk of decreased vitamin B12 levels. In a randomized trial of patients with T2DM treated with insulin plus metformin or placebo, patients started on metformin had an increased risk of vitamin B12 deficiency, defined as a vitamin B12 level of less than 150 pmol/L (absolute risk increase of 7.2%, NNH [number needed to harm] 13.8 at 4.3 years) compared with patients in the control group.[16] The clinical implications of this are less clear, as studies have not assessed clinical outcomes. Should a patient on metformin therapy have symptoms concerning for vitamin B12 deficiency, including macrocytic anemia, cognitive impairment, or neuropathy, vitamin B12 testing should be performed.

Metformin can safely be used in combination with all other diabetic medications.

Sulfonylureas

Sulfonylureas (SUs), including glyburide, glimepiride and glipizide, are very frequently prescribed in the management of T2DM. There are several reasons for this, including the familiarity and comfort providers have using these medications given their long history on the market. In addition, these medications are inexpensive and thus financially available to most patients. And finally, these medications are available in convenient dosing regimens, as most are available in once daily dosing.

SUs lower blood glucose through increased insulin release from the pancreatic beta cells. Being aware of this mechanism of action is key in understanding some of the issues that arise when using these medications. Because there is an increase in insulin, these medications can result in hypoglycemia and weight gain. As well, because the mechanism of action is dependent on functional pancreatic beta-cells these medications may have waning activity over time as a patient's diabetes progresses and beta-cell failure develops.

The increased cardiovascular disease risk with SU therapy has been discussed for years and remains unclear. Much of the data indicating an increased risk is based on observational studies. A recent meta-analysis performed regarding this question found an increased risk of cardiovascular mortality with use of SUs (relative risk [RR] 1.27), but it should be noted that of the 33 studies included in the meta-analysis, only 13 were randomized controlled trials, and on analysis of these studies alone, there was no increase in cardiovascular risk.[17]

SUs are expected to lower HbA1c by approximately 1%, both when used as mono-therapy and when added to metformin.[18,19] They can be used safely with many other diabetes medications. SUs are commonly used in combination with insulin sensitizers metformin and thiazolidinediones. They can be used cautiously in combination with other medications that result in increased insulin secretion. This includes basal insulin, although with any of these combinations patients' risk of hypoglycemia is increased. SU should not be used in combination with meglitinides, which have a similar mechanism of action, or with prandial insulin.

Dipeptidyl-Peptidase 4 Inhibitors

Dipeptidyl-peptidase 4 (DPP-4) inhibitors are a new class of oral diabetes medications. Medications in this class include sitagliptin, saxagliptin, linagliptin, and alogliptin. These medications act through the incretin pathway, augmenting levels of intestinal hormones that are released when an individual eats. DPP-4 is present throughout the body on various cells, and inactivates the incretin hormone glucagon-like peptide 1 (GLP-1). GLP-1 has many effects on metabolism, including release of insulin in response to food intake, slowing of gastric emptying, and a sensation of satiety. Therefore DPP-4 inhibitors, via increased GLP-1 levels, result in improved blood sugar control. By virtue of the mechanism of action, these agents will not result in hypoglycemia, as they only augment insulin release in the setting of oral intake. These medications are also weight neutral.

Blood glucose lowering with these agents is likely slightly less than with other commonly prescribed diabetes medications. In a comparative effectiveness trial, metformin monotherapy resulted in more HbA1c lowering than DPP-4 monotherapy,[19] with DPP-4 inhibitors lowering HbA1c by approximately 0.5%. DPP-4 inhibitors are more often considered for add-on therapy, where they perform as well as other typical second-line medications. A meta-analysis of randomized controlled trials comparing SUs and DPP-4 inhibitors, with the majority of the studies included using these agents as add-on therapy to metformin, found similar blood glucose lowering for both groups.[20] DPP-4 inhibitors were not associated with weight gain, in contrast to SUs, which were associated with a 1.6 kg increase in weight. Importantly, DPP-4 inhibitors were associated with lower rates of reported hypoglycemia (odds ratio [OR] 0.13), total adverse effects (OR 0.79), and cardiovascular events (OR 0.53), although it should be noted these were trials of overall short duration with only a few trials reporting CV events, and this last benefit needs more study.

In general, DPP-4 inhibitors are well tolerated. There is ongoing study regarding a potential risk of pancreatitis with these medications, although if there is a risk, it is likely low, with an estimated NNH of 1940 per year in 1 recent meta-analysis.[21] Recently, an association with severe arthralgias was identified.[22] This is a relatively new class of medications, and therefore the possibility of additional adverse effects with long-term therapy may only become evident after years of postmarketing surveillance. One significant barrier to use of these agents is cost. Although metformin and SUs are typically affordable medications, DPP-4 inhibitors are costly, with no generic alternatives available.

DPP-4 inhibitors are rarely used as monotherapy, largely due to their modest HbA1c-lowering effects. They can safely be used with other oral medications. DPP-4 inhibitors can safely be used in patients on basal insulin, but should be discontinued if prandial insulin is added to a patient's medication regimen. And finally, given that these medications are acting on the incretin hormone pathway, they should not be prescribed in combination GLP-1 analogs, which also act on this pathway.

Thiazolidinediones

Thiazolidinediones (TZD) are a class of diabetes medications that act on the peroxisome-proliferator-activated receptor gamma, which is a nuclear transcription factor. When rosiglitazone and pioglitazone were initially released, they were commonly prescribed for the treatment of T2DM. Benefits of these medications include consistent HbA1c reduction and no risk of hypoglycemia. Unfortunately, with postmarketing surveillance, concern arose regarding the cardiovascular safety of rosiglitazone, with a meta-analysis identifying an increased risk of myocardial infarction,[23] and prescribing in the United States became limited for a number of years. However, in May of 2014, the FDA mandated Risk Evaluation and Mitigation Strategy, which was created to regulate rosiglitazone use in response to the noted safety concerns, was revised based on reanalysis of the available data. This led to the conclusion that rosiglitazone was not in fact associated with increased CV risk compared with standard diabetes treatment.[24] At this time, neither special provider training nor patient registries are required for prescribing rosiglitazone.

Regardless of the risk of myocardial infarction, the TZDs have been found to have several other adverse effects including edema and, likely related to this, an increased risk of heart failure exacerbation.[25] Another risk associated with TZD is an increased risk of fracture, particularly in postmenopausal women. Pioglitazone has been associated with an increased risk of bladder cancer as well; a recent meta-analysis found an increased risk based in both randomized controlled trials (OR 2.51) and observational trials (OR 1.21), with increased risk associated with total dose and duration of therapy.[26]

Given the multiple potential adverse effects of these medications and lingering concern regarding cardiovascular safety, these medications are typically used as third-line oral agents. They can safely be used with other blood sugar-lowering therapies and insulin (**Table 3**).

Sodium-Glucose Cotransporter 2 Inhibitors

The newest medications to treat T2DM are the sodium-glucose cotransporter 2 (SGLT2) inhibitors. Medications in this class include canagliflozin, dapagliflozin, and empagliflozin. These agents act by blocking SGLT2, which is typically responsible for reabsorbing 90% of the glucose in the urine.[27] They decrease both fasting and postprandial blood sugar values, and result in an HbA1c reduction between 0.5% and 1%. Other favorable characteristics of these medications include weight loss, as much as 2 to 4 kg when used as monotherapy, and modest reductions in systolic blood pressure, on the order of 1 to 8 mm Hg.[27] When used as monotherapy, hypoglycemia related to these agents is rare, but if used in combination with other agents that can cause hypoglycemia, such as insulin or SUs, it can occur.

Genital mycotic infections have consistently been found to be more common with use of SGLT2 inhibitors, in the form of *Candida* balanitis or vulvovaginitis. It is less clear if there is an increased risk of urinary tract infections. Postmarketing case reports of euglycemic diabetic ketoacidosis in the setting of SGLT2 inhibitor therapy led to the FDA adding this to the medication labeling. In addition, the FDA added potential risk of

Table 3
Oral medication summary

Drug Class	Approximate HbA1c Decrease (a)	Pros	Cons	Safety in Renal Insufficiency	Cost
Metformin	1%	Reduction in CV and all-cause death Weight neutral/loss No hypoglycemia	Gastrointestinal adverse effects	Use with caution; do not initiate with eGFR <45 mL/min/1.73 m^2	Low
Sulfonylurea	1%	Provider comfort	Risk of hypoglycemia Weight gain	Use with caution; risk of hypoglycemia increases	Low
DPP-4 Inhibitors	0.5%	No hypoglycemia Weight neutral	Lack of long-term safety data	Linagliptin best; dose reduce other agents	High
Thiazolidinediones	1%	No hypoglycemia	Edema Increased risk of CHF exacerbation Questions regarding CV safety	No dose adjustments required	Low
SGLT2 Inhibitors	0.5%	No hypoglycemia Potential reduction in CV and all-cause death	Gential *Candida* infections Lack of long-term safety data	Canagliflozin, empagliflozin contraindicated at eGFR <45 mL/min/1.73 m^2, dapagliflozin at eGFR of <60 mL/min/1.73 m^2	High

Adapted from Bennett WL, Maruthur NM, Singh S, et al. Comparative effectiveness and safety of medications for type 2 diabetes: an update including new drugs and 2-drug combinations. Ann Intern Med 2011;154(9):602–13.

bone fracture and is performing postmarketing surveillance of these medications for potential risk of bladder cancer (www.FDA.gov). Further study is required to evaluate these potential risks.

A recent study of empagliflozin in patients with cardiovascular disease in addition to T2DM had the exciting finding of reduced rates of cardiovascular events and all-cause death when this medication was added to patients' standard diabetic care,[28] including statins, antihypertensive medications, and additional diabetes medications including insulin and metformin. The primary outcome (CV death, nonfatal myocardial infarction and CVAs) was less common in the empagliflozin group compared to placebo (HR 0.86), with the estimated number of patients needed to treat for 3 years to prevent 1 death being 39.

SGLT2 inhibitors are best used in combination with other agents and can be used in combination with metformin, SUs, TZDs, DPP4 inhibitors, and basal insulin. The cost of these medications is likely to be a barrier for many patients.

INJECTABLE AGENTS
Glucagon-Like Peptide-1 Receptor Agonists

Additional medications in the incretin class include the injectable GLP-1 receptor agonists (GLP-1RAs). As previously described, GLP-1 is an incretin hormone produced by cells of the intestinal mucosa in response to food intake. Unlike the DPP-4 inhibitors, which increase endogenous levels of GLP-1, the GLP-1RAs achieve supraphysiologic levels of GLP-1 activity. In addition to the increased insulin secretion in response to food intake and slowed gastric emptying, which attenuates the post-meal glucose rise, similar to the DPP-4 inhibitors, the GLP-1RAs also promote satiety with resultant weight loss.[29]

There are currently 5 GLP-1 RAs available for use in the United States: exenatide, liraglutide, exenatide ER, albiglutide, and dulaglutide (**Table 4**). They differ in dosing schedule: once daily, twice daily, or once weekly, with the main clinical difference among the medications being the rate of adverse effects, particularly nausea. When used as second- or third-line agents, the GLP-1 RAs achieve 0.6% to 1.9% HbA1c lowering. Numerous head-to-head trials have compared the different GLP-1 RAs. In general, the long-acting GLP-1 RAs have greater HbA1C lowering when compared with the once or twice-daily formulations; however, these differences are small. There was similar weight loss seen in all groups. There was no significant difference in efficacy among the three once-weekly formulations.[30]

Given the effect of the GLP-1 RAs to decrease postprandial glucose excursions, they may be an alternative to prandial insulin for patients who are not well controlled on basal insulin alone. Several of the GLP-1 RAs have been studied in combination with basal insulin. Twice-daily exenatide added to basal insulin results in lower HbA1C with lower insulin doses compared with placebo. There was weight loss in

Table 4
Summary of currently available GLP-1 receptor agonists

Medication	Dose	HbA1C Lowering	Weight Loss	Rate of Nausea
Exenatide[41]	5–10 μg twice daily	0.7%–0.9%	1.1–2.7 kg	8%–44%
Exenatide QW[42]	2 mg weekly	1.3%–1.6%	Not noted	9.3%–27.0%
Liraglutide[43]	0.6–1.8 mg daily	1.0%–1.5%	1.0–2.8 kg	7.5%–34.6%
Albiglutide[44]	30–50 mg weekly	0.6%–0.9%	0.4–1.2 kg	11.1%
Dulaglutide[45]	0.75–1.5 mg weekly	0.7%–1.6%	+0.2–3.2 kg	12.4%–21.1%

the exenatide group, compared with weight gain in the placebo group, with no difference in hypoglycemia versus placebo.[31] Similar results were seen for patients not well controlled on glargine, who were randomized to once-weekly albiglutide or lispro 3 times daily. Both treatments were effective at lowering HbA1C and reducing the dose of glargine, but the albiglutide groups had significant weight loss compared to weight gain with the lispro group. There were more hypoglycemia events with the lispro group.[32]

There are no published results from studies of long-term cardiovascular outcomes with the GLP-1 RAs, although several are studies are underway.[33,34] Several studies have found a decrease in systolic blood pressure with exenatide, liraglutide, and dulagluti, but not with albiglutide.[35,36] A recent epidemiologic study found a lower incidence of heart failure, myocardial infarction, and stroke for patients who had received prescriptions for exenatide twice daily versus those who were treated with other diabetes agents.[37]

Nausea is the most common adverse effect with the GLP-1 RAs, ranging from 11% to 44% depending on the clinical study, with the lower rates of nausea with the longer-acting formulations.[38] Similar to the DPP-4 inhibitors, GLP-1 RAs act only to augment insulin secretion when glucose is elevated; thus risk of hypoglycemia is low and is typically only seen when used in combination with an SU. The provider should be aware of this increased risk of hypoglycemia and adjust the patient's diabetes regimen accordingly. As was noted for the DPP-4 inhibitors, there have been reports of acute pancreatitis with the GLP-1 RAs, and these medications are not recommended for use in patients with a history of pancreatitis. However, a meta-analysis of 60 clinical trials involving different GLP-1RA and DPP-4 inhibitors found no increased risk of pancreatitis, so this relationship remains unclear. Long-term outcome studies are needed to more definitively answer this question.[39] Medullary thyroid cancer (MTC) has been observed in rodents treated with liraglutide, which has resulted in a black box warning for all of the incretins. However, a recent meta-analysis found no increased risk of thyroid cancer with liraglutide or exenatide.[40] These medication should be avoided in patients with a history of MTC or a family history of MTC or MTC syndromes.

GLP-1 RAs should be considered for patients not well controlled with lifestyle and metformin, or for those who are unable to tolerate metformin as a first line agent. They are likely to be most beneficial for obese patients, given their positive effect on body weight or when minimizing hypoglycemia is a primary goal.[9,10] They are not recommended for use as monotherapy, but they can be used in combination with most oral medications. The exceptions would be combined use with the DPP-4 inhibitors, as noted earlier, due to duplicate mechanism of actions, and use with the SGLT2 inhibitors because of a lack of data.[38]

Basal Insulin

T2DM is a progressive disease, and many patients will require insulin for treatment at some time in their disease course. For patients not well controlled on 2 oral agents, some may benefit from addition of a third agent, but if HbA1C is greater than 9.5%, basal insulin has been shown to have more effective glucose lowering.[46] Insulin should also be considered early in treatment for patients with symptomatic hyperglycemia, who would benefit from more rapid glucose control. For many patients, adding insulin may be safer and more cost-effective than intensifying oral medications.[47]

There are several options for basal insulin, all of which are equally efficacious at lowering HbA1C. A 2009 Cochrane Review comparing Neutral Protamin Hagedorn (NPH) with the basal analogs glargine and detemir found no clinically significant difference in HbA1c levels among the insulins. Moreover, there was no difference in rates of severe hypoglycemia, although there was a lower risk of symptomatic and nocturnal hypoglycemia with the analogs.[48] NPH has the benefit of a lower cost when compared with glargine and detemir; however, it does require twice-daily dosing. A study comparing glargine and detemir found no difference in HbA1C lowering, but many patients on detemir did require higher insulin doses and twice-daily dosing to achieve the same HbA1C lowering as glargine.[49]

The initial goal of basal insulin is not rapid glycemic control, but rather helping the patient establish a routine with once-daily injections, while avoiding hypoglycemia. Basal insulin is typically started at 10 U once daily or 0.1 to 0.2 U/kg/d depending on degree of hyperglycemia. Once-daily basal insulin is typically administered at night, to better suppress hepatic glucose production. Patients can self-titrate their dose by 2 to 4 U weekly to achieve target fasting blood glucose, generally between 80 to 130 mg/dL, although this should be individualized for each patient.[50,51] If NPH is used as the basal insulin, the dose should be divided into 70% before breakfast and 30% before dinner.

Once patients are taking more than 50 to 60 U of basal insulin, dividing the dose to reduce the volume may help improve absorption and efficacy. A concentrated form of glargine is now available, glargine U-300, which is 3 times more concentrated than U-100 glargine and thus delivers the same amount of insulin in one-third the volume. This may be another option for patients requiring higher volumes of insulin. Dosing conversion from U-100 is 1:1, with no dose adjustment needed. It is supplied in pen form.

The newest basal insulin on the market is insulin degludec. This is an ultralong-acting basal insulin, with a duration of 42 hours. The benefit of this basal insulin is there is more flexibility in timing. It does not need to be taken at the same time every day, which may be useful for patients with variable schedules, such as shift workers. The dosing conversion from other basal insulins is 1:1, and it is dosed once daily. It does take approximately 3 days to achieve steady state, so patients and providers should be aware that blood sugars may run higher for the first few days after starting the medication.[52]

Basal insulin can be used in combination with all oral medications, as well as the injectable GLP-1 RAs. It should be used with caution when combined with SUs, due to increased risk of hypoglycemia.

Prandial Insulin

When patients have persistently elevated HbA1C despite fasting blood glucoses that are at goal, or when basal insulin dose is greater than 0.5 U/kg/d, providers should consider starting prandial insulin.[50] Currently available options for prandial insulin include regular human insulin and the rapid-acting insulin analogs (RAAs) aspart, glulisine, and lispro, which have quicker absorption and shorter duration of action. Similar to studies of the long-acting human versus analog insulins, there is no significant difference in blood sugar control between regular human insulin and the RAAs, and no increased risk of hypoglycemia with regular insulin compared with the rapid-acting analog insulins.[53,54] There is also no evidence that the RAAs provide any advantage over human insulin when it comes to preventing diabetes-related vascular complications. The analogs provide a more physiologic insulin profile, but no study has shown this to be beneficial with regards to HbA1c levels or long-term outcomes. However, their more rapid onset provides convenience with mealtime dosing, which is a benefit for many patients.

When starting prandial insulin, once-daily dosing before the largest meal of the day is a reasonable starting point. Typical dose is 4 U, 0.1 U/kg or 10% of the basal dose before the meal. If HbA1C is less than 8%, basal insulin dose should be decreased by a similar amount. If a single dose of prandial insulin is not adequate to achieve glycemic control, additional prandial doses can be added.[50] When adding prandial insulin, most oral agents should be discontinued in order to avoid hypoglycemia. Metformin can safely be continued.

Concentrated Insulins

For patients with significant insulin resistance, defined as requiring more than 500 U of insulin daily, concentrated regular insulin is an option. This allows for fewer injections, as well as lower insulin volumes, which may improve insulin absorption. The time to peak following injection for U-500 insulin is similar to regular human insulin, with a duration of action similar to NPH. Given these pharmacokinetics of insulin U-500, it provides both basal and prandial coverage, allowing the patient to take a single type of insulin in fewer injections.[55] The transition from U-100 insulin to concentrated U-500 insulin can be intimidating for providers, but a recent study showed that this can be safely and effectively done utilizing a twice-daily dosing algorithm. Patients can be initially started on injections before breakfast (60% of total dose) and before dinner (40% of total dose). Based on premeal blood sugars, insulin doses can be safely adjusted to achieve glucose targets. Overall, patients on U-500 insulin show a significant decrease in HbA1C, although this is typically associated with weight gain.[55,56]

SPECIAL POPULATIONS
Renal Dysfunction

T2DM is one of the leading causes of chronic kidney disease. As such, providers are often faced with adjusting diabetes regimens in the setting of decreased renal function. Although many diabetes medications can be safely used in renal disease, dose adjustments are often needed, as well as discontinuation of some medications if chronic kidney disease (CKD) should progress.

As previously discussed, FDA labeling suggests metformin should be discontinued for males with creatinine $\geq$ 1.5 or females with creatinine $\geq$ 1.4. Fortunately, there is increasing acceptance that this concern may be overstated, and it is likely safe to prescribe metformin in the setting of mild renal insufficiency (refer to **Table 2**). Similar to metformin, caution needs to be taken when prescribing SUs to patients with renal insufficiency. These medications are renally cleared; therefore, patients with renal insufficiency are at a higher risk of drug-related hypoglycemia. The SU with the lowest risk of hypoglycemia in the setting of renal insufficiency is glipizide.[57]

With the exception of linagliptin, the DPP-4 inhibitors are also renally cleared. They can safely be used in patients with renal insufficiency, although dosing adjustments are needed. Because linagliptin is not extensively metabolized and excreted 80% in the feces, it can safely be used in patients with decreased renal clearance without dose adjustment. TZDs are not renally cleared, so it can be safely used in renal disease without dose adjustment. However, in CKD stage 4 to 5, the risk of fluid retention and metabolic bone disease with TZDs does need to be considered, given the increased risk of these conditions with end stage renal disease (ESRD).[58] The SGLT-2 inhibitors are not effective in patients with significant renal insufficiency. Canagliflozin and empagliflozin are contraindicated in patients with estimated glomerular filtration rate (eGFR) less than 45 mL/min/1.73 m^2, and dapagliflozin at a eGFR of less than 60 mL/min/1.73 m^2.

Among the GLP-1 RAs, albiglutide does not require dosing adjustment and is safe to use in CKD. There is limited experience with liraglutide and dulaglutide in CKD, so although no specific dose adjustments are recommended, it is advised that one exercise caution with their use in patients with renal impairment. Exenatide is not recommended for use in patients with stage 4 or 5 CKD. No dosage adjustment is needed for stage 1 to 3 CKD. Insulin is safe to use in CKD, with appropriate dose adjustments to avoid hypoglycemia. See **Table 5** for summary.

Elderly Patients

With elderly patients, glycemic targets typically need to be adjusted. Increased mortality is seen with HbA1C values less than 6.0% and above 9.0%.[59] Guidelines recommend HbA1C between 7.5% and 9.0% for elderly patients, depending on their comorbidities.[60] In addition, elderly patients are more at risk from adverse events related to their medications. Metformin is considered a good option for elderly patients. If a second agent is needed, glipizide is a reasonable choice, because of the lower risk of hypoglycemia. The DPP-4 inhibitors, with their low rates of adverse events, are another good choice. TZDs should not be used because of the risk of heart failure and fractures. The nausea and weight loss associated with GLP-1 RAs could also be problematic for elderly patients, so these should be avoided as well. SGLT-2 inhibitors increase risk of genital yeast infections, and could worsen urinary incontinence, so they are not a good choice for elderly patients. Insulin can safely be used, although dosing should be conservative in order to avoid hypoglycemia. See **Table 6** for summary.

Other Pharmacologic Therapies for Reduction of Macrovascular Complication

In addition to blood sugar-lowering therapies, there are several other important therapies to consider in patients with T2DM to reduce their risk of cardiovascular disease and stroke. These include antihypertensive therapy, statin medications, and low-dose aspirin.

Blood pressure medications should be initiated for systolic blood pressure greater than 140 or diastolic blood pressure greater than 90. The American Diabetes Association (ADA) recommends using an angiotensin-converting enzyme (ACE) inhibitor or an angiotensin receptor blocker (ARB) as first-line therapy, whereas the Joint National Committee recommends initiation of treatment with any first-line blood pressure medication (including ACE inhibitors, ARBs, thiazide-type diuretics, or calcium channel blockers).[61,62]

Both the American Heart Association and American Diabetes Association guidelines recommend statin therapy for primary prevention in all diabetic patients age 40 years

Table 5 Use of diabetes medications in chronic kidney disease	
Medication	**Considerations in CKD**
Metformin	Decrease dose by 50% for GFR <45, discontinue for GFR <30
Sulfonylurea	Glipizide safe to use with caution, no dose adjustment needed
TZDs	Safe to use, no dose adjustment needed
DPP-4 inhibitors	Linagliptin safe to use without dose adjustment; others require decreased dose
SGLT-2 inhibitors	Do not use with GFR <45 (GFR <60 for dapagliflozin)
GLP-1RA	Albiglutide safe to use without dose adjustment, exenatide contraindicated with GGR <30, others should be used with caution

Table 6
Use of diabetes medications in elderly patients

Medications	Consideration for Elderly
Metformin	Dose adjustment for renal disease
Sulfonylurea	Glipizide only due to lower risk of hypoglycemia
DPP-4 inhibitors	Low risk of adverse effects
TZDs	Avoid due to heart failure and fracture risk
GLP-1RAs	Avoid due to nausea and weight loss
SGLT-2 inhibitors	Avoid due to risk of mycotic infections and urinary incontinence
Insulin	Safe to use, conservative dosing to avoid hypoglycemia

and older.[62,63] In choosing which statin to use, it is recommended that the provider calculates the patient's 10 year risk of ateriosclerotic cardiovascular disease (ASCVD, refer to http://my.americanheart.org), and if at least 7.5%, use a high-potency statin such as atorvastatin 80 mg daily or rosuvastatin 20 g daily. If risk is less than 7.5%, a moderate dose statin will likely provide adequate CVD risk reduction.

Aspirin has a modest benefit in reduction of cardiovascular events in the general population and is recommended for primary prevention in all patients, including diabetics, with a 10-year ASCVD risk of greater than 10%.[62] In general, this degree of risk is seen in men greater than 50 years of age and women greater than 60 years of age with an additional cardiovascular risk factors such as high blood pressure. The most common dose used for this indication in the United States is 81 mg daily, as there is no evidence that a higher dose would offer additional benefit.

SUMMARY

T2DM is a common condition encountered in primary care, and there are a number of pharmacologic therapies to be considered in its management. For glycemic control, there are convincing data that metformin is the optimal first-line therapy for the majority of patients, but if additional medications are needed, there are many issues to consider. In order to make informed and patient-centered decisions regarding additional therapies, one must consider not only the medications' effects on blood sugar lowering, but also effects on weight, risk of hypoglycemia, costs, and what routes of administration (oral vs injection) are acceptable to the patient. Additional important patient factors to consider are renal function and the patient's ability to manage hypoglycemia-related side effects. And finally, when considering pharmacologic therapy for T2DM, it is critical not to overlook important therapies that reduce the risk of cardiovascular disease, independent of blood sugar lowering, agents including statins, antihypertensives, and aspirin.

REFERENCES

1. 2014 National Diabetes Statistics Report. 2014. Available at: http://www.cdc.gov/diabetes/data/statistics/2014statisticsreport.html. Accessed September 1, 2015.

2. Zhuo X, Zhang P, Barker L, et al. The lifetime cost of diabetes and its implications for diabetes prevention. Diabetes Care 2014;37(9):2557–64.

3. Intensive blood-glucose control with sulphonylureas or insulin compared with conventional treatment and risk of complications in patients with type 2 diabetes

(UKPDS 33). UK Prospective Diabetes Study (UKPDS) Group. Lancet 1998; 352(9131):837–53.

4. Holman RR, Paul SK, Bethel MA, et al. 10-year follow-up of intensive glucose control in type 2 diabetes. N Engl J Med 2008;359(15):1577–89.

5. Effect of intensive blood-glucose control with metformin on complications in overweight patients with type 2 diabetes (UKPDS 34). UK Prospective Diabetes Study (UKPDS) Group. Lancet 1998;352(9131):854–65.

6. Gerstein HC, Miller ME, Byington RP, et al. Effects of intensive glucose lowering in type 2 diabetes. N Engl J Med 2008;358(24):2545–59.

7. Patel A, MacMahon S, Chalmers J, et al. Intensive blood glucose control and vascular outcomes in patients with type 2 diabetes. N Engl J Med 2008; 358(24):2560–72.

8. Duckworth W, Abraira C, Moritz T, et al. Glucose control and vascular complications in veterans with type 2 diabetes. N Engl J Med 2009;360(2): 129–39.

9. Inzucchi SE, Bergenstal RM, Buse JB, et al. Management of hyperglycemia in type 2 diabetes: a patient-centered approach: position statement of the American Diabetes Association (ADA) and the European Association for the Study of Diabetes (EASD). Diabetes Care 2012;35(6):1364–79.

10. Garber AJ, Abrahamson MJ, Barzilay JI, et al. AACE comprehensive diabetes management algorithm 2013. Endocr Pract 2013;19(2):327–36.

11. United Kingdom Prospective Diabetes Study (UKPDS). 13: Relative efficacy of randomly allocated diet, sulphonylurea, insulin, or metformin in patients with newly diagnosed non-insulin dependent diabetes followed for three years. BMJ 1995;310(6972):83–8.

12. Inzucchi SE, Lipska KJ, Mayo H, et al. Metformin in patients with type 2 diabetes and kidney disease: a systematic review. JAMA 2014;312(24):2668–75.

13. Salpeter SR, Greyber E, Pasternak GA, et al. Risk of fatal and nonfatal lactic acidosis with metformin use in type 2 diabetes mellitus. Cochrane Database Syst Rev 2010;(4):CD002967.

14. Zhang X, Harmsen WS, Mettler TA, et al. Continuation of metformin use after a diagnosis of cirrhosis significantly improves survival of patients with diabetes. Hepatology 2014;60(6):2008–16.

15. Moreno G, Mangione CM, Kimbro L, et al. Guidelines abstracted from the American Geriatrics Society Guidelines for Improving the Care of Older Adults with Diabetes Mellitus: 2013 update. J Am Geriatr Soc 2013;61(11):2020–6.

16. de Jager J, Kooy A, Lehert P, et al. Long term treatment with metformin in patients with type 2 diabetes and risk of vitamin B-12 deficiency: randomised placebo controlled trial. BMJ 2010;340:c2181.

17. Phung OJ, Schwartzman E, Allen RW, et al. Sulphonylureas and risk of cardiovascular disease: systematic review and meta-analysis. Diabet Med 2013;30(10): 1160–71.

18. Bolen S, Feldman L, Vassy J, et al. Systematic review: comparative effectiveness and safety of oral medications for type 2 diabetes mellitus. Ann Intern Med 2007; 147(6):386–99.

19. Bennett WL, Maruthur NM, Singh S, et al. Comparative effectiveness and safety of medications for type 2 diabetes: an update including new drugs and 2-drug combinations. Ann Intern Med 2011;154(9):602–13.

20. Zhang Y, Hong J, Chi J, et al. Head-to-head comparison of dipeptidyl peptidase-IV inhibitors and sulfonylureas - a meta-analysis from randomized clinical trials. Diabetes Metab Res Rev 2014;30(3):241–56.

21. Abbas AS, Dehbi HM, Ray KK. Cardiovascular and non-cardiovascular safety of dipeptidyl peptidase-4 inhibition: a meta-analysis of randomised controlled cardiovascular outcome trials. Diabetes Obes Metab 2015;18(3):295–9.

22. FDA Drug Safety Communication: FDA warns that DPP-4 inhibitors for type 2 diabetes may cause severe joint pain. 2015. Available at: http://www.fda.gov/Drugs/DrugSafety/ucm459579.htm. Accessed October 14, 2015.

23. Nissen SE, Wolski K. Rosiglitazone revisited: an updated meta-analysis of risk for myocardial infarction and cardiovascular mortality. Arch Intern Med 2010; 170(14):1191–201.

24. FDA approves Avandia (rosiglitzone) label update, lifts restriction on patient access. 2014. Available at: http://us.gsk.com/en-us/media/press-releases/2014/fda-approves-avandia-rosiglitazone-label-update-lifts-restrictions-on-patient-access/. Accessed October 15, 2015.

25. Consoli A, Formoso G. Do thiazolidinediones still have a role in treatment of type 2 diabetes mellitus? Diabetes Obes Metab 2013;15(11):967–77.

26. Turner RM, Kwok CS, Chen-Turner C, et al. Thiazolidinediones and associated risk of bladder cancer: a systematic review and meta-analysis. Br J Clin Pharmacol 2014;78(2):258–73.

27. Vivian E. Sodium-glucose cotransporter 2 inhibitors in the treatment of type 2 diabetes mellitus. Diabetes Educ 2015;41(1 Suppl):5S–18S.

28. Zinman B, Wanner C, Lachin JM, et al. Empagliflozin, cardiovascular outcomes, and mortality in type 2 diabetes. N Engl J Med 2015;373(22):2117–28.

29. Baggio LL, Drucker DJ. Biology of incretins: GLP-1 and GIP. Gastroenterology 2007;132(6):2131–57.

30. Trujillo JM, Nuffer W, Ellis SL. GLP-1 receptor agonists: a review of head-to-head clinical studies. Ther Adv Endocrinol Metab 2015;6(1):19–28.

31. Buse JB, Bergenstal RM, Glass LC, et al. Use of twice-daily exenatide in Basal insulin-treated patients with type 2 diabetes: a randomized, controlled trial. Ann Intern Med 2011;154(2):103–12.

32. Rosenstock J, Fonseca VA, Gross JL, et al. Advancing basal insulin replacement in type 2 diabetes inadequately controlled with insulin glargine plus oral agents: a comparison of adding albiglutide, a weekly GLP-1 receptor agonist, versus thrice-daily prandial insulin lispro. Diabetes Care 2014;37(8):2317–25.

33. Marso SP, Poulter NR, Nissen SE, et al. Design of the liraglutide effect and action in diabetes: evaluation of cardiovascular outcome results (LEADER) trial. Am Heart J 2013;166(5):823–30.e5.

34. Tibble CA, Cavaiola TS, Henry RR. Longer acting GLP-1 receptor agonists and the potential for improved cardiovascular outcomes. Expert Rev Endocrinol Metab 2013;8(3):247–59.

35. Ferdinand KC, White WB, Calhoun DA, et al. Effects of the once-weekly glucagon-like peptide-1 receptor agonist dulaglutide on ambulatory blood pressure and heart rate in patients with type 2 diabetes mellitus. Hypertension 2014; 64(4):731–7.

36. Karagiannis T, Liakos A, Bekiari E, et al. Efficacy and safety of once-weekly glucagon-like peptide 1 receptor agonists for the management of type 2 diabetes: a systematic review and meta-analysis of randomized controlled trials. Diabetes Obes Metab 2015;17(11):1065–74.

37. Paul SK, Klein K, Maggs D, et al. The association of the treatment with glucagon-like peptide-1 receptor agonist exenatide or insulin with cardiovascular outcomes in patients with type 2 diabetes: a retrospective observational study. Cardiovasc Diabetol 2015;14:10.

38. Prasad-Reddy L, Isaacs D. A clinical review of GLP-1 receptor agonists: efficacy and safety in diabetes and beyond. Drugs Context 2015;4:212283.

39. Li L, Shen J, Bala MM, et al. Incretin treatment and risk of pancreatitis in patients with type 2 diabetes mellitus: systematic review and meta-analysis of randomised and non-randomised studies. BMJ 2014;348:g2366.

40. Alves C, Batel-Marques F, Macedo AF. A meta-analysis of serious adverse events reported with exenatide and liraglutide: acute pancreatitis and cancer. Diabetes Res Clin Pract 2012;98(2):271–84.

41. Byetta [package insert]. San Diego, CA: Amylin Pharmaceuticals; 2009.

42. Bydureon [package insert]. Wlimington, DE: AstraZeneca Pharmaceuticals; 2015.

43. Victoza [package insert]. Plainsboro, NJ: Novo Nordik; 2015.

44. Tanzeum [package insert]. Wilmington, DE: GlaxoSmithKline; 2015.

45. Trulicity [package insert]. Indianapolis, IN: Eli Lilly; 2014.

46. Rosenstock J, Sugimoto D, Strange P, et al. Triple therapy in type 2 diabetes: insulin glargine or rosiglitazone added to combination therapy of sulfonylurea plus metformin in insulin-naive patients. Diabetes Care 2006;29(3):554–9.

47. Schwartz S, Sievers R, Strange P, et al. Insulin 70/30 mix plus metformin versus triple oral therapy in the treatment of type 2 diabetes after failure of two oral drugs: efficacy, safety, and cost analysis. Diabetes Care 2003;26(8):2238–43.

48. Horvath K, Jeitler K, Berghold A, et al. Long-acting insulin analogues versus NPH insulin (human isophane insulin) for type 2 diabetes mellitus. Cochrane Database Syst Rev 2007;(2):CD005613.

49. Swinnen SG, Simon AC, Holleman F, et al. Insulin detemir versus insulin glargine for type 2 diabetes mellitus. Cochrane Database Syst Rev 2011;(7):CD006383.

50. Inzucchi SE, Bergenstal RM, Buse JB, et al. Management of hyperglycemia in type 2 diabetes, 2015: a patient-centered approach: update to a position statement of the American Diabetes Association and the European Association for the Study of Diabetes. Diabetes Care 2015;38(1):140–9.

51. American Diabetes Association. (6) Glycemic targets. Diabetes Care 2015; 38(Suppl):S33–40.

52. Vora J, Cariou B, Evans M, et al. Clinical use of insulin degludec. Diabetes Res Clin Pract 2015;109(1):19–31.

53. Mannucci E, Monami M, Marchionni N. Short-acting insulin analogues vs. regular human insulin in type 2 diabetes: a meta-analysis. Diabetes Obes Metab 2009; 11:53–9.

54. Davidson MB. Insulin analogs–is there a compelling case to use them? No! Diabetes Care 2014;37(6):1771–4.

55. Lane WS, Cochran EK, Jackson JA, et al. High-dose insulin therapy: is it time for U-500 insulin? Endocr Pract 2009;15(1):71–9.

56. Hood RC, Arakaki RF, Wysham C, et al. Two treatment approaches for human regular u-500 insulin in patients with type 2 diabetes not achieving adequate glycemic control on high-dose u-100 insulin therapy with or without oral agents: a randomized, titration-to-target clinical trial. Endocr Pract 2015;21(7):782–93.

57. Scheen AJ. Pharmacokinetic considerations for the treatment of diabetes in patients with chronic kidney disease. Expert Opin Drug Metab Toxicol 2013;9(5): 529–50.

58. Nogueira C, Souto SB, Vinha E, et al. Oral glucose lowering drugs in type 2 diabetic patients with chronic kidney disease. Hormones (Athens) 2013;12(4):483–94.

59. Huang ES, Liu JY, Moffet HH, et al. Glycemic control, complications, and death in older diabetic patients: the diabetes and aging study. Diabetes Care 2011;34(6): 1329–36.
60. Bansal N, Dhaliwal R, Weinstock RS. Management of diabetes in the elderly. Med Clin North Am 2015;99(2):351–77.
61. James PA, Oparil S, Carter BL, et al. 2014 evidence-based guideline for the management of high blood pressure in adults: report from the panel members appointed to the Eighth Joint National Committee (JNC 8). JAMA 2014;311(5): 507–20.
62. American Diabetes Association. (8) Cardiovascular disease and risk management. Diabetes Care 2015;38(Suppl):S49–57.
63. Stone NJ, Robinson JG, Lichtenstein AH, et al. 2013 ACC/AHA guideline on the treatment of blood cholesterol to reduce atherosclerotic cardiovascular risk in adults: a report of the American College of Cardiology/American Heart Association Task Force on Practice Guidelines. J Am Coll Cardiol 2014;63(25 Pt B): 2889–934.

Update in Hypertension Therapy

Leonard A. Mankin, MD

KEYWORDS

- Hypertension • Blood pressure • Therapy • Antihypertensives
- Blood pressure goals • Spironolactone • SGLT-2 inhibitors

KEY POINTS

- Targets for blood pressure control, traditionally less than 140/90 mm Hg, should be reduced to less than 120 mm Hg systolic in patients more than 50 years of age at very high risk for cardiovascular events.
- With few exceptions, first-line therapy for hypertension should be selected from one of 4 classes: thiazide diuretics, dihydropyridine calcium channel blockers, angiotensin-converting enzyme (ACE) inhibitors, or angiotensin receptor blockers (ARBs).
- When blood pressure is not controlled on a low dose of a single agent, adding a second agent is more effective than simply increasing the dose of monotherapy.
- ACE inhibitors seem to be superior to ARBs with regard to overall mortality and should be chosen preferentially. ACE inhibitors and ARBs should not be used in combination because of increased adverse events without appreciable benefits.
- Spironolactone is a particularly potent agent for blood pressure reduction in patients with refractory hypertension.

INTRODUCTION

Hypertension affects about 1 in every 3 adults in the United States and more than 1 billion people worldwide, and the prevalence is projected to increase by 60% by 2025.[1–3] It is the leading global risk factor for mortality, accounting for about 1 out of every 8 deaths worldwide. Hypertension results in an average loss of life of 5 years, and those living with hypertension are more often burdened with morbidities of congestive heart failure, chronic kidney disease, neurologic deficits from stroke, and vision loss.[4]

CLINICAL QUESTION: WHAT ARE THE APPROPRIATE TARGETS FOR BLOOD PRESSURE CONTROL?

Reducing chronically increased blood pressure using medications clearly reduces the incidence of coronary artery disease, stroke, congestive heart failure, and chronic

Department of Graduate Medical Education, Legacy Health, 1200 Northwest 23rd Avenue, Portland, OR 97210, USA
E-mail address: LMANKIN@LHS.ORG

Med Clin N Am 100 (2016) 665–693
http://dx.doi.org/10.1016/j.mcna.2016.03.005   medical.theclinics.com
0025-7125/16/$ – see front matter © 2016 Elsevier Inc. All rights reserved.

kidney disease.[5–7] Epidemiologic evidence suggests a profound increase in cardiovascular mortality with increasing blood pressure greater than systolic pressures of 115 mm Hg.[8] For the past 3 decades, physicians have settled on a target blood pressure of less than 140/90 mm Hg based on a preponderance of epidemiologic studies. However, most randomized controlled trials have not shown convincing benefits for blood pressure reduction below a systolic target of 150 mm Hg.

Several trials have examined the question of the most appropriate systolic targets for blood pressure in different age and risk categories. A Cochrane Review in 2009 examined outcomes differences between groups treated to standard blood pressure targets (<140–160/90–100 mm Hg) versus more intensive control (<135/85).[9] The investigators identified 7 randomized trials involving more than 22,000 subjects. Despite significant blood pressure differences, there were no differences in outcomes between the groups. In addition, subgroup analyses did not reveal differences among higher risk patients such as those with diabetes mellitus or chronic kidney disease.

The AASK (African American Study of Kidney Disease and Hypertension) trial examined 1094 African American patients with chronic kidney disease, comparing a standard blood pressure target (<140 mm Hg systolic) with a more aggressive blood pressure goal (<130 mm Hg systolic).[10] Despite significant differences in blood pressure achieved between the two groups, there were no differences in the end point of progression of chronic kidney disease or mortality over roughly a decade of follow-up.

The ACCORD (Action to Control Cardiovascular Risk in Diabetes) trial was a randomized controlled trial of adults with diabetes and hypertension who were at very high risk for cardiovascular events.[11] The investigators enrolled 4733 patients and followed them over approximately 5 years to determine whether pursuing a more aggressive blood pressure target (<120 mm Hg) would result in fewer important cardiovascular events compared with the traditional systolic blood pressure target (<140 mm Hg). The study failed to show improvement in the primary composite end point of nonfatal myocardial infarction, nonfatal stroke, or cardiovascular death. The investigators noted a significant reduction in stroke rate with aggressive blood pressure control, but the number needed to treat was large (~450 over 5 years) to prevent a single event. These small gains came with a cost: increased serious adverse events were significantly more common; namely hypotension, electrolyte disturbances, and worsening of serum creatinine levels.

The paucity of evidence supporting more aggressive blood pressure control led the National Expert Panel (JNC 8) to recommend a less stringent target blood pressure of less than 150/90 mm Hg in adults more than age 60 years in their 2014 guidelines.[12] The group continued to recommend a target blood pressure of less than 140/90 mm Hg in younger adults, although this the recommendation of less than 140/90 mm Hg emanated from expert opinion in the absence of randomized trials. The JNC 8 conclusions raised a great deal of debate about appropriate blood pressure targets and left physicians and patients with much uncertainty.

In 2015, the National Heart, Lung, and Blood Institute released results of the Systolic Blood Pressure Intervention Trial (SPRINT), a randomized controlled, open-label trial of intensive versus standard blood pressure control in nondiabetic adults more than 50 years of age.[13] In the trial, 9361 patients at high risk for cardiovascular events were randomly assigned to standard (<140 mm Hg) versus aggressive (<120 mm Hg) control of blood pressure. Average starting blood pressure in the trial was 139.7 mm Hg, and participants were seen monthly for medication adjustments until their blood pressure target had been reached. The investigators achieved mean systolic blood pressures of 134.6 mm Hg in the standard group and 121.5 mm Hg in the intensive treatment group using an average of 1.8 and 2.8 antihypertensive medications, respectively.

In contrast with AASK[10] and ACCORD,[11] SPRINT was stopped well ahead of the expected completion date (mean average follow-up, 3.26 years) because of striking differences in outcomes favoring aggressive control. Subjects assigned to the aggressive control group experienced a 38% relative risk reduction for congestive heart failure, a 43% relative risk reduction for cardiovascular mortality, and a 27% relative reduction for overall death (**Table 1**).

Hypotension, syncope, electrolyte disturbances, and acute worsening of renal function were observed more frequently in the aggressively managed group. Because of the shortened duration of the study, it is not clear whether the acute changes in glomerular filtration rate (GFR) likely caused by the effects of increased use of diuretics and angiotensin-converting enzyme (ACE) or angiotensin receptor blockers (ARBs), will have lasting detrimental effects on renal function. Patients in the study with chronic kidney disease at baseline did not experience significant declines in renal function.

Up to this point, several trials have shown cardiovascular benefits with treatment of systolic blood pressure less than 150 mm Hg in the elderly.[14–16] SPRINT included a large number of geriatric patients, with 28% of the participants 75 years of age or older. The beneficial effects of aggressive control were seen equally in this older subset of patients. Orthostatic changes and falls are expected at a higher rate among geriatric patients with multiple comorbidities. However, falls were not increased with intensive control, and orthostatic hypotension was observed more frequently in the standard control group.

A systematic review and meta-analysis of randomized trials examining greater versus lesser intensity of blood pressure reduction, more inclusive than the 2009 Cochrane Review,[9] was published shortly after SPRINT.[17] In about 45,000 participants, achieving average blood pressure of 133/76 mm Hg was linked to significant reduction in cardiovascular events, myocardial infarction, stroke, albuminuria, and retinopathy protection compared with subjects with average blood pressure of 140/81 mm Hg.

The JNC 8 guidelines of 2014[12] recommended a less stringent blood pressure target in patients aged 60 years or older, straying from the traditional target of less than 140/90 mm Hg. The core of investigators cited lack of definitive evidence for benefit

Table 1
Primary and secondary outcomes

Outcomes	Intensive Treatment, n (%) (n = 4678)	Standard Treatment, n (%) (n = 4683)	Hazard Ratio (95% CI)	P Value	NNT Over 3.26 y
Primary outcome[a]	243 (5.2)	319 (6.8)	0.75 (0.64–0.89)	<.001	61
Heart failure	62 (1.3)	100 (2.1)	0.62 (0.45–0.84)	.002	125
CV mortality	37 (0.8)	65 (1.4)	0.57 (0.38–0.85)	.005	172
All-cause mortality	155 (3.3)	210 (4.5)	0.73 (0.60–0.90)	.003	90
MI	97 (2.1)	116 (2.5)	0.83 (0.64–1.09)	.19	NS
Stroke	62 (1.3)	70 (1.5)	0.89 (0.63–1.25)	.50	NS

Abbreviations: CI, confidence interval; CV, cardiovascular; MI, myocardial infarction; NNT, number needed to treat.
[a] Myocardial infarction, acute coronary syndrome not resulting in myocardial infarction, stroke, acute decompensated heart failure, or death from cardiovascular causes.

of blood pressure treatment below a level of 150/90 mm Hg, with dissenters among the JNC 8 group publishing their reservations about this change in a subsequent editorial.[18] The SPRINT findings lend support to the argument that blood pressure targets should head the opposite direction, with goal pressures less than 140 mm Hg, or perhaps lower still. The results of SPRINT should be carefully weighed in the context of current guidelines.

The results from SPRINT are striking and clinically important. Aggressive blood pressure reduction to a target of 120 mm Hg decreases the incidence of acute decompensated heart failure and death for nondiabetic adults age more than 50 years of age who are at high risk for cardiovascular events. Achieving these results in clinical practice will prove more challenging. The most recent figures suggest that clinicians are achieving blood pressure control to less than 140/90 mm Hg in slightly more than half of hypertensive adults.[2] It will take a paradigm shift in the attitudes of both physicians and the public to make progress toward achieving these more aggressive blood pressure targets.

It is important to consider that the SPRINT investigators enrolled patients who were at very high risk for cardiovascular events. Most adults had a 10-year risk for a major event of greater than 20%. Patients at high risk stand to gain the most from an intervention such as aggressive blood pressure reduction. It is not clear that these findings can be extrapolated to lower risk patients, who are less likely to gain the same degree of benefit but would still be exposed to the same amount of risk from adverse events. Several questions remain unanswered. Specifically, what targets should clinicians aim for in patients with diabetes, prior stroke, and in adult patients with lower risk profiles than those studied in SPRINT, including those less than 50 years old? Further studies are needed to fine tune the approach to these patient subsets. For now, SPRINT helps answer an important clinical question in a high-risk cohort of patients.

CLINICAL BOTTOM LINE

A systolic blood pressure target less than 120 mm Hg is appropriate in patients more than 50 years of age who are at high risk for cardiovascular events, provided it can be attained with minimal adverse effects.

CLINICAL QUESTION: WHAT IS THE BEST INITIAL AGENT FOR ESSENTIAL HYPERTENSION?

According to the 2014 JNC 8 guidelines,[12] for nonblack individuals, the first drug chosen for hypertension should be a thiazide diuretic, a dihydropyridine calcium channel blocker, an ACE inhibitor, or an ARB. Each of these drug classes have shown similar efficacy in reducing all-cause mortality and cardiovascular, cerebrovascular, and renal outcomes. Among the thiazide diuretics, chlorthalidone has the greatest evidence for event reduction and should be the preferred agent in this class.[19,20] β-Blockers are no longer recommended as first-line agents for hypertension because of their failure to reduce cardiovascular events compared with other agents.[12] Recommendations for initial therapy among specific subgroups are listed in **Table 2**.

Certain patient subsets deserve mention, as follows.

DIABETES

Although the JNC 8 guidelines do not specify which of the 3 initial agents should be selected in patients with diabetes, the American Diabetes Association recommends treatment with an ACE inhibitor or ARB for initial therapy for hypertension.[21]

Table 2 Initial monotherapy	
General Population	
Nonblack	THZD, ACE inhibitor, ARB, or CCB
Black	THZD or CCB
CKD	
Nonblack	ACE inhibitor or ARB
Black	ACE inhibitor or ARB
Diabetes	
Nonblack	ACE inhibitor or ARB
Black	THZD or CCB[a]

Abbreviations: ACE, angiotensin-converting enzyme; ARB, angiotensin receptor blocker; CCB, calcium channel blocker; CKD, chronic kidney disease; THZD, thiazide-type diuretic.
   [a] Black patients with both diabetes and CKD should receive an ACE inhibitor or an ARB.
   Adapted with special permission from Treatment Guidelines from The Medical Letter, May 2014; Vol. 12 (141):31. www.medicalletter.org.

SYSTOLIC HEART FAILURE

According to the 2013 American College of Cardiology Foundation/American Heart Association guidelines, ACE inhibitors should be included as first-line therapy for patients with systolic heart failure to reduce morbidity and mortality.[22] ARBs should serve as initial therapy in patients who are intolerant to ACE inhibitors. β-Blockers with evidence of mortality reduction (carvedilol, bisoprolol, and sustained-release metoprolol) may be used as initial therapy for patients who are unable to take either an ACE inhibitor or an ARB.

BLACK PATIENTS

Recommendations for initial therapy in black patients comes from the ALLHAT (Antihypertensive and Lipid Lowering Treatment to Prevent Heart Attack Trial), in which thiazide diuretics and calcium channel blockers were superior to ACE inhibitors in a prespecified subset. In ALLHAT, black patients on ACE inhibitors were less likely to have controlled blood pressure and were 51% more likely to experience a stroke.[23] As an exception, black patients with chronic kidney disease should receive ACE inhibitors as first-line therapy because of improved renal outcomes in this subset.[24]

CHRONIC KIDNEY DISEASE

Patients aged 18 to 75 years with kidney disease should initially receive an ACE inhibitor or an ARB, regardless of race, diabetes status, or presence of proteinuria.

   For patients who are unable to achieve adequate blood pressure control with a single agent, medications should be added beginning with other first-line agents until patients are on a thiazide diuretic, dihydropyridine calcium channel blocker, and an ACE or an ARB. Agents from other classes may then be added if blood pressures remain higher than the desired target. **Tables 3–8** list the currently available antihypertensive agents available in the United States.

CLINICAL QUESTION: DOUBLE THE DOSE OF ANTIHYPERTENSIVE, OR ADD A SECOND AGENT?

It is clear that achieving proper blood pressure targets plays the largest role in reducing cardiovascular events. In patients with hypertension that is not controlled

Table 3
Diuretics

Drug[b]	Some Available Oral Formulations	Usual Maintenance Dosage[c]	Pregnancy Category[d]	Frequent or Severe Adverse Effects[e]	Cost ($)[f]
Thiazide Type					
Chlorthalidone: generic	25, 50 mg tabs	12.5–25 mg once/d	B	Hyperuricemia, hypokalemia, hypomagnesemia, hyperglycemia, hyponatremia, hypercalcemia, hypercholesterolemia, hypertriglyceridemia, pancreatitis, rash and other allergic reactions, photosensitivity reactions	6.60
Chlorothiazide: generic	250, 500 mg tabs	125–500 mg once/d	C		2.60
Diuril (Salix)	250 mg/5 mL susp				16.70
Hydrochlorothiazide: generic	12.5 mg caps; 12.5, 25, 50 mg tabs	12.5–50 mg once/d	B		8.40
Microzide (Actavis)	12.5 mg caps				35.10
Indapamide: generic	1.25, 2.5 mg tabs	1.25–2.5 mg once/d	B		6.90
Metolazone: generic	2.5, 5 mg tabs	2.5–5 mg once/d	B		24.70
Zaroxolyn (UCB)					83.10
Loop					
Bumetanide[a]: generic	0.5, 1, 2 mg tabs	0.5–2 mg once/d or divided BID	C	Dehydration, circulatory collapse, hypokalemia, hyponatremia, hypomagnesemia, hyperglycemia, metabolic alkalosis, hyperuricemia, blood dyscrasias, rash, hypercholesterolemia, hypertriglyceridemia	13.40
Ethacrynic acid[a]: *Edecrin* (Valeant)	25 mg tabs	50–200 mg once/d or divided BID	B		484.20
Furosemide: generic	20, 40, 80 tabs; 10 mg/mL, 40 mg/5 mL soln	20–80 mg once/d or divided BID	C		1.20
Lasix (Sanofi)	20, 40, 80 mg tabs				13.20
Torsemide: generic	5, 10, 20, 100 mg tabs	5–10 mg once/d	B		9.00
Demadex (Meda)					53.10

Potassium Sparing

Drug	Forms	Dosage	Preg.	Adverse Effects	Cost
Amiloride: generic	5 mg tabs	5–10 mg once/d	B	Hyperkalemia, GI disturbances, rash, headache	23.90
Triamterene[a]: *Dyrenium* (WellSpring)	50, 100 mg caps	50–150 mg once/d or divided BID	C	Hyperkalemia, GI disturbances, nephrolithiasis	99.60
Aldosterone Antagonists					
Eplerenone: generic *Inspra* (Pfizer)	25, 50 mg tabs	50 mg once/d or BID	B	Hyperkalemia, hyponatremia	94.20 174.60
Spironolactone: generic *Aldactone* (Pfizer)	25, 50, 100 mg tabs	50–100 mg once/d or divided BID	C	Hyperkalemia, hyponatremia, mastodynia, gynecomastia, menstrual abnormalities, GI disturbances, rash	6.20 68.10

Abbreviations: BID, twice a day; caps, capsules; GI, gastrointestinal; soln, solution; susp, suspension; tabs, tablets.
[a] Not US Food and Drug Administration (FDA)–approved for treatment of hypertension.
[b] Diuretics are not recommended for treatment of gestational hypertension.
[c] Dosage adjustments may be needed for renal or hepatic impairment.
[d] FDA pregnancy categories: A, controlled studies show no risk; B, no evidence of risk in animals; no human studies; C, risk cannot be ruled out; D, positive evidence of risk; X, contraindicated during pregnancy.
[e] Class effects. Some may not have been reported with every drug in the class. In addition to the adverse effects listed, antihypertensive drugs may interact adversely with other drugs.
[f] Approximate wholesale acquisition cost (WAC) for 30 days' treatment at the lowest recommended dosage. Source: Analy$ource Monthly (selected from FDB MedKnowledge) April 5, 2014. Reprinted with permission by FDB, Inc. All rights reserved. 2014. www.fdbhealth.com/policies/drug-pricing-policy. Actual retail prices may be higher.
Adapted with special permission from Treatment Guidelines from The Medical Letter, May 2014; Vol. 12 (141):31. www.medicalletter.org.

Table 4
Renin-angiotensin system inhibitors

Drug	Some Available Oral Formulations	Usual Maintenance Dosage[a]	Pregnancy Category[b,c]	Frequent or Severe Adverse Effects[d]	Cost[e]
ACE Inhibitors					
Benazepril: generic *Lotensin* (Novartis)	5, 10, 20, 40 mg tabs	20–80 mg once/d or divided BID	D	Cough, hypotension (particularly with diuretic use or volume depletion), rash, acute renal failure in patients with bilateral renal artery stenosis or stenosis of the artery to a solitary kidney, angioedema, hyperkalemia (particularly if also taking potassium supplements or potassium-sparing diuretics), mild to moderate loss of taste, hepatotoxicity, pancreatitis, blood dyscrasias and renal damage (particularly in patients with renal dysfunction)	$3.60
Captopril: generic	12.5, 25, 50, 100 mg tabs	25–50 mg BID or TID	D		57.30
Enalapril: generic *Vasotec* (Valeant)	2.5, 5, 10, 20 mg tabs	2.5–40 mg once/d or divided BID	D		22.80
			D		3.00
Fosinopril: generic	10, 20, 40 mg tabs	10–80 mg once/d or divided BID	D		135.50
					7.80
Lisinopril: generic *Zestril* (AstraZeneca) *Prinivil* (Merck)	2.5, 5, 10, 20, 30, 40 mg tabs 5, 10, 20 mg tabs	10–40 mg once/d	D		2.80
					39.60
					38.10
Moexipril: generic *Univasc* (UCB)	7.5, 15 mg tabs	7.5–30 mg once/d or divided BID	D		27.00
					78.00
Perindopril: generic *Aceon* (Xoma)	2, 4, 8 mg tabs	4–8 mg once/d or divided BID	D		19.80
					73.20
Quinapril: generic *Accupril* (Pfizer)	5, 10, 20, 40 mg tabs	10–80 mg once/d or divided BID	D		20.70
					74.10
Ramipril: generic *Altace* (Pfizer)	1.25, 2.5, 5, 10 mg caps	2.5–20 mg once/d or divided BID	D		5.70
					91.20
Trandolapril: generic *Mavik* (Abbvie)	1, 2, 4 mg tabs	1–8 mg once/d or divided BID	D		12.00
					52.50

ARBs					
Azilsartan: *Edarbi* (Arbor)	40, 80 mg tabs	80 mg once/d	D	Similar to ACE inhibitors; seldom cause cough, rarely cause angioedema and rhabdomyomas	118.00
Candesartan: generic; *Atacand* (AstraZeneca)	4, 8, 16, 32 mg tabs	8–32 mg once/d or divided BID	D		77.60 / 88.10
Eprosartan: generic; *Teveten* (Abbvie)	400, 600 mg tabs	400–800 mg once/d or divided BID	D		82.20 / 98.10
Irbesartan: generic; *Avapro* (Sanofi)	75, 150, 300 mg tabs	150–300 mg once/d	D		12.70 / 106.00
Losartan: generic; *Cozaar* (Merck)	25, 50, 100 mg labs	25–100 mg once/d or divided BID	D		3.60 / 63.90
Olmesartan: *Benicar* (Daiichi Sankyo)	5, 20, 40 mg tabs	20–40 mg once/d	D		106.80
Telmisartan: generic; *Micardis* (Boehringer Ingelheim)	20, 40, 68 mg tabs	20–80 mg once/d	D		115.70 / 147.20
Valsartan: *Diovan* (Novartis)	40, 80, 160, 320 mg tabs	80–320 mg once/d	D		129.00
Direct Renin Inhibitor (DRI)					
Aliskiren: *Tekturna* (Novartis)	150, 300 mg tabs	150–300 mg once/d	D	Same as ARBs, but can also cause GI effects such as diarrhea	115.30

Abbreviation: ARB, angiotensin receptor blocker.

a Dosage adjustments may be needed for renal or hepatic impairment.

b ACE inhibitors, ARBs, and aliskiren are classified as category D during the second and third trimesters. Drugs that act on the renin-angiotensin system can cause fetal and neonatal morbidity and death.

c FDA pregnancy categories: A, controlled studies show no risk; B, no evidence of risk in animals; no human studies; C, risk cannot be ruled out; D, positive evidence of risk; X, contraindicated during pregnancy.

d In addition to the adverse effects listed, antihypertensive drugs may interact adversely with other drugs.

e Approximate WAC for 30 days' treatment at the lowest recommended dosage. Source: Analy$ource monthly (selected from FDB Medknowledge) April 5, 2014.

Reprinted with permission by FDB, Inc. All rights reserved. 2014. www.fdbhealth.com/policies/drug-pricing-policy. Actual retail prices may be higher.

Adapted with special permission from Treatment Guidelines from The Medical Letter, May 2014; Vol. 12 (141):31. www.medicalletter.org.

Table 5
Calcium channel blockers

Drug	Some Available Oral Formulations	Usual Maintenance Dosage[a]	Pregnancy Category[b]	Frequent or Severe Adverse Effects[c]	Cost ($)[d]
Dihydropyridines					
Amlodipine[e]: generic	2.5, 5, 10 mg tabs	2.5–10 mg once/d	C	Dizziness, headache, peripheral edema (more than with verapamil and diltiazem, more common in women), flushing, tachycardia, rash, gingival hyperplasia	4.80
Norvasc (Pfizer)					94.50
Felodipine: generic	2.5, 5, 10 mg ER tabs	2.5–10 mg once/d	C		32.40
Isradipine: generic	2.5, 5 mg caps	5–10 mg divided BID	C		42.30
Nicardipine: generic ER	20, 30 mg caps	60–120 mg divided TID	C		58.50
Cardene SR (EKR)	30, 60 mg ER caps	60–120 mg divided BID			99.70
Nifedipine[f]: extended release, generic	30, 60, 90 mg ER tabs	30–90 mg once/d	C		27.90
Adalat CC (Bayer)					42.30
Procardia XL (Pfizer)					94.20
Nisoldipine: generic	8.5, 17, 20, 25.5, 30, 34, 40 mg ER tabs	17–34 mg once/d	C		182.70
Sular (Shionogi)	8.5, 17, 34 mg ER tabs				396.90

Nondihydropyridines					
Diltiazem[f] generic (ER)	180, 240, 300, 360, 420 mg ER tabs	120–540 mg once/d	C	Dizziness, headache, edema, constipation (especially verapamil), AV block, bradycardia, heart failure, lupuslike rash with diltiazem	106.77
Cardizem LA (Abbvie)	120, 180, 240, 300, 360, 420 mg ER tabs				114.10
generic (ER)	120, 180, 240, 300, 360 mg ER caps	120–540 mg once/d			19.40
Taztia XT[g] (Actavis)					24.40
Tiazac[h] (Valeant)					39.30
generic (continuous-delivery)	120, 180, 240, 300, 360 mg ER caps	180–360 mg once/d			27.30
Cardizem CD (Valeant)					320.30
Cartia XT[i] (Actavis)					27.90
Dilt-CD[i] (Apotex)					27.90
Verapamil (ER)	—	120–480 mg once/d or divided BID	C		—
generic (tabs)	120, 180, 240 mg ER tabs				23.30
generic (caps)	120, 180, 240, 360 mg ER caps				24.00
Calan SR (Pfizer) ER (once/d)	120, 180, 240 mg SR tabs	—			93.30
Covera-HS (Pfizer)	180, 240 mg ER tabs	180–480 mg once/d			64.20
Verelan (Elan) generic	120, 180, 240, 360 mg SR caps	120–480 mg once/d			144.30
					22.80
Verelan PM (Elan) generic	100, 200, 300 mg ER caps	200–400 mg once/d			150.60
					60.30

Abbreviations: AV, atrioventricular; ER, extended release; SR, sustained release.

a Dosage adjustments may be needed for renal or hepatic impairment.

b FDA pregnancy categories: A, controlled studies show no risk; B, no evidence of risk in animals; no human studies; C, risk cannot be ruled out; D, positive evidence of risk; X, contraindicated during pregnancy.

c In addition to the adverse effects listed, antihypertensive drugs may interact adversely with other drugs.

d Approximate WAC for 30 days' treatment at the lowest recommended dosage. Source: Analy$ource Monthly (selected from FDB MedKnowledge) April 5, 2014. Reprinted with permission by FDB, Inc. All rights reserved. 2014. www.fdbhealth.com/policies/drug-pricing-policy. Actual retail prices may be higher.

e Amlodipine is also available in combination with atorvastatin (*Caduet*, and generics).

f Immediate-release formulation is not recommended for treatment of hypertension.

g *Dilacor XR* (Actavis) is also available in 120, 180, 240 mg ER capsules.

h Also available in 420 mg ER caps.

i Not available in 360 mg ER caps.

Adapted with special permission from Treatment Guidelines from The Medical Letter, May 2014; Vol. 12 (141):31. www.medicalletter.org.

Table 6

Beta-adrenergic blockers

Drug	Some Available Oral Formulations	Usual Maintenance Dosage[a]	Pregnancy Category[b]	Frequent or Severe Adverse Effects[c]	Cost ($)[d]
Atenolol[e]: generic Tenormin (AstraZeneca)	25, 50, 100 mg tabs	50–100 mg once/d	D	Fatigue, depression, bradycardia, erectile dysfunction, decreased exercise tolerance, heart failure, worsening of peripheral arterial insufficiency, may aggravate allergic reactions, bronchospasm, may mask symptoms of and delay recovery from hypoglycemia, Raynaud phenomenon, insomnia, vivid dreams or hallucinations, acute mental disorder, increased serum triglyceride level, decreased HDL cholesterol level, increased incidence of diabetes, sudden withdrawal may lead to exacerbation of angina and myocardial infarction or precipitate thyroid storm	1.50
					47.10
Betaxolol[e]: generic	10, 20 mg tabs	5–20 mg once/d	C		12.80
Bisoprolol[e]: generic Zebeta (Teva)	5, 10 mg tabs	5–20 mg once/d	C		25.50
					134.90
Metoprolol[e]: generic ER generic	25, 50, 100 mg tabs 25, 50, 100, 200 mg ER tabs	100–450 mg divided BID or TID 25–400 mg once/d	C		2.40
					22.00
Toprol-XL (AstraZeneca)	—	—			35.70
Nadolol: generic Corgard (Pfizer)	20, 40, 80 mg tabs	40–320 mg once/d	C		95.60
					117.90
Propranolol: generic ER generic	10, 20, 40, 60, 80 mg tabs 60, 80, 120, 160 mg ER caps	80–240 mg divided BID 60–240 mg once/d	C		3.60
					47.00
Inderal LA (Akrimax)	—	—			315.60
InnoPran XL (GSK)	80, 120 mg ER caps	80–120 mg once/d			395.30
Timolol: generic	5, 10, 20 mg tabs	20–60 mg divided BID	C		39.60

β-Blockers with Intrinsic Sympathomimetic Activity

Acebutolol[e]: generic Sectral (Promius)	200, 400 mg caps	200–1200 mg once/d or divided BID	B	Similar to other beta-adrenergic blocking drugs, but with less resting bradycardia and lipid changes; acebutolol has been associated with a positive antinuclear antibody test and occasional drug-induced lupus	8.10 108.60
Penbutolol: Levatol (Auxilium)	20 mg tabs	10–80 mg once/d	C		50.85
Pindolol: generic	5, 10 mg tabs	10–60 mg divided BID	B		52.20

β-Blockers with α-Blocking Activity

Carvedilol: generic	3.125, 6.25, 12.5, 25 mg tabs	12.5–50 mg divided BID	C	Similar to other beta-adrenergic blocking drugs, but more orthostatic hypotension: hepatotoxicity with labetalol	6.40
Coreg (GSK) ER	10, 20, 40, 60 mg ER caps	20–80 mg once/d			159.60
Coreg CR (GSK)	100, 200, 300 mg tabs	200–1200 mg divided BID	C		160.70
Labetalol: generic	100, 200 mg tabs	—			21.00
Trandate (Prometheus)					37.20

β-Blockers with Vasodilating Nitric Oxide-mediated Activity

Nebivolol: Bystolic (Forest)	2.5, 5, 10, 20 mg tabs	5–40 mg once/d	C	Similar to other beta-adrenergic blocking drugs, but may not cause impotence, and may improve erectile dysfunction	78.70

Abbreviations: HDL, high-density lipoprotein; TID, 3 times a day.

a Dosage adjustments may be needed for renal or hepatic impairment.

b FDA pregnancy categories: A, controlled studies show no risk; B, no evidence of risk in animals; no human studies; C, risk cannot be ruled out; D, positive evidence of risk; X, contraindicated during pregnancy.

c In addition to the adverse effects listed, antihypertensive drugs may interact adversely with other drugs.

d Approximate WAC for 30 days' treatment at the lowest recommended dosage. Source: Analy$ource Monthly (selected from FDB MedKnowledge) April 5, 2014. Reprinted with permission by FDB. Inc. All rights reserved. 2014. www.fdbhealth.com/policies/drug-pricing-policy. Actual retail prices may be higher.

e Cardioselective.

Adapted with special permission from Treatment Guidelines from The Medical Letter, May 2014; Vol. 12 (141):31. www.medicalletter.org.

Table 7
Alpha-adrenergic blockers and other antihypertensives

Drug	Some Available Oral Formulations	Usual Maintenance Dosage[b]	Pregnancy Category[c]	Frequent or Severe Adverse Effects[d]	Cost ($)[e]
Alpha-adrenergic Blockers					
Doxazosin: generic	1, 2, 4, 8 mg tabs	1–16 mg once/d	C	Syncope with first dose (less likely with terazosin and doxazosin), dizziness and vertigo, headache, palpitations, fluid retention, drowsiness, weakness, anticholinergic effects, priapism, thrombocytopenia, atrial fibrillation	16.20
Cardura (Pfizer) ER					65.40
Cardura XL[a]	4, 8 mg ER tabs	4–8 mg once/d	C		75.50
Prazosin: generic	1, 2, 5 mg caps	6–20 mg divided BID or TID	C		30.30
Minipress (Pfizer)					139.50
Terazosin: generic	1, 2, 5, 10 mg caps	1–20 mg once/d or divided BID	C		4.60
Central Alpha-adrenergic Agonists					
Clonidine: generic	0.1, 0.2, 0.3 mg tabs	0.2–0.6 mg divided BID or TID	C	CNS reactions similar to methyldopa, but more sedation and dry mouth; bradycardia, heart block, rebound hypertension (less likely with patch), contact dermatitis from patch	3.60
Catapres (Boehringer Ingelheim)					111.00
Guanfacine: generic	1, 2 mg tabs	1–3 mg once/d[f]	B	Similar to clonidine but milder	8.30
Tenex (Promius)					72.00
Methyldopa: generic	250, 500 mg tabs	500 mg–2 g divided BID or 4 times a day	B	Sedation, fatigue, depression, dry mouth, orthostatic hypotension, bradycardia, heart block, autoimmune disorders (including colitis, hepatitis), hepatic necrosis, Coombs-positive lupuslike syndrome, thrombocytopenia, red cell aplasia, impotence, hemolytic anemia	9.00

Direct Vasodilators

Drug	Dosage form	Dosage	Pregnancy category	Adverse effects	Price
Hydralazine: generic	10, 25, 50, 100 mg tabs	40–200 mg divided BID or 4 times a day	C	Tachycardia, aggravation of angina, headache, dizziness, fluid retention, nasal congestion, lupuslike syndrome, hepatitis	22.60
Minoxidil: generic	2.5, 10 mg tabs	5–40 mg once/d or divided BID	C	Tachycardia, aggravation of angina, marked fluid retention, pericardial effusion, hair growth on face and body	20.10

Abbreviations: CNS, central nervous system; ER, extended release.

[a] Not FDA-approved for treatment of hypertension.
[b] Dosage adjustments may be needed for renal or hepatic impairment.
[c] FDA pregnancy categories: A, controlled studies show no risk; B, no evidence of risk in animals, no human studies; C, risk cannot be ruled out; D, positive evidence of risk; X, contraindicated during pregnancy.
[d] In addition to the adverse effects listed, antihypertensive drugs may interact adversely with other drugs.
[e] Approximate WAC for 30 days' treatment at the lowest recommended dosage. Source: Analy$ource Monthly (selected from FDB MedKnowledge) April 5, 2014. Reprinted with permission by FDB, Inc. All rights reserved. 2014. www.fdbhealth.com/policies/drug-pricing-policy. Actual retail prices may be higher.
[f] The first dose is 1 mg at bed time.

Adapted with special permission from Treatment Guidelines from The Medical Letter, May 2014; Vol. 12 (141):31. www.medicalletter.org.

Table 8
Some combination products

Drug	Some Oral Formulations	Cost ($)[a]
ACE Inhibitors and Diuretics		
Benazepril/HCTZ generic	5/6.25, 10/12.5, 20/12.5, 20/25 mg tabs	48.60
Captopril/HCTZ generic	25/15, 25/25, 50/15, 50/25 mg tabs	8.70
Enalapril/HCTZ generic	5/12.5, 10/25 mg tabs	14.70
Vaseretic (Valeant)	10/25 mg tabs	168.60
Fosinopril/HCTZ generic	10/12.5, 20/12.5 mg tabs	32.40
Lisinopril/HCTZ generic	10/12.5, 20/12.5, 20/25 mg tabs	5.70
Zestoretic (AstraZeneca)		43.80
Moexipril/HCTZ generic	7.5/12.5, 15/12.5, 15/25 mg tabs	27.00
Uniretic (UCB)		75.00
Quinapril/HCTZ generic	10/12.5, 20/12.5, 20/25 mg tabs	30.30
Accuretic (Pfizer)		72.00
ARBs and Diuretics		
Azilsartan/chlorthalidone	40/12.5, 40/25 mg tabs	111.30
Edarbyclor (Arbor)		
Candesartan/HCTZ generic	16/12.5, 32/12.5, 32/25 mg tabs	94.40
Atacand HCT (AstraZeneca)		119.10
Eprosartan/HCTZ	600/12.5, 600/25 mg tabs	134.10
Teveten HCT (Abbvie)		
Irbesartan/HCTZ generic	150/12.5, 300/12.5 mg tabs	21.60
Avalide (Sanofi)		141.00
Losartan/HCTZ generic	50/12.5, 100/12.5, 100/25 mg tabs	9.30
Hyzaar (Merck)		94.80
Olmesartan/HCTZ	20/12.5, 40/12.5, 40/25 mg tabs	106.80
Benicar HCT (Daiichi Sankyo)		
Telmisartan/HCTZ generic	40/12.5, 80/12.5, 80/25 mg tabs	120.90
Micardis HCT (Boehringer Ingelheim)		147.20
Valsartan/HCTZ generic	80/12.5, 160/12.5, 160/25, 320/12.5,	104.00
Diovan HCT (Novartis)	320/25 mg tabs	104.70
Direct Renin Inhibitor and Diuretic		
Aliskiren/HCTZ	150/12.5, 150/25, 300/12.5, 300/25 mg	114.30
Tekturna HCT (Novartis)	tabs	
Beta-Adrenergic Blockers and Diuretics		
Atenolol/chlorthalidone generic	50/25, 100/25 mg tabs	4.10
Tenoretic (AstraZeneca)		51.60
Bisoprolol/HCTZ generic	2.5/6.25, 5/6.25, 10/6.25 mg tabs	6.10
Ziac (Duramed/Barr)		134.70
Metoprolol/HCTZ generic	50/25, 100/25, 100/50 mg tabs	27.90
Lopressor HCT (Validus)	50/25 mg tabs	62.10
Nadolol/bendroflumethiazide generic	40/5, 80/5 mg tabs	55.80
Corzide (Pfizer)		121.80
Calcium Channel Blockers and ACE Inhibitors		
Amlodipine/benazepril generic	2.5/10, 5/10, 5/20,5/40	40.90

(continued on next page)

Table 8
(continued)

Drug	Some Oral Formulations	Cost ($)[a]
Lotrel (Novartis)	10/20, 10/40 mg caps	157.80
Verapamil ER/trandolapril Tarka (Abbvie)	180/2, 240/1, 240/2, 240/4 mg tabs	127.20
Calcium Channel Blockers and ARBs		
Amlodipine/telmisartan: generic Twynsta (Boehringer Ingelheim)	5/40, 5/80, 10/40, 10/80 mg tabs	127.30 158.40
Amlodipine/valsartan Exforge (Novartis)	5/160, 5/320, 10/160, 10/320 mg tabs	151.90
Amlodipine/olmesartan Azor (Daiichi Sankyo)	5/20, 5/40, 10/20, 10/40 mg tabs	133.20
Calcium Channel Blocker and Direct Renin Inhibitor		
Amplodipine/aliskiren Tekamlo (Novartis)	5/150, 10/150, 5/300, 10/300 mg tabs	114.00
Diuretic Combinations		
HCTZ/spironolactone generic	25/25 mg tabs	30.20
Aldactazide (Pharmacia)	25/25, 50/50 mg tabs	39.90
HCTZ/triamterene generic	25/37.5, 50/75 mg tabs, 25/37.5, 25/50 mg caps	6.40
Dyazide (GSK)	25/37.5 mg caps	37.80
Maxzide (Mylan)	25/37.5, 50/75 mg tabs	40.50
HCTZ/amiloride generic	50/5 mg tabs	8.10
Central Alpha-Adrenergic Agonist and Diuretic		
Clonidine/chlorthalidone Clorpres (Mylan)	0.1/15, 0.2/15, 0.3/15 mg tabs	59.40
Triple Drug Combinations		
Aliskiren/amlodipine/HCTZ Amturnide (Novartis)	150/5/12.5, 300/5/12.5, 300/5/25, 300/10/12.5, 300/10/25 mg tabs	103.70
Valsartan/amlodipine/HCTZ Exforge HCT (Novartis)	160/5/12.5, 160/5/25, 160/10/12.5, 160/10/25, 320/10/25 mg tabs	151.90
Olmesartan/amlodipine/HCTZ Tribenzor (Daiichi Sankyo)	20/5/12.5, 40/5/12.5, 40/5/25, 40/10/12.5, 40/10/25 mg tabs	133.20

Abbreviation: HCTZ, hydrochlorothiazide.

[a] Approximate WAC for 30 of the lowest strength tablets or capsules. Source: Analy$ource monthly (selected from FDB MedKnowledge) April 5, 2014. Reprinted with permission by FDB, Inc. All rights reserved. 2014. www.fdbhealth.com/policies/drug-pricing-policy. Actual retail prices may be higher.

Adapted with special permission from Treatment Guidelines from The Medical Letter, May 2014; Vol. 12 (141):31. www.medicalletter.org.

with a low dose of a single agent, a long-standing question is whether clinicians should continue to increase the dose of the initial agent or add a second agent. A meta-analysis reviewed blood pressure reductions of 11,000 patients included in 42 randomized trials comparing monotherapy with escalation of dose against combination therapy.[25] Overall, combination therapy resulted in a 5-fold greater reduction in blood pressure compared with combination therapy. Fixed-dose combinations of antihypertensive agents are becoming increasingly available, improve compliance compared with the individual components given separately, and reduce overall costs of therapy.[26–28] In major randomized trials of blood pressure reduction resulting in cardiovascular benefits, at least 75% of included patients required 2 or more medications to achieve a target blood pressure of less than 140/90 mm Hg.[29,30]

CLINICAL BOTTOM LINE

For most patients with hypertension that is not controlled on a low dose of a single agent, switching to combination therapy rather than increasing the dosage is the most effective approach for reaching blood pressure targets.

CLINICAL QUESTION: DOES TIMING MATTER?

Blood pressure fluctuates diurnally, and epidemiologic studies have shown a preponderance of angina, myocardial infarction, and stroke during the early morning hours.[31] Studies of ambulatory blood pressure reveal that most individuals with or without hypertension experience a reduction in blood pressure of 10% to 20% during the nighttime, a phenomenon known as dipping. Absence of a dipping pattern at night as well as nocturnal hypertension have been linked to increased risk of cardiovascular morbidity and mortality.[32,33] In patients with refractory hypertension, the usual course is to increase the dose of an existing medication or add an additional agent. In lieu of these strategies, recent investigations have assessed changing the timing of blood pressure medication administration to try to address nighttime blood pressures without adding medications or adjusting dosage, a process known as chronotherapy.

Two studies examined the effects of administration of at least 1 antihypertensive medication at nighttime compared with conventional morning-only dosing.[34,35] The first enrolled 448 type 2 diabetics with hypertension and randomly assigned them to receive their usual blood pressure medications in the morning, or to have at least 1 of their medications moved to bedtime administration.[34] The study did not call for any dose adjustments in medication at baseline, just a change in timing.

Over a follow-up period of 5.4 years, taking at least 1 blood pressure medication at night resulted in significant improvements in sleeping systolic pressure (115.0 vs 122.4 mm Hg; $P<.001$) and controlled ambulatory blood pressure (62.5% vs 50.9%; $P = .013$), and (most impressively) cardiovascular events were reduced by about two-thirds (54.2 vs 19.8 events per 1000 patients; $P<.001$). There were no differences in the number or types of antihypertensive medications used between the two groups. Based on these results, the American Diabetes Association recommends (grade A) that patients with diabetes and hypertension on multiple medications have at least 1 medication administered at nighttime.[36]

The second study of identical design followed 661 patients with hypertension and chronic kidney disease over a period of 5.4 years.[35] Once again, nighttime administration of at least 1 blood pressure agent resulted in a significantly greater percentage of patients with controlled ambulatory blood pressures (56% vs 45%; $P = .003$) and a vast reduction in cardiovascular events (adjusted hazard ratio [HR], 0.31; 95% confidence interval [CI], 0.21–0.46; $P<.001$).

CLINICAL BOTTOM LINE

Timing of blood pressure medications may have an important effect on ambulatory and nighttime blood pressures as well as cardiovascular events. Although further studies are needed to confirm these findings, it is reasonable to consider changing 1 or more morning blood pressure medications to evening administration in patients with uncontrolled hypertension.

CLINICAL QUESTION: ANGIOTENSIN-CONVERTING ENZYME VERSUS ANGIOTENSIN RECEPTOR BLOCKER VERSUS BOTH?

Both ACE inhibitors and ARBs target the renin-angiotensin-aldosterone system (RAAS) and are reasonable first-line agents for blood pressure control. Both classes of medication have been shown to reduce progression of kidney disease in patients with diabetes and evidence of proteinuria. In addition, both ACE inhibitors and ARBs have proven efficacy for reduction of symptoms, cardiovascular events, and mortality in patients with systolic heart failure. An important question arises: are these drugs interchangeable?

There have been a few direct comparison trials involving about 11,000 patients. In a systematic review of those trials, the two classes had similar efficacy on blood pressure with no differences seen in mortality or cardiovascular events.[37] Withdrawal from drug because of adverse events was seen more often with ACE inhibitors, primarily related to presence of a dry cough, with a number needed to treat with an ARB of 55 over 4.1 years to see 1 fewer drug withdrawal event.

However, a couple of recent meta-analyses examined the performance of each of these drug classes versus placebo on a much larger scale.[38,39] In a collection of nearly 160,000 patients randomized to receive an RAAS drug versus placebo, there was an overall 5% reduction in all-cause mortality and a 7% reduction in cardiovascular mortality.[38] When separated by drug class, it became apparent that the entire reduction was accounted for by the ACE inhibitor class, with an overall reduction in all-cause mortality of 10% with ACE inhibition, with no significant reduction in trials of ARBs versus placebo.

A second meta-analysis assessed studies of ACE or ARB versus placebo in 56,704 patients with diabetes.[39] ACE inhibitor usage resulted in a 13% risk reduction in all-cause mortality, a 17% risk reduction in cardiovascular mortality, and a 14% reduction in major cardiovascular events. In contrast, using ARBs did not significantly affect all-cause mortality, cardiovascular mortality, or serious cardiovascular events. Although imperfect, this large volume of indirect comparison evidence is highly suggestive of a greater benefit with use of ACE inhibitors compared with ARBs for hypertension control.

CLINICAL BOTTOM LINE

When selecting a RAAS inhibitor for hypertension, ACE inhibitors should remain the drugs of choice.

CLINICAL QUESTION: IS THERE A ROLE FOR COMBINATION ANGIOTENSIN-CONVERTING ENZYME AND ANGIOTENSIN RECEPTOR BLOCKER THERAPY?

Diabetic nephropathy is the leading cause of end-stage renal disease in the United States, and individuals with proteinuria are at the highest risk.[40,41] Both ACE inhibitors and ARBs have been proved to delay the onset of proteinuria as well as to postpone the development of proteinuric renal failure.[42,43] The degree of reduction in proteinuria directly correlates with the magnitude of benefit from these agents.[41] Combination therapy with both ACE inhibitors and ARBs has been shown to provide further reduction in proteinuria beyond that of either agent alone.[44] Both ACE inhibitors and ARBs have also been shown to reduce cardiovascular morbidity and mortality in patients with heart failure, left ventricular dysfunction, vascular disease, or high-risk diabetes without heart failure.[45–48]

Two trials investigated combining ACE inhibitors and ARBs in management of patients with congestive heart failure.[49,50] The Val-HeFT (Valsartan Heart Failure Trial) trial randomized patients with systolic heart failure on traditional medications to receive the ARB valsartan or placebo.[49] Ninety-three percent of the participants were taking an ACE inhibitor during enrollment. The investigators discovered a significant reduction in heart failure symptoms and hospitalizations among patients on dual therapy. Safety concerns emerged from the trial, with post hoc analysis showing increased cardiovascular mortality among patients taking the combination of valsartan, an ACE inhibitor, and a β-blocker. Renal impairment and dizziness were also more common in patients receiving valsartan therapy.

The CHARM-Added trial involved 2548 patients with symptomatic systolic heart failure on ACE inhibitors who were then randomized to receive candesartan or placebo.[50] The primary outcome examined was a composite end point of cardiovascular death or hospitalization for congestive heart failure. The primary outcome was significantly reduced with combination therapy with ACE and candesartan after a median of 41 months of follow-up. Unlike the Val-HeFT study, patients experienced benefit while on β-blockers as well. Once again, worsening of serum creatinine levels and hyperkalemia occurred more frequently with the combination of ACE and ARB therapy.

These observations have led investigators to study the effects of combined RAAS inhibition for both the reduction of cardiovascular events and for nephroprotection. In the ONTARGET trial, investigators randomized 25,620 patients with vascular disease or high-risk diabetes to ramipril, telmisartan, or a combination of the two drugs.[51] The primary composite outcome measured was death from cardiovascular causes, myocardial infarction, stroke, or hospitalization for heart failure. After 56 months of follow-up, there was no difference in primary event rates between the three groups. Combination therapy did result in increased rates of hypotensive symptoms, syncope, acute kidney injury, and hyperkalemia.

The NEPHRON-D trial randomly assigned 1448 patients with diabetes, chronic kidney disease, and significant proteinuria (urine albumin/creatinine ratio >300) to therapy with losartan and lisinopril versus losartan alone.[52] The primary end point measured was a combination of decline in GFR greater than 30 mL/min, new-onset end-stage renal disease, or death. After a mean follow-up of 2.2 years, the two groups did not differ in development of the primary end point despite a significantly greater reduction in albuminuria in the combination therapy group. The study was halted prematurely because of a significant increase in serious adverse events with combination therapy, specifically acute kidney injury and hyperkalemia.

A third major randomized controlled trial of dual RAAS inhibition was the ALTITUDE study, which used aliskiren, a direct renin inhibitor.[53] The investigator compared the effects of aliskiren versus placebo in 8606 diabetic patients with baseline proteinuria or cardiovascular disease. All of the subjects were already taking an ACE inhibitor or an ARB. The primary outcomes measured were important cardiovascular and renal events. Once again, the study was halted early (mean follow-up, 32 months) because of a lack of cardiovascular and renal benefits with a clear increase in adverse events, primarily hyperkalemia and hypotension.

CLINICAL BOTTOM LINE

RAAS inhibitors should never be combined for treatment of hypertension because of an excess of adverse effects without additional cardiovascular or renal benefits.

CLINICAL QUESTION: WHEN SHOULD ADDITION OF SPIRONOLACTONE BE CONSIDERED?

Spironolactone, a potassium-sparing diuretic, is a highly effective but seldom used agent for hypertension. Two separate meta-analyses of spironolactone trials showed an average blood pressure reduction of 17 to 20 mm Hg over 4 to 9 mm Hg, with the largest reductions seen in patients with systolic blood pressure greater than 150 mm Hg at baseline.[54,55] Refractory hypertension is defined as blood pressure that remains greater than 140/90 mm Hg despite adherence to an antihypertensive regimen of 3 or more drugs with at least 1 of those agents being a diuretic. Approximately 12% of all hypertensives have refractory hypertension, which corresponds with about 9 million people in the United States.[56] In a study of 175 patients with refractory hypertension on a mean of 4 blood pressure medications, addition of spironolactone resulted in a reduction of blood pressure by an average of 16/9 mm Hg, with about half of the patients on the medication achieving a goal blood pressure of less than 140/90 mm Hg.[57]

CLINICAL BOTTOM LINE

For patients with hypertension that is refractory to 3 or more medications, including a diuretic, spironolactone is an excellent adjunctive agent for blood pressure control. Patients should be monitored carefully for hyperkalemia.

CLINICAL QUESTION: MY PATIENT HAS GOUT AND HYPERTENSION. ANY SPECIAL CONSIDERATIONS?

Hypertension is a common comorbidity in patients with gout. According to the US National Health and Nutrition Survey of 2007 to 2008, hypertension is present in 74% of patients with gout.[58] Certain antihypertensive medications, such as thiazide diuretics, β-blockers, and ACE inhibitors, induce hyperuricemia, whereas other medications, such as losartan and dihydropyridine calcium antagonists, reduce serum uric acid levels.[59–61] A nested case-control study focused on 24,768 people with gout and compared them with 50,000 controls in a general practice setting.[62] As shown in **Table 9**, gout was diagnosed more frequently in patients on drugs that promote hyperuricemia, and followed a consistent pattern according to a drug's tendency to increase or decrease serum uric acid level.

CLINICAL BOTTOM LINE

For hypertensive patients with gout, losartan and calcium channel blockers are preferred agents because of their urate level–reducing properties. Diuretics pose the greatest risk for inducing gout flares.

Table 9 New Diagnosis of gout according to anti-hypertensive drug or class	
Antihypertensive	RR of New Diagnosis of Gout
Losartan	0.81 (0.70–0.94)
Calcium antagonists	0.87 (0.82–0.93)
ACE inhibitors	1.24 (1.17–1.32)
Nonlosartan ARBs	1.29 (1.16–1.43)
Beta-antagonists	1.48 (1.40–1.57)
Diuretics	2.36 (2.21–2.52)

Abbreviation: RR, Relative risk.

CLINICAL QUESTION: ARE THERE ANY NEW DRUGS AVAILABLE FOR TREATMENT OF HYPERTENSION?

The sodium-glucose cotransporter 2 (SGLT-2) inhibitors (canagliflozin, dapagliflozin, empagliflozin) are a novel class of agents that have gained widespread use in type 2 diabetes since their approval in 2013. These drugs selectively inhibit glucose reabsorption in the proximal renal tubules, resulting in significant glucosuria, with a resultant osmotic diuresis, weight loss, and blood pressure reduction.[63] Although not approved specifically for hypertension, a meta-analysis of studies of the SGLT-2 inhibitors in about 13,000 diabetic patients revealed average blood pressure reduction of 4.0/1.6 mm Hg.[64] Although it is not certain why blood pressure declines, proposed mechanisms include diuresis, nephron remodeling, reduction of arterial stiffness, and weight loss.[65]

A recent analysis of 7020 diabetic patients with established cardiovascular disease randomized to empagliflozin therapy versus placebo revealed significant reductions in hospitalization for heart failure as well as cardiovascular and all-cause mortality.[66] Empagliflozin was generally well tolerated, with the most common adverse effect of a higher incidence of genital area infections.

CLINICAL BOTTOM LINE

The SGLT-2 inhibitors seem to be useful adjuncts for blood pressure control in patients with type 2 diabetes, especially those with concomitant cardiovascular disease.

CLINICAL QUESTION: WHAT LIFESTYLE MODIFICATIONS ARE REASONABLE FOR MANAGEMENT OF HYPERTENSION?

Blood pressure reduction can be achieved by both pharmacologic and nonpharmacologic means, and, for many patients, maximal medical therapy proves insufficient for controlling blood pressure to desired targets. Several lifestyle interventions can produce important and dramatic decreases in blood pressure, with weight reduction the most potent mediator among them.[5] **Table 10** summarizes the impact of several lifestyle approaches.[5,67]

CLINICAL BOTTOM LINE

Lifestyle modifications can have a major impact on blood pressure control, and should be discussed with all patients before initiating pharmacologic interventions.

Table 10 Lifestyle interventions for hypertension	
Intervention	Average Systolic BP Reduction (mm Hg)
Weight Reduction	5–20 per 10 kg weight loss
DASH diet	8–14
Dietary sodium restriction (<2.4 g/d)	2–8
Increased physical activity	4–9
Moderation of alcohol	2–4
Vegetarian diet	5

Abbreviations: BP, blood pressure; DASH, Dietary approaches to stop hypertension.

CLINICAL QUESTION: WHAT NONPHARMACOLOGIC METHODS ARE REASONABLE FOR MANAGEMENT OF HYPERTENSION?

There has long been an interest in nonpharmacologic therapies to reduce blood pressure. However, there are few properly conducted large randomized placebo-controlled trials to definitively support use of most nonpharmacologic treatments. Although there may be merit to several of these listed interventions, at present there is insufficient evidence to recommend acupuncture, yoga, classical music, prayer, biofeedback, controlled breathing devices, herbal products, or supplements to reliably reduce blood pressure. **Table 11** highlights a few interventions that have reasonable evidence to be considered as adjuncts to major lifestyle modifications and pharmacologic agents.

Dark Chocolate

Two meta-analyses of 15 to 20 randomized trials of varying quantities of dark chocolate versus placebo have found a blood pressure reduction of approximately 3/2 mm Hg.[68,69]

Tea

A meta-analysis of 25 randomized trials involving 1476 subjects showed that regular consumption of tea resulted in average blood pressure reduction of 1.8/1.4 mm Hg, with green tea having a more pronounced effect than black tea.[70] Although acute intake of caffeine (200–300 mg) results in an abrupt increase in blood pressure of 8.1/5.7 mm Hg, chronic coffee consumption does not seem to cause persistent increases in blood pressure readings.[71–73]

Massage

A systematic review of 24 trials involving 1962 subjects randomized to massage therapy compared with placebo or antihypertensive medications found significant blood pressure reductions with massage, although the methodological quality of the studies was assessed as poor.[74]

Tai Chi

A 2008 review of 26 studies of tai chi including 1087 patients in randomized controlled trials showed a consistent benefit of tai chi for blood pressure.[75] A recent randomized controlled trial of 266 older Chinese adults with hypertension found significant reduction in blood pressure at the end of a 12-month study period, although the blood pressure difference may be accounted for by loss of greater than 1 unit of body mass index in the tai chi participants.[76]

Table 11
Nonpharmacologic interventions for hypertension

Intervention	Average BP Reduction (mm Hg)
Dark chocolate	2.8–3.2/2.0–2.2
Tea consumption	1.8/1.4
Green tea	2.1/1.7
Black tea	1.4/1.1
Massage therapy	6.9/3.6
Tai chi	8.1/4.6

CLINICAL QUESTION: ARE THERE EFFECTIVE PROCEDURAL APPROACHES TO HYPERTENSION MANAGEMENT?

Procedural approaches to hypertension management have generated a lot of interest in the past decade, with particular focus on 2 procedures: radiofrequency denervation of the renal arteries and electrical stimulation of the carotid baroreceptors. Early, unblinded trials of renal denervation therapy resulted in impressive reductions in blood pressure, with improvement extending out to 3 years of follow-up.[77,78] The procedure was generally safe and well tolerated. However, a well-designed, blinded, multicenter randomized trial (SYMPLICITY-HTN-3) failed to corroborate these findings, stemming the tide of enthusiasm for this approach.[79] Further studies are needed to elucidate whether there is a role for renal denervation therapy in certain subsets of patients with refractory hypertension.

Electrostimulation of the carotid baroreflex system through a surgically implantable device has been shown to reduce blood pressure for sustained periods, but at the expense of a high rate of surgical complications.[80,81] Further studies are needed to determine whether this procedure will provide lasting control of blood pressure at an acceptable level of risk.

CLINICAL BOTTOM LINE

There are no convincing data to support the safety and efficacy of procedural approaches for the management of high blood pressure.

REFERENCES

1. Lim SS, Vos T, Flaxman AD, et al. A comparative risk assessment of burden of disease and injury attributable to 67 risk factors and risk factor clusters in 21 regions, 1990-2010: a systematic analysis for the Global Burden of Disease Study 2010. Lancet 2012;380:2224–60.
2. Nwankwo T, Yoon SS, Burt V, et al. Hypertension among adults in the United States: National Health and Nutrition Examination Survey, 2011-2012. NCHS Data Brief 2013;133:1–8.
3. Kearney PM, Whelton M, Reynolds K, et al. Global burden of hypertension: analysis of worldwide data. Lancet 2005;365:217–23.
4. Lloyd-Jones D, Adams R, Carnethon M, et al. Heart disease and stroke statistics–2009 update: a report from the American Heart Association Statistics Committee and Stroke Statistics Subcommittee. Circulation 2009;119:e21–181.
5. Chobanian AV, Bakris GL, Black HR, et al. The seventh report of the Joint National Committee on Prevention, Detection, Evaluation, and Treatment of High Blood Pressure: the JNC 7 report. JAMA 2003;289:2560–72.
6. Neal B, MacMahon S, Chapman N, Blood Pressure Lowering Treatment Trialists' Collaboration. Effects of ACE inhibitors, calcium antagonists, and other blood-pressure-lowering drugs: results of prospectively designed overviews of randomised trials. Blood Pressure Lowering Treatment Trialists' Collaboration. Lancet 2000;356:1955–64.
7. Psaty BM, Smith NL, Siscovick DS, et al. Health outcomes associated with antihypertensive therapies used as first-line agents. A systematic review and meta-analysis. JAMA 1997;277:739–45.
8. Law MR, Morris JK, Wald NJ. Use of blood pressure lowering drugs in the prevention of cardiovascular disease: meta-analysis of 147 randomised trials in the

context of expectations from prospective epidemiological studies. BMJ 2009; 338:b1665.

9. Arguedas JA, Perez MI, Wright JM. Treatment blood pressure targets for hypertension. Cochrane Database Syst Rev 2009;(3):CD004349.

10. Appel LJ, Wright JT Jr, Greene T, et al. Intensive blood-pressure control in hypertensive chronic kidney disease. N Engl J Med 2010;363:918–29.

11. ACCORD Study Group, Cushman WC, Evans GW, Byington RP, et al. Effects of intensive blood-pressure control in type 2 diabetes mellitus. N Engl J Med 2010;362:1575–85.

12. James PA, Oparil S, Carter BL, et al. 2014 evidence-based guideline for the management of high blood pressure in adults: report from the panel members appointed to the Eighth Joint National Committee (JNC 8). JAMA 2014;311:507–20.

13. SPRINT Research Group, Wright JT Jr, Williamson JD, Whelton PK, et al. A randomized trial of intensive versus standard blood-pressure control. N Engl J Med 2015;373:2103–16.

14. Beckett NS, Peters R, Fletcher AE, et al. Treatment of hypertension in patients 80 years of age or older. N Engl J Med 2008;358:1887–98.

15. Prevention of stroke by antihypertensive drug treatment in older persons with isolated systolic hypertension. Final results of the Systolic Hypertension in the Elderly Program (SHEP). SHEP Cooperative Research Group. JAMA 1991;265: 3255–64.

16. Staessen JA, Fagard R, Thijs L, et al. Randomised double-blind comparison of placebo and active treatment for older patients with isolated systolic hypertension. The Systolic Hypertension in Europe (Syst-Eur) Trial Investigators. Lancet 1997;350:757–64.

17. Brunström M, Carlberg B. Lower blood pressure targets: to whom do they apply? Lancet 2015;387(10017):405–6.

18. Wright JT Jr, Fine LJ, Lackland DT, et al. Evidence supporting a systolic blood pressure goal of less than 150 mm Hg in patients aged 60 years or older: the minority view. Ann Intern Med 2014;160(7):499–503.

19. Kostis JB, Cabrera J, Cheng JQ. Association between chlorthalidone treatment of systolic hypertension and long-term survival. JAMA 2011;306:2588–93.

20. Wright JT Jr, Probstfield JL, Cushman WC, et al. ALLHAT findings revisited in the context of subsequent analyses, other trials, and meta-analyses. Arch Intern Med 2009;169:832–42.

21. American Diabetes Association. Standards of medical care in diabetes–2015. Diabetes Care 2015;38(Suppl 1):S1–93.

22. Yancy CW, Jessup M, Bozkurt B, et al. 2013 ACCF/AHA guideline for the management of heart failure: executive summary: a report of the American College of Cardiology Foundation/American Heart Association Task Force on Practice Guidelines. Circulation 2013;128(16):1810–52.

23. Leenen FH, Nwachuku CE, Black HR, et al. Clinical events in high-risk hypertensive patients randomly assigned to calcium channel blocker versus angiotensin-converting enzyme inhibitor in the antihypertensive and lipid-lowering treatment to prevent heart attack trial. Hypertension 2006;48(3):374–84.

24. Wright JT Jr, Bakris G, Greene T, et al. Effect of blood pressure lowering and antihypertensive drug class on progression of hypertensive kidney disease: results from the AASK trial. JAMA 2002;288(19):2421–31.

25. Wald DS, Law M, Morris JK, et al. Combination therapy versus monotherapy in reducing blood pressure: meta-analysis on 11,000 participants from 42 trials. Am J Med 2009;122:290–300.

26. Gupta AK, Arshad S, Poulter NR. Compliance, safety, and effectiveness of fixed-dose combinations of antihypertensive agents: a meta-analysis. Hypertension 2010;55:399–407.

27. Yang W, Chang J, Kahler KH, et al. Evaluation of compliance and health care utilization in patients treated with single pill vs. free combination antihypertensives. Curr Med Res Opin 2010;26:2065–76.

28. Aagren M, Luo W. Association between glycemic control and short-term healthcare costs among commercially insured diabetes patients in the United States. J Med Econ 2011;14:108–14.

29. Gradman AH, Basile JN, Carter BL, et al. Combination therapy in hypertension. J Am Soc Hypertens 2010;4(1):42–50.

30. Corrao G, Parodi A, Zambon A, et al. Reduced discontinuation of antihypertensive treatment by two-drug combination as first step. Evidence from daily life practice. J Hypertens 2010;28(7):1584–90.

31. Smolensky MH, Portaluppi F. Chronopharmacology and chronotherapy of cardiovascular medications: relevance to prevention and treatment of coronary heart disease. Am J Med 1999;137(4):S14–24.

32. Friedman O, Logan AG. Can nocturnal hypertension predict cardiovascular risk? Integr Blood Press Control 2009;2:25–37.

33. Fagard RH, Celis H, Thijs L, et al. Daytime and nighttime blood pressure as predictors of death and cause-specific cardiovascular events in hypertension. Hypertension 2008;51(1):55–61.

34. Hermida RC, Ayala DE, Mojón A, et al. Influence of time of day of blood pressure-lowering treatment on cardiovascular risk in hypertensive patients with type 2 diabetes. Diabetes Care 2011;34(6):1270–6.

35. Hermida RC, Ayala DE, Mojón A, et al. Bedtime dosing of antihypertensive medications reduces cardiovascular risk in CKD. J Am Soc Nephrol 2011;22:2313–21.

36. American Diabetes Association. Standards of medical care in diabetes–2013. Diabetes Care 2013;36(Suppl 1):S11–66.

37. Li EC, Heran BS, Wright JM. Angiotensin converting enzyme (ACE) inhibitors versus angiotensin receptor blockers for primary hypertension. Cochrane Database Syst Rev 2014;(8):CD009096.

38. van Vark LC, Bertrand M, Akkerhuis KM, et al. Angiotensin-converting enzyme inhibitors reduce mortality in hypertension: a meta-analysis of randomized clinical trials of renin-angiotensin-aldosterone system inhibitors involving 158,998 patients. Eur Heart J 2012;33(16):2088–97.

39. Cheng J, Zhang W, Zhang X. Effect of angiotensin-converting enzyme inhibitors and angiotensin II receptor blockers on all-cause mortality, cardiovascular deaths, and cardiovascular events in patients with diabetes mellitus: a meta-analysis. JAMA Intern Med 2014;174(5):773–85.

40. United States Renal Data System. 2015 USRDS annual data report: Epidemiology of kidney disease in the United States. Bethesda (MD): National Institutes of Health, National Institute of Diabetes and Digestive and Kidney Diseases; 2015.

41. de Zeeuw D, Remuzzi G, Parving HH, et al. Proteinuria, a target for renoprotection in patients with type 2 diabetic nephropathy: lessons from RENAAL. Kidney Int 2004;65:2309–20.

42. Lewis EJ, Hunsicker LG, Bain RP, et al. The effect of angiotensin-converting-enzyme inhibition on diabetic nephropathy. The Collaborative Study Group. N Engl J Med 1993;329:1456–62.

43. Lewis EJ, Hunsicker LG, Clarke WR, et al. Renoprotective effect of the angiotensin-receptor antagonist irbesartan in patients with nephropathy due to type 2 diabetes. N Engl J Med 2001;345:851–60.
44. Kunz R, Friedrich C, Wolbers M, et al. Meta-analysis: effect of monotherapy and combination therapy with inhibitors of the renin angiotensin system on proteinuria in renal disease. Ann Intern Med 2008;148:30–48.
45. Effect of enalapril on survival in patients with reduced left ventricular ejection fractions and congestive heart failure. The SOLVD Investigators. N Engl J Med 1991; 325:293–302.
46. Pfeffer MA, Braunwald E, Moyé LA, et al. Effect of captopril on mortality and morbidity in patients with left ventricular dysfunction after myocardial infarction. Results of the survival and ventricular enlargement trial. The SAVE Investigators. N Engl J Med 1992;327:669–77.
47. Yusuf S, Sleight P, Pogue J, et al. Effects of an angiotensin-converting-enzyme inhibitor, ramipril, on cardiovascular events in high-risk patients. The Heart Outcomes Prevention Evaluation Study Investigators. N Engl J Med 2000;342: 145–53.
48. Effects of ramipril on cardiovascular and microvascular outcomes in people with diabetes mellitus: results of the HOPE study and MICRO-HOPE substudy. Heart Outcomes Prevention Evaluation Study Investigators. Lancet 2000;355:253–9.
49. Cohn JN, Tognoni G, Valsartan Heart Failure Trial Investigators. A randomized trial of the angiotensin-receptor blocker valsartan in chronic heart failure. N Engl J Med 2001;345:1667–75.
50. McMurray JJ, Ostergren J, Swedberg K, et al. Effects of candesartan in patients with chronic heart failure and reduced left-ventricular systolic function taking angiotensin-converting-enzyme inhibitors: the CHARM-Added trial. Lancet 2003;362(9386):767–71.
51. ONTARGET Investigators, Yusuf S, Teo KK, Pogue J, et al. Telmisartan, ramipril, or both in patients at high risk for vascular events. N Engl J Med 2008;358: 1547–59.
52. Fried LF, Emanuele N, Zhang JH, et al. Combined angiotensin inhibition for the treatment of diabetic nephropathy. N Engl J Med 2013;369:1892–903.
53. Parving HH, Brenner BM, McMurray JJ, et al. Cardiorenal end points in a trial of aliskiren for type 2 diabetes. N Engl J Med 2012;367:2204–13.
54. Batterink J, Stabler SN, Tejani AM, et al. Spironolactone for hypertension. Cochrane Database Syst Rev 2010;(8):CD008169.
55. Liu G, Zheng XX, Xu YL, et al. Effect of aldosterone antagonists on blood pressure in patients with resistant hypertension: a meta-analysis. J Hum Hypertens 2015;29:159–66.
56. Pimenta E, Calhoun DA. Resistant hypertension: incidence, prevalence, and prognosis. Circulation 2012;125(13):1594–6.
57. de Souza F, Muxfeldt E, Fiszman R, et al. Efficacy of spironolactone therapy in patients with true resistant hypertension. Hypertension 2010;55:147–52.
58. Zhu Y, Pandya BJ, Choi HK. Prevalence of gout and hyperuricemia in the US general population: the National Health and Nutrition Examination Survey 2007-2008. Arthritis Rheum 2011;63(10):3136–41.
59. Reyes AJ. Cardiovascular drugs and serum uric acid. Cardiovasc Drugs Ther 2003;17:397–414.
60. Burnier M, Waeber B, Brunner HR. Clinical pharmacology of the angiotensin II receptor antagonist losartan potassium in healthy subjects. J Hypertens Suppl 1995;13:S23–8.

61. Ruilope LM, Kirwan BA, de Brouwer S, et al. Uric acid and other renal function parameters in patients with stable angina pectoris participating in the ACTION trial: impact of nifedipine GITS (gastro-intestinal therapeutic system) and relation to outcome. J Hypertens 2007;25:1711–8.

62. Choi HK, Soriano LC, Zhang Y, et al. Antihypertensive drugs and risk of incident gout among patients with hypertension: population based case-control study. BMJ 2012;344:d8190.

63. Oliva RV, Bakris GL. Blood pressure effects of sodium-glucose co-transport 2 (SGLT2) inhibitors. J Am Soc Hypertens 2014;8(5):330–9.

64. Baker WL, Smyth LR, Riche DM, et al. Effects of sodium-glucose co-transporter 2 inhibitors on blood pressure: a systematic review and meta-analysis. J Am Soc Hypertens 2014;8:262–75.

65. Maliha G, Townsend RR. SGLT2 inhibitors: their potential reduction in blood pressure. J Am Soc Hypertens 2015;9(1):48–53.

66. Zinman B, Wanner C, Lachin JM, et al. Empagliflozin, cardiovascular outcomes, and mortality in type 2 diabetes. N Engl J Med 2015;373:2117–28.

67. Yokoyama Y, Nishimura K, Barnard ND, et al. Vegetarian diets and blood pressure: a meta-analysis. JAMA Intern Med 2014;174:577–87.

68. Ried K, Sullivan TR, Fakler P, et al. Effect of cocoa on blood pressure. Cochrane Database Syst Rev 2012;(8):CD008893.

69. Ried K, Sullivan T, Fakler P, et al. Does chocolate reduce blood pressure? A meta-analysis. BMC Med 2010;8:39.

70. Liu G, Mi XN, Zheng XX, et al. Effects of tea intake on blood pressure: a meta-analysis of randomised controlled trials. Br J Nut 2014;112(7):1043–54.

71. Mesas AE, Leon-Muñoz LM, Rodriguez-Artalejo F, et al. The effect of coffee on blood pressure and cardiovascular disease in hypertensive individuals: a systematic review and meta-analysis. Am J Clin Nutr 2011;94(4):1113–26.

72. Jee SH, He J, Whelton PK, et al. The effect of chronic coffee drinking on blood pressure: a meta-analysis of controlled clinical trials. Hypertension 1999;33: 647–52.

73. Geleijnse JM. Habitual coffee consumption and blood pressure: an epidemiological perspective. Vasc Health Risk Manag 2008;4(5):963–70.

74. Xiong XJ, Li SJ, Zhang YQ. Massage therapy for essential hypertension: a systematic review. J Hum Hypertens 2015;29(3):143–51.

75. Yeh GY, Wang C, Wayne PM, et al. The effect of tai chi exercise on blood pressure: a systematic review. Prev Cardiol 2008;11(2):82–9.

76. Sun J, Buys N. Community-based mind-body meditative tai chi program and its effects on improvement of blood pressure, weight, renal function, serum lipoprotein, and quality of life in Chinese Adults with hypertension. Am J Cardiol 2015; 116(7):1076–81.

77. Krum H, Schlaich M, Whitbourn R, et al. Catheter-based renal sympathetic denervation for resistant hypertension: a multicentre safety and proof-of-principle cohort study. Lancet 2009;373:1275–81.

78. Symplicity HTN-2 Investigators, Esler MD, Krum H, Sobotka PA, et al. Renal sympathetic denervation in patients with treatment-resistant hypertension (The Symplicity HTN-2 Trial): a randomised controlled trial. Lancet 2010;376:1903–9.

79. Bhatt DL, Kandzari DE, O'Neill WW, et al. A controlled trial of renal denervation for resistant hypertension. N Engl J Med 2014;370:1393–401.

80. Heusser K, Tank J, Engeli S, Diedrich A. Carotid baroreceptor stimulation, sympathetic activity, baroreflex function, and blood pressure in hypertensive patients. Hypertension 2010;55:619–26.

81. Bisognano JD, Bakris G, Nadim MK, et al. Baroreflex activation therapy lowers blood pressure in patients with resistant hypertension: results from the double-blind, randomized, placebo-controlled Rheos pivotal trial. J Am Coll Cardiol 2011;58:765–73.

Pharmacologic Therapies in Anticoagulation

Joana Lima Ferreira, MD[a],*, Joyce E. Wipf, MD[b]

KEYWORDS

- Anticoagulation • Venous thromboembolism • Atrial fibrillation • Warfarin
- Direct oral anticoagulants • Heparin

KEY POINTS

- Anticoagulants are beneficial for prevention and treatment of venous thromboembolism and stroke prevention in atrial fibrillation.
- Approach to antithrombotic therapy varies according to indication, patient's bleeding risk, presence of comorbidities, cost, and patient's preference.
- The development of new target-specific oral agents is changing the landscape of anticoagulation therapy; data are evolving on indications, drug interactions, and relative efficacy and risks versus vitamin K antagonists and other anticoagulants.
- Understanding the pharmacology of different anticoagulants is required to adequately treat patients while minimizing risk of serious complications.

INTRODUCTION

Venous thromboembolism (VTE), a common condition affecting hospitalized and ambulatory patients, is associated with significant morbidity, mortality, and health care costs.[1] The etiology of VTE is usually multifactorial, resulting from risk factors that either predisposes to venous stasis, vascular wall injury, and/or hypercoagulability (eg, thrombophilia, pregnancy, cancer).

Normal hemostasis is achieved through a complex interplay between vascular endothelium, platelets, coagulation factors, and natural anticoagulants.[2] The anticoagulant drugs act by inhibiting, directly or indirectly, specific coagulation factors to prevent thrombus formation (**Fig. 1**). Different classes of anticoagulants have been approved for prevention and treatment of thromboembolic events, including deep venous thrombosis (DVT), pulmonary embolism (PE), stroke prevention in patients with atrial fibrillation (AF), or thrombus formation in patients with mechanical heart valves.

[a] Division of General Internal Medicine, Department of Medicine, University of Washington Medical Center, 1959 North East Pacific Street, Box 356429, Seattle, WA 98195, USA; [b] Department of Medicine, Center of Excellence in Primary Care Education, Seattle VA Puget Sound Health Care System, University of Washington, 1660 South Columbian Way (S-123-CoE), Seattle, WA 98108, USA
* Corresponding author.
E-mail address: limaferr@uw.edu

Med Clin N Am 100 (2016) 695–718
http://dx.doi.org/10.1016/j.mcna.2016.03.007
0025-7125/16/$ – see front matter
medical.theclinics.com

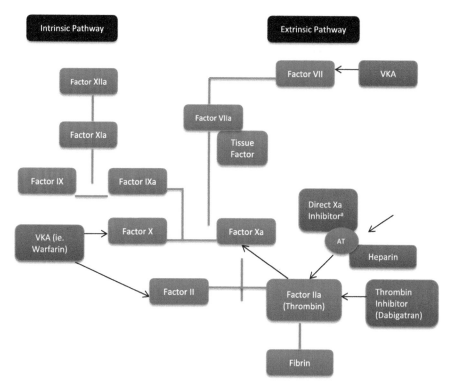

Fig. 1. Coagulation cascade and therapeutic targets of the anticoagulant drugs. [a] Rivaroxaban, apixaban, edoxaban. AT, antithrombin; VKA, vitamin K antagonist.

The vitamin K antagonists (VKA), such as warfarin, have been the standard of care for more than 50 years in long-term oral anticoagulation therapy for most of the indications above. Parenteral anticoagulants, such as unfractionated heparin (UFH) and low molecular weight heparin (LMWH), also have an important and established role in the anticoagulation treatment in both inpatient and outpatient settings.[1] However, these medications have several limitations. The VKAs have a narrow therapeutic index, wide interpatient and intrapatient variability due to genetic mutations as well as multiple food and drug interactions, thus requiring frequent monitoring to enhance its efficacy and safety.[3] The LMWHs have more predictable pharmacokinetics but the need for parenteral application and high cost are limitations.

In the hopes to overcome these issues, researchers have worked for many years on the development of safe oral drugs that would provide same or superior benefits as the VKAs without the need for frequent monitoring. These drugs were initially referred as "new" oral anticoagulants (NOACs), but as time passes preference has been to call them "direct" oral anticoagulants (DOACs) or target-specific oral anticoagulants (TSOAC), which more accurately reflects their mechanism of action.[4] In 2010, the US Food and Drug Administration (FDA) approved the direct thrombin inhibitor dabigatran for the prevention of thromboembolic complications in patients with AF. In the following years, 3 direct factor Xa inhibitors (rivaroxaban, apixaban, and edoxaban) were approved for treatment of AF and venous thromboembolism. Since then, other DOAC drugs are in development and/or pending approval process by the FDA.

Despite justifiable excitement for new anticoagulant options with potential to simplify management, initial speculation that DOACs would completely replace the use of VKAs is not proving feasible. Clinical experience has shown that many patients, especially those with compliance issues and/or funding limitations, might still benefit by a less expensive drug that has compliance monitored by blood tests.[5] Hypercoagulability resulting from missed doses is a black box warning on all DOACs, thus nonadherence to medication regimens is an essential consideration in selection of anticoagulant. Some conditions, such as mechanical valves, require VKA or heparin anticoagulation given improved efficacy over DOACs. Pregnant patients were excluded from the randomized trials with DOACs, and therefore their safety, efficacy, and teratogenic risk during pregnancy are unknown. Other valid questions with DOACs are comparative safety and benefit (vs noninferiority with VKA), risk of bleeding, limited availability of antidote for reversing anticoagulation, and choice of DOAC agent. We discuss the current evidence, recognizing the published literature and postapproval clinical experience are in rapid evolution.

This article reviews the pharmacology of the main anticoagulant classes (VKAs, direct oral anticoagulants, and heparins) and their indications based on evidence-based data available in the literature. Although important for the prevention and treatment of arterial thromboembolism, the antiplatelet drugs are not in the scope of this review and hence are not covered here.

CLINICAL APPLICATION
Prevention of Stroke in Patients with Atrial Fibrillation

AF is a common supraventricular tachyarrhythmia with higher prevalence in the elderly population (one-third of patients affected are >80 years old). Stroke complications of AF ultimately lead to significant morbidity and mortality.[6] Valvular AF (mitral valve disease) is associated with an 18-fold increased risk of stroke versus age-matched controls in sinus rhythm. Nonvalvular AF is associated with a fivefold overall increase risk of stroke. Risk stratification for individual patients with nonvalvular heart disease may indicate higher or lower risk. The decision regarding anticoagulation treatment for stroke prevention in nonvalvular AF should be based on individual stroke and bleeding risk, patient preference, and treatment cost irrespective of whether the AF pattern is paroxysmal, persistent, or permanent. Two main risk score tools have been validated in several cohorts. The $CHADS_2$ risk score (Congestive heart failure, Hypertension, Age ≥ 75 years old, Diabetes, prior Stroke or transient ischemic attack [TIA] [doubled]) has been used extensively in the literature and clinical practice. Anticoagulation is recommended for $CHADS_2$ score of 1 or more. Most recently the CHA_2DS_2VASc score (Congestive heart failure, Hypertension, Age ≥ 75 [doubled], Diabetes, Prior Stroke or TIA or thromboembolism [doubled], Vascular disease, Age 65–74 years, Sex category) has been shown to more accurately discriminate patients who are truly low risk and for whom physicians could consider withholding anticoagulation (CHA_2DS_2VASc score of 0–1).[7] Several tools exist for calculation of bleeding risk, with example described later in this article; however, utility is mainly for identification of modifiable risk factors.

Warfarin has been the mainstay anticoagulant treatment for AF for many years and has provided significant reduction of stroke events in patients with AF. However, given the challenges associated with its dosage, monitoring, and major bleeding complications, the direct oral anticoagulants have been replacing warfarin in many countries, including the United States. Several randomized controlled trials have been conducted to compare the efficacy and safety of warfarin against different DOACs (**Table 1**), largely noninferiority trials.

The 2014 American Heart Association/American College of Cardiology/Heart Rhythm Society Guideline for the management of patients with AF recommends oral anticoagulant therapy with warfarin (goal international normalized ratio [INR] 2.0–3.0. target 2.5), dabigatran, rivaroxaban, apixaban, or edoxaban in patients with nonvalvular AF with prior stroke, TIA, or a CHA_2DS_2-VASc score of 2 or greater.[6] Higher targets are used for warfarin management of mechanical heart valves. DOACs are not indicated for mechanical valves as less efficacious in that setting.

Treatment of Deep Vein Thrombosis and Pulmonary Embolism

The clinical suspicion of DVT and PE is best managed with the use of diagnostic algorithms that include a (1) risk score to predict the pretest probability (eg, DVT or PE Wells score), (2) plasma D-dimer, and (3) imaging test (eg, lower extremity duplex, computed tomography pulmonary angiography). Based on results of the applied risk score, the diagnosis of VTE will be classified as "unlikely" or "likely." In patients "unlikely" to have VTE, a negative D-dimer will rule out this diagnosis without the need for further imaging tests. Patients "likely" to have VTE or a positive D-dimer should be referred for image testing. The usual D-dimer threshold is 500 µg/L, however the age-adjusted D-dimer threshold for patients older than 50 years was proposed to decrease the number of false-positive D-dimer results and consequently decrease the need of radiation exposure related to computed tomography. The age-adjusted D-dimer threshold can be calculated by multiplying the patient's age by 10 in µg/L (**Table 2**).[8] Ongoing focused research of D-dimer level variation by age, gender, cancer diagnosis, and other factors are highly anticipated to further inform algorithms on risk and imaging indications.

Once the diagnosis of acute DVT and/or PE is confirmed, there should be no delay in the initiation of anticoagulation therapy. It is important to achieve full anticoagulation as quickly as possible, and given the challenges with unfractionated heparin and partial thromboplastin time (PTT) monitoring for dose adjustments, LMWH is typically used even in the hospitalized setting, unless surgery is likely. Traditionally, the acute treatment of VTE is achieved with a parental anticoagulant drug (LMWH, UFH, fondaparinux), which will be used as a bridge to an oral anticoagulant or for the total duration of anticoagulation. The American College of Chest Physicians (ACCP) guidelines recommend at least 3 months of anticoagulation treatment for provoked VTE and extended therapy (indefinitely) for unprovoked or cancer-associated VTE if patients have low to moderate bleeding risk.[9,10] The direct oral anticoagulants dabigatran, rivaroxaban, apixaban, and edoxaban have been approved for the treatment of VTE in the United States based on studies that have shown noninferiority of these drugs in comparison with standard VKA therapy. Furthermore, episodes of hemorrhagic complications (especially intracranial hemorrhage) occurred less frequently with DOACs, with the exception of gastrointestinal bleeding incidence, which was increased with dabigatran.[5] Based on these results, the 2016 ACCP guidelines are now recommending the DOACs over the VKAs as initial and long-term/extended therapy for treatment of DVT/PE in patients without cancer. Dabigatran and edoxaban still require initial parenteral therapy, whereas rivaroxaban and apixaban can be used from the start without bridging.[10]

Patients with acute PE associated with hypotension should be monitored closely in an intensive care unit and be offered systemically administered thrombolytic therapy, if low to moderate bleeding risk. Those patients should be treated with UFH infusion rather than an oral anticoagulant until close to discharge from the hospital.[10]

Table 1
Direct oral anticoagulants

	Direct "Targeted" Oral Anticoagulants			
	Dabigatran	Rivaroxaban	Apixaban	Edoxaban
Mechanism of action	Direct thrombin inhibitor	Direct factor Xa inhibitor	Direct factor Xa inhibitor	Direct factor Xa inhibitor
Study	REL-Y[31] Nonvalvular Atrial Fibrillation (NVAF) RE-COVER[68] for VTE (venous thromboembolism)	ROCKET[66]; NVAF EINSTEIN[67] ×2	ARISTOTLE[69] NVAF VTE AMPLIFY[70]	ENGAGE[71] study ×2 VTE, NVAF
All noninferiority trials vs warfarin, no studies comparing DOACs directly with each other				
Food and Drug Administration (FDA)-approved indications	NVAF (10/2010) VTE (4/2014)	NVAF (11/2011) VTE (11/2012) Orthopedics Hip and Knee Total Joint Replacement	NVAF (12/2012) VTE (8/2014) Orthopedics Hip and Knee Total Joint Replacement	NVAF (1/08/15) VTE (1/08/2015) – after 5–10 d Heparin
Time in Therapeutic Range of Warfarin arm (TTR) (goal at least 65%–70%)	64%	55%	62%	65%
Bleeding risk vs warfarin	Approved dose similar risk (Relative Risk 1.01) Higher rate gastrointestinal (GI) bleed	Approved dose similar Higher rate GI bleed	Lower risk (Hazard ratio 0.7) Higher rate GI bleed	Lower risk overall (Hazard ratio 0.81)
Reduction in clotting vs warfarin	Hazard ratio 0.75 stroke	Similar	Hemorrhagic stroke hazard ratio 0.5 NS diff other CVA	Similar stroke risk at higher of 2 doses studied; similar VTE rates
Contraindications/Dose adjustments	Mechanical valves Creatinine clearance (CC)<30	CC<15 (Dose adjust if <50 dose adjust); liver disease Partial renal clearance	CC<30 Dose adjust for creatinine <2.5 Liver disease	CC<30 or >95 Dose adjust CC 30–50

(continued on next page)

Table 1
(continued)

	Direct "Targeted" Oral Anticoagulants			
	Dabigatran	**Rivaroxaban**	**Apixaban**	**Edoxaban**
Potential drug interactions/ medication contraindications (data are emerging)	Dual (P-glycoprotein inducers [P-gp]) interacting and/or CYP3A4 drugs (examples: carbamazepine, diltiazem, phenytoin, rifampin) Nonsteroidal anti-inflammatory drugs (NSAIDs), other anticoagulants	Dual (P-gp) interacting and/or CYP3A4 drugs (examples: carbamazepine, diltiazem, phenytoin, rifampin) NSAIDs, other anticoagulants	Dual (P-gp) interacting and/or CYP3A4 drugs (examples: carbamazepine, diltiazem, phenytoin, rifampin) NSAIDs, other anticoagulants	Dual (P-gp) interacting and/or CYP3A4 drugs (examples: carbamazepine, diltiazem, phenytoin, rifampin) NSAIDs, other anticoagulants
Elimination half-life	12–17 h 15–34 h, renal impairment	5–12 h 11–19 h, elderly 10 h, hepatic impairment 9–10 h, renal impairment	7 h (2.5 mg oral) 15 h (5 mg oral) 9 h, Obesity	10–14 h
Side effects/black box warnings	GI common; increased risk stroke/systemic embolism (SE) if suddenly stop medication. Analysis 7 studies: Significantly increased risk Myocardial infarction/ acute coronary syndrome (odds ratio 1.33) →relative contraindication. Precautions elderly. Black box warnings: Premature discontinuation risk; spinal and epidural hematomas with neuraxial anesthesia and spinal puncture.	Hepatic (lower dose approved than studied) Increased risk stroke/SE if suddenly stop medication Box box warnings: Spinal and epidural hematomas with neuraxial anesthesia or spinal puncture; Discontinuation risk.	Hypersensitivity (latter <1%) Increased risk stroke/SE if suddenly stop medication Black box warnings: Discontinuation risk; Neuraxial anesthesia or spinal puncture increases risk of spinal and epidural hematomas.	Bleeding, anemia Hypercoagulable if stop suddenly Black box warnings: 1. Increased stroke risk atrial fibrillation in patients with high CC >95. 2. Premature discontinuation risk. 3. Epidural or spinal hematomas, increased risk with neuraxial anesthesia or spinal puncture.
Antidote	YES: Idarucizumab FDA approval fall 2015.	Antidotes in testing	Antidotes in testing	NO

Data from Randomized trials, Micromedex.

Table 2	
D-dimer thresholds based on patient's age	
Patient's Age	**Value**
<50 y	500 μg/L
>50 y	Patient's age × 10 in μg/L

Data from van der Hulle T, Dronkers CEA, Huisman MV, et al. Current standings in diagnostic management of acute venous thromboembolism: still rough around the edges. Blood Reviews 2016;30(1):21–6.

Cancer-Associated Venous Thromboembolism

Active cancer is a strong risk factor for the development and recurrence of VTE, especially when patients are hospitalized. Most patients with cancer have additional risk factors, such as older age, medical comorbidities, and immobility due to surgery or diminished performance status. At the same time, cancer-related features, such as primary site, stage, and its treatment (chemotherapy, antiangiogenic agents, hormonal therapy, erythropoiesis-stimulating agents) can increase the risk of VTE even further.[11,12]

The American Society of Clinical Oncology has developed evidence-based clinical practice guidelines for prophylaxis and treatment of VTE in patients with cancer. The most recent version, completed in 2014, states that most hospitalized patients with active cancer should receive thromboprophylaxis throughout hospitalization in the absence of bleeding or other contraindications. Patients admitted for major cancer surgery should have prophylaxis started before the procedure and continued for at least 7 to 10 days or up to 4 weeks in patients submitted to major abdominal or pelvic surgery. Although routine thromboprophylaxis is not recommended for ambulatory patients, it can be considered for highly select high-risk patients, such as patients with multiple myeloma on treatment with antiangiogenic agents.[13]

The LMWHs (enoxaparin, dalteparin) are the anticoagulant drugs of choice for acute treatment of cancer-associated venous thromboembolism (CAT). The CLOT trial has been the main reference to support this recommendation since it demonstrated that dalteparin for the first 3 months was more effective than VKAs in preventing VTE recurrence in this population without increasing the risk of bleeding.[14,15] The VKAs might still have a role in patients with inactive cancer or in those with severe renal failure. The currently available data are insufficient to make evidence-based recommendations on the use of DOACs in this setting. Therefore, clinical trials in which they are directly compared with LMWH are needed to clarify their role.[11]

Venous Thromboembolism Prophylaxis

Hospitalization of acutely ill medical patients and surgical procedures significantly increase the risk of VTE, especially in the setting of prior history of DVT/PE, active cancer, or orthopedic surgery. The occurrence of events is not limited to the hospitalization period and in fact is higher during the first months after discharge. An observational study analyzing medical records from Worcester residents diagnosed with possible VTE showed that 73.7% of patients developed VTE in the outpatient setting. A substantial proportion of these patients had undergone surgery (23.1%) or hospitalization (36.8%) in the preceding 3 months.[16] This highlights the need to discuss the indications for extended prophylaxis beyond hospital stay. Although studies have shown a benefit to extend thromboprophylaxis in patients undergoing orthopedic surgeries (total hip and knee arthroplasty), this practice is not recommended in acutely ill medical patients due to the increased episodes of major bleeding.[17,18]

Acutely Ill Medical Patients

Prophylactic anticoagulation in acutely ill, hospitalized medical patients has been shown to significantly reduce the incidence of symptomatic VTE and fatal PE. The ninth ACCP guidelines published in 2012 recommend prophylaxis with LMWH, low-dose UFH (LUFH), or fondaparinux for acutely ill hospitalized patients at increased risk of thrombosis determined by the Padua Prediction Score (**Table 3**). Patients with active bleeding or at risk for major bleeding should receive mechanical prophylaxis with sequential compression devices.[18]

Two direct oral anticoagulants have been evaluated for the prevention of VTE in acutely ill medical patients. Two Phase III trials have compared extended use of the DOACs apixaban (ADOPT trial)[19] and rivaroxaban (MAGELLAN trial)[20] to standard dose enoxaparin LMWH. Both trials have shown that although these drugs are noninferior to enoxaparin in reducing VTE at day 10, they do significantly increase the risk of major bleeding. Efficacies of dabigatran and edoxaban have not been studied in this setting but the factor Xa inhibitor betrixaban is currently being compared with enoxaparin in the phase II APEX trial. At this point, none of the DOACs are approved for VTE prophylaxis in acutely ill medical patients.[1,21]

Orthopedic Patients

Major orthopedic surgery (total hip arthroplasty and total knee arthroplasty) carries the highest risk for VTE among all surgical subspecialties.[5] Multiple studies have shown that this risk can be effectively and safely decreased with a variety of thromboprophylactic approaches. The 2012 ACCP guidelines recommend prevention of VTE during the perioperative period with one of the following drugs: LMWH, UFH, fondaparinux, VKAs, and aspirin. The preference, however, is to use LMWH over the other alternative agents for a minimum of 10 to 14 days, and ideally for up to 35 days from the day of major orthopedic surgery. Most recently, randomized trials have shown noninferiority of the DOACs (apixaban, dabigatran, rivaroxaban) in comparison with LMWH, making their use an attractive alternative to conventional anticoagulation.[21] The use of apixaban or dabigatran can be considered in patients who decline parenteral or mechanical prophylaxis. Although studies comparing rivaroxaban with enoxaparin showed a potential superiority of the former in decreasing the incidence of VTE in this population, the ACCP guidelines recommend using this agent only if the other 2 DOACs are not available based on data indicating increased bleeding risk with rivaroxaban.[17,21,22]

Table 3 Padua prediction score	
Points	**Patient's Comorbidities**
3	Active cancer, previous VTE, reduced mobility, thrombophilia
2	Recent (<1 mo) trauma and/or surgery
1	Age ≥70 y, heart and/or respiratory failure, acute myocardial infarction or ischemic stroke, acute infection and/or rheumatologic disorder, obesity (BMI ≥30), ongoing hormonal treatment

Patients with ≥4 points were considered high risk.
Abbreviations: BMI, body mass index; VTE, venous thromboembolism.
Data from Kahn SR, Lim W, Dunn AS, et al. Prevention of VTE in nonsurgical patients: antithrombotic therapy and prevention of thrombosis, 9th ed: American College of Chest Physicians evidence-based clinical practice guidelines. Chest 2012;141(2 Suppl):e195S–226S.

Nonorthopedic Surgical Patients

The indication and duration of anticoagulation for prevention of VTE in patients submitted to general, gynecologic, colorectal, bariatric, cardiovascular, or plastic surgery should be tailored to individual risk based on both patient-specific and procedure-specific risk factors.[23] Several models for risk stratification have been developed; however, most of them have important limitations and have not been extensively validated. The authors of the ninth edition of the ACCP guidelines used the Rogers and the Caprini risk score models to stratify patients into very low, low, moderate, and high risk. Based on their recommendations, patients at moderate and high risk for VTE who have no significant risk of bleeding should receive prophylactic anticoagulation with either LMWH or low-dose unfractionated heparin. For patients at high risk for VTE submitted to abdominal or pelvic surgery for cancer, the recommendation is to use LMWH for an extended period of time (4 weeks after the procedure).[23,24]

PRACTICAL RECOMMENDATIONS
Periprocedural Management of Anticoagulation

The need for bridging therapy and timing for postoperative anticoagulation is determined based on assessment of thromboembolism risk against the risk of bleeding during and after the procedure. Although common practice has been to offer bridging to most patients on anticoagulation, most recent studies have questioned its universal use given bleeding complications. Guidelines have been developed to avoid bridging in patients at low risk of thrombosis and providing it to patients at moderate to high risk.[25,26] The BRIDGE trial published in 2015 demonstrated that in patients with AF, interruption of warfarin for an elective operation or invasive procedure without bridging anticoagulation was noninferior to perioperative bridging with LMWH for the prevention of thromboembolism and was associated with decreased risk of major bleeding.[27]

A patient's risk of thrombosis when off anticoagulation depends on the condition for which the drug is prescribed, timing from initial event, and comorbidities that lead to a hypercoagulable state. The risk of bleeding in the perioperative period will be mainly determined by the type (considering the amount of blood loss) and location of procedure (sites where a small hemorrhage can have serious consequences or where bleeding cannot be seen).[26]

The recommendations for perioperative management of warfarin are well established. The bridging therapy drugs recommended in this situation are either LMWH or UFH. The increasing use of direct oral anticoagulants (eg, dabigatran, rivaroxaban), however, has decreased the need to use heparin as bridging therapy given its rapid rate of elimination and quick onset of action.[28] The exception to this rule is patients with renal failure who will require a longer period of time to clear the drug once they are stopped.

A special situation is spinal epidural injection for patients on DOACs. Limited manufacturer guidance is available; our practice is to hold the DOAC 36 hours before the procedure, and if no procedural bleeding complications, resume 12 to 24 hours after the procedure.

Switching Between Anticoagulants

Transition from one anticoagulant drug to the other should be well planned and closely followed so as to maintain its efficacy while minimizing the risk of bleeding (**Table 4**).[1,29]

Choice of Anticoagulant

The landscape of anticoagulation is changing with the introduction of the target-specific oral anticoagulants, which are rapidly replacing warfarin for several indications. These

Table 4
Switching between anticoagulants

Switching to a DOAC	Switching from a DOAC

From warfarin:
  Warfarin should be discontinued and DOAC started when INR is ≤2.5
	To warfarin:
	  DOAC and warfarin should be administered concomitantly until INR in therapeutic range

From parental anticoagulant:
  LMWH: DOAC should be started 0–2 h before the time the next schedule dose of LMWH was due
Continuous UFH: start DOAC 0–2 h after discontinuation of intravenous infusion
	To parenteral anticoagulant:
	  First dose of parenteral anticoagulant should be given at the time the next DOAC dose would be taken

Switching from one DOAC to another: Start the new drug at previous drug next scheduled dose	

Abbreviations: DOAC, direct oral anticoagulant; INR, international normalized ratio; LMWH, low molecular weight heparin; UFH, unfractionated heparin.

Adapted from Gomez-Outes A, Suarez-Gea ML, Lecumberri R, et al. Direct-acting oral anticoagulants: pharmacology, indications, management, and future perspectives. Eur J Haematol 2015;95(5):398; and Ferns SJ, Naccarelli GV. New oral anticoagulants: their role in stroke prevention in high-risk patients with atrial fibrillation. Med Clin North Am 2015;99(4):769.

agents became attractive in clinical practice given several advantages over warfarin, including predictable pharmacokinetics allowing administration of fixed doses without routine coagulation laboratory monitoring, less food or drug-drug interactions, evidence of same efficacy with decreased intracranial hemorrhage, and rapid onset/offset of action eliminating the need for initial treatment with a parenteral anticoagulant in patients with acute thrombosis or need for "bridging" in the perioperative period.[3,30] Yet caution and informed decision making require discussion of about current lack of antidote to reverse anticoagulation for DOACs other than dabigatran, higher risk of gastrointestinal bleeding, hypercoagulability when missed doses, and dose adjustments or contraindications with renal insufficiency, liver disease, and emerging recognition of drug interactions with DOACs. Data are lacking on DOAC teratogenicity and are not approved for use during pregnancy. Dabigatran may have higher risk of cardiovascular events based on the REL-Y study with 1.3 relative risk,[31] and ACCP 2012 guidelines do not recommend in patients with known coronary artery disease.

The current challenge for physicians is how to personalize therapy for individuals who require long-term anticoagulation treatment (**Table 5**). One approach is to determine if the patient is a candidate for one of the DOACs before automatically starting patients on warfarin. The factors that will influence this decision are evidence of efficacy on the specific indication, presence of renal and/or liver failure, compliance ability, cost (copayments), physicians experience with the new drugs, and patient's preference.

The DOACs have been approved in the United States for different indications, including stroke prevention in nonvalvular AF, acute VTE treatment, secondary VTE prevention, and VTE prevention in major orthopedic surgery.[5,32–34] On the other hand, current evidence is insufficient to recommend the use of DOACs over warfarin in patients requiring anticoagulation for mechanical heart valves, antiphospholipid syndrome (APS), and heparin-induced thrombocytopenia (HIT).[11] There is also no sufficient evidence to choose these agents over LMWH in patients with cancer-associated thrombosis.[14] Several studies exploring the efficacy and safety of these

Table 5
Anticoagulant choices based on clinical scenario

Approved Indications	Warfarin	Dabigatran	Rivaroxaban	Apixaban	Edoxaban	LMWH
Nonvalvular AF[6]	¶	¶	¶	¶	¶	
VTE prophylaxis (major orthopedic surgery)	¶		¶	¶		¶
VTE treatment[9]	¶	¶	¶	¶	¶	¶
Special situations						
Mechanical valve, valvular AF	¶					
Cancer related VTE						¶
Poor compliance	¶					
Renal failure						
CrCl 30–50 mL/min	¶		¶	¶		¶
CrCl <30 mL/min	¶					
Liver failure	¶					
Pregnancy						¶

Abbreviations: AF, atrial fibrillation; CrCl, creatinine clearance; VTE, venous thromboembolism.

Adapted from Weitz JI, Gross PL. New oral anticoagulants: which one should my patient use? Hematology Am Soc Hematol Educ Program 2012;2012:539; and Garcia DA. The target-specific oral anticoagulants: practical considerations. Hematology Am Soc Hematol Educ Program 2014;1:511.

drugs in different settings are under way and physicians should continue to look for changes in recommendations in the near future.[11]

The DOACs are contraindicated in patients with severe renal failure given renal excretion is the main route of clearance for dabigatran and contributes variably to clearance of the factor Xa inhibitors. The use of DOACs in patients with severe hepatic failure also should be avoided, as these patients were excluded from most large phase III clinical trials.[5]

Noncompliant patients should either be offered/continue on warfarin or not receive any anticoagulation. The DOACs are not a good option in this situation due to rapid loss of effect after a missing dose and inability to assess its efficacy via laboratory monitoring.

Finally, the cost associated with treatment should be taken into consideration, as high copayments might be a reason for noncompliance.

VITAMIN K ANTAGONISTS

The VKAs, also known as coumarins, have been the mainstay of oral anticoagulant therapy for more than 5 decades. Warfarin is by far the most widely used one and, for this reason, its name has been commonly used interchangeably with VKAs. The other VKAs (acenocoumarol, phenprocoumon, and fluindione) have been less commonly used in clinical practice and/or mentioned in the American literature.

Pharmacology

The mechanism of action of the VKAs involves inhibition of the vitamin K epoxide reductase complex that promotes the cyclic conversion of oxidized vitamin K to its reduced form. The decreased amount of reduced vitamin K will then impair the gamma carboxylation of vitamin K–dependent coagulation factors II, VII, IX, and X in the liver. Without carboxylation, these factors will lose the ability to bind to cofactors on the phospholipid membranes and consequently its procoagulant effect.[35]

The same way, the VKAs inhibit the carboxylation of the natural anticoagulants protein C and S leading to a transient early prothrombotic effect, which is attributed to the shorter half-life of protein C in comparison with factor II.[36] This prothrombotic effect can be particularly serious in patients with inherited protein C deficiency and in rare cases can manifest as skin necrosis.[2,35]

Warfarin is well absorbed by the gastrointestinal tract, reaches peak concentration in the blood 90 minutes after oral intake, circulates bound to albumin, and eventually accumulates in the liver where it is going to be primarily metabolized by the CYP2C9 enzyme of the cytochrome P450 system.

One of the major challenges for providers treating patients with warfarin is the significant interpatient and intrapatient variability in the dose required for optimal anticoagulation therapy. Numerous studies have shown that different genetic and environmental factors can modulate the anticoagulant effects of warfarin.[2,35] Genetic mutations in the cytochrome P450 enzyme and factor IX propeptide will result in increased half-life and potentially higher risk for bleeding complications. On the other hand, mutations on the vitamin K oxide reductase enzyme gene can lead to variable sensitivity to inhibition by warfarin and potentially explain why some individuals can be resistant to this drug.[35] The following are the most recognized environmental factors associated with warfarin pharmacokinetics and pharmacodynamics:

- Diet rich in vitamin K (green vegetables or vitamin K supplements)
- Concomitant use of drugs and/or herbal medicines that interfere with the metabolism of VKAs
- Reduced vitamin K stores (malnutrition, use of broad-spectrum antibiotics, malabsorptive conditions)
- Comorbid conditions (eg, liver and renal failure)

Dosage

The initial and maintenance doses of VKA should be individualized for different factors related to the patient as well as for the specific indication for anticoagulation. The decision regarding what initial dose to use and the ability to maintain the patient in the desired therapeutic range is of utmost importance for treatment outcomes, including effective antithrombotic therapy and decreased risk of bleeding. Maintaining the patient on a stable therapeutic range can be challenging and requires a comprehensive and organized system, including an experienced provider, consistent follow-up, reliable prothrombin time (PT)/INR monitoring, and appropriate patient education and frequent communication.

It is important to notice that the initial effect of warfarin will be reflected in the INR approximately 2 to 3 days after the first dose. The full antithrombotic effect, however, only occurs a few days later given the longer half-life (60–72 hours) of the coagulation factor II (thrombin) in comparison with the other 3 vitamin K–dependent factors. For this reason, patients at higher thrombotic risk (DVT, PE) should receive concomitant treatment with a rapid anticoagulant drug, such as UFH or LMWH. Both the ACCP and the British Committee for Standards in Haematology current guidelines recommend to continue the anticoagulant used for "bridging" to warfarin for at least 5 days and until the INR is at therapeutic range for at least 24 hours, whichever is the longer.[37,38] To decrease the time to therapeutic range, the VKA should be started on day 1 or 2 of heparin therapy.[39]

The appropriate initial dose of warfarin should be based on patient's clinical characteristics (age, weight, nutritional status) as well as presence of organ dysfunctions (**Table 6**). If not already available, additional blood tests should be ordered to rule out renal or liver failure before initiation of the VKA. Women in childbearing age should also have a pregnancy test done because of potential teratogenic effects of warfarin. If indicated, genetic and serologic tests can be done to rule out thrombophilia and APS, given these conditions might require higher therapeutic goals and prolonged treatment time.

Pharmacogenetic testing to assess for mutations related to warfarin metabolism and target molecules (CYP2C9 and VKORC1) has been the subject of several studies in the hope that a more accurate algorithm for VKA dosing could be developed. Observational studies have demonstrated an association between the previously mentioned gene mutations and variations in warfarin dose requirement.[40] However, subsequent small clinical trials were unable to determine the clinical utility of warfarin dosing based on genotype-guided algorithms. In attempt to answer this question, the COAG (Clarification of Optimal Anticoagulation through Genetics), a multicenter, double-blind randomized controlled trial compared a genotype-guided warfarin dosing strategy with a clinically based dose strategy. The results published in 2013 showed no significant difference in the percentage of time in the therapeutic range (INR 2–3) between the 2 groups, from the completion of the intervention period (day 4–5 of treatment) through day 28. There was also no significant difference of secondary outcomes, namely any INR of 4 or higher, major bleeding events, or recurrent thromboembolism in the first 4 weeks of treatment.[41]

Monitoring and Maintenance Dose

The INR is the test used to adjust the warfarin dose toward the range recommended for its indication. The time in the therapeutic INR range (TTR) has been used to assess the efficacy and risk of bleeding associated with VKA treatment as well as to compare quality of dose adjustment between different settings (primary care clinic, anticoagulation clinic, or self-monitoring/dosing). The TTR can be calculated by different methods, the most simple being calculating the number of INRs in range divided by the total number of INR tests.[37,42,43]

The ability to maintain a patient within the narrow therapeutic range is challenging and influenced by patient compliance, addition or discontinuation of other medications, dietary vitamin K ingestion, fluctuations in clinical status of comorbid conditions, and the quality of dose adjustment decisions.

The INR is usually measured daily for hospitalized patients initiated on a VKA until the targeted therapeutic range has been achieved and maintained for at least 2 consecutive days. In the outpatient setting, the INR can be initially checked every

Table 6	
Initial dose of warfarin based on patients' clinical characteristics	
Patient Population	**Initial Dose (Days 1 and 2)**
Otherwise healthy adults	5 mg daily[a]
Older patients (woman >70 and man >80) Comorbidities (malnutrition, ESLD, CKD, or CHF) Concomitant drugs known to increase warfarin sensitivity	2.5–5 mg daily

Abbreviations: CHF, chronic heart failure; CKD, chronic kidney disease; ESLD, end-stage liver disease.

[a] 2012 ACCP guideline: 10 mg daily may be considered.

2 to 3 days and then reduced to intervals of 4 to 6 weeks once a stable dose is found. This interval, however, should be reduced if medications known to interact with warfarin are added on or discontinued, if patients develop new medical problems (especially kidney, liver, or heart failure), and in any other situations in which there is concern of potential factors affecting INR stability.

Adverse Events

The most common and concerning adverse event related to warfarin therapy is bleeding. Most investigators report those events as minor or major bleeding. The latter usually refers to life-threatening/fatal bleeds (eg, intracranial or retroperitoneal hemorrhage) or bleeding requiring hospitalization and/or blood transfusions.[37]

The bleeding risk is mostly influenced by the intensity of warfarin therapy but also by the patient's prior history of bleeding, age, and comorbidities. The benefits of thromboprophylaxis should always be balanced against the individual risk of bleeding. To help with this equation, various bleeding risk stratification scores have been proposed. The HAS-BLED risk score (**Table 7**) was originally developed to estimate the 1-year risk for major bleeding in patients receiving antithrombotic therapy for AF.[44] Subsequent studies have validated the HAS-BLED risk score in different cohorts (eg, VTE population, patients treated with non-VKA oral anticoagulants), as well as demonstrated its better predictive value when compared with other bleeding-risk scores.[45,46] Important to mention that the 2012 ACCP guidelines recommend against the routine use of bleeding-risk scores as the only criteria to withhold VKA therapy.[39] Expert opinion suggests that more than a tool to exclude high-risk patients from anticoagulation, the HAS-BLED score should be used by clinicians to improve reversible risk factors in attempt to reduce the bleeding risk.[45]

Table 7
HAS-BLED clinical bleeding risk score

Letter	Clinical Characteristic	Definition	Points
H	Hypertension	Uncontrolled, >160 mm Hg systolic	1
A	Abnormal renal and liver function	Abnormal renal function: serum creatinine ≥200 μmol/L, chronic dialysis or renal transplantation	1 or 2
		Abnormal liver function: cirrhosis or biochemical evidence of significant hepatic derangement (Bb >2× upper limit of normal, AST/ALT/Alkaline phosphatase >3× upper limit of normal)	
S	Stroke	Previous history, particularly lacunar	1
B	Bleeding	Bleeding history or predisposition	1
L	Labile INRs	TTR <60%	1
E	Elderly	Age >65 y	1
D	Drugs or alcohol	Drugs: antiplatelet agents, NSAIDs	1 or 2
		Ethanol abuse: ≥8 units/wk	

According to the final score, patients are subdivided into 3 categories: 0, low risk; 1–2, moderate risk; ≥3, high risk. Refer to the text for further details in how to apply the score to clinical practice.

Abbreviations: ALT, alanine aminotransferase; AST, aspartate aminotransferase; Bb, total bilirubin; INR, international normalized ration; NSAID, nonsteroidal anti-inflammatory drugs; TTR, time in therapeutic range.

Data from Zhu W, He W, Guo L, et al. The HAS-BLED score for predicting major bleeding risk in anticoagulated patients with atrial fibrillation: a systematic review and meta-analysis. Clin Cardiol 2015;38(9):555–61.

Reversal of Anticoagulation Effect and Management of Bleeding

Different strategies can be used to reverse warfarin anticoagulant effect and the decision on which one to use will mostly depend on the urgency of reversal and severity of the bleeding (**Table 8**). Patient assessment including bleeding versus thrombotic risk as well as the presence of comorbidities should be taken into account before choosing a specific strategy.[38,39] Goldstein and colleagues[47] demonstrated in a multicenter randomized trial that 4-factor prothrombin complex concentrate (coagulation factors II, VII, IX, X) is superior to plasma for rapid INR reversal and effective hemostasis in patients needing urgent surgical or invasive procedures.

Contraindications

The following are the conditions listed as contraindications for use of warfarin therapy by the FDA[48]:

- Active bleeding or blood dyscrasias
- Obstetric: pregnancy, threatened abortion, eclampsia, and preeclampsia
- Recent or contemplated surgery of the central nervous system, eye, or traumatic surgery resulting in large open surfaces
- Unsupervised patients with conditions associated with potential of noncompliance
- Spinal puncture and other diagnostic/therapeutic procedures with potential for uncontrollable bleeding
- Hypersensitivity to warfarin or to any other components of this product
- Malignant hypertension

Drug Interactions

A large number of medications interact with the VKAs by different mechanisms and with different effects on INR. Medications can potentiate the effect of warfarin increasing the risk of bleeding or inhibit it decreasing its efficacy in the prevention of thromboembolic events. Other medications, such as aspirin and nonsteroidal

Table 8
Reversal of VKA anticoagulant effect based on American College of Physicians and the British Committee for Standards in Haematology current guidelines

Clinical Presentation	INR	Management in Addition to Holding VKA
Supratherapeutic INR without bleeding	4.5–10 >10	• No vitamin K recommended • Oral vitamin K (1–5 mg)[a]
Minor bleeding	Any	IV Vitamin K (1–3 mg)[a]
Major bleeding	Any	• 4-F PCC + IV vitamin K (5–10 mg)[a] • FFP should be used only if PCC not available
Surgery		
Elective/nonurgent	—	Consider oral vitamin K
Urgent	—	4-F PCC + IV vitamin K

Abbreviations: 4-F PCC, 4-factor prothrombin complex concentrate; FFP, fresh frozen plasma; INR, international normalized ratio; IV, intravenous.

[a] Repeat doses of vitamin K can be given every 24h or earlier until bleeding controlled or INR back to therapeutic range.

Data from Keeling D, Baglin T, Tait C, et al. Guidelines on oral anticoagulation with warfarin - fourth edition. Br J Haematol 2011;154(3):311–24; and Holbrook A, Schulman S, Witt DM, et al. Evidence-based management of anticoagulant therapy: antithrombotic therapy and prevention of thrombosis, 9th ed: American College of Chest Physicians evidence-based clinical practice guidelines. Chest 2012;141(2 Suppl):e152S–84S.

anti-inflammatory drugs (NSAIDs) can increase the risk of bleeding without affecting the INR. Physicians should consult their institution's pharmacist or use available Web tools to search for possible interactions when introducing new drugs. The same way, patients should be encouraged to discuss with their providers the safety of using any over-the-counter medications or supplements.[37]

DIRECT ORAL ANTICOAGULANTS

The target-specific oral anticoagulants, including direct thrombin inhibitors, such as dabigatran, and direct factor Xa inhibitors, such as rivaroxaban, apixaban, and edoxaban, have emerged as a new generation of anticoagulants. They act by decreasing the enzymatic activity of the correspondent procoagulant enzymes. These medications have been proved to be as effective as the VKAs in several indications while causing less intracranial bleeding and not requiring frequent monitoring given its reliable pharmacokinetics and lack of significant food and drug-drug interactions.[5,49]

Dabigatran Etexilate

Dabigatran is a direct thrombin inhibitor able to bind to free thrombin as well as to clot-bound thrombin with high specificity and affinity. Inhibition of thrombin will have a negative effect on thrombus formation by reducing the conversion of fibrinogen to fibrin, thrombin generation, and platelet activation. The drug capsules have tartaric acid added to them to facilitate the intestinal absorption of dabigatran, which is enhanced in a low pH. The peak plasma concentration occurs approximately 2 hours after ingestion and the mean half-life averages 8 hours when patients take the medications while fasting. Dabigatran is predominantly eliminated by the kidneys ($\sim$80%) and differently from the other DOACs can be eliminated from the blood by hemodialysis. The renal clearance of dabigatran is in linear relationship with the creatinine clearance. Therefore, dabigatran should be used with caution in patients with renal failure and is contraindicated in patients with a creatinine clearance less than 30 mL/min.[29,50]

Rivaroxaban

This direct factor Xa inhibitor has the ability to act both on free factor Xa and factor Xa within the prothrombinase complex. Although this drug has high oral bioavailability, patients need to take higher doses with food to improve its absorption. Plasma peak levels were found 3 hours after ingestion in healthy volunteers and the plasma half-life is approximately 8 hours. Impaired renal function results in prolonged half-life and increased effect of the drug. Rivaroxaban is therefore contraindicated in patients with a creatinine clearance less than 15 mL/min and should have its therapeutic dose of 20 mg daily decreased to 15 mg daily in patients with creatinine clearance of 15 to 50 mL/min. The use of rivaroxaban in patients with cirrhosis CHILD B and C is not recommended given reduced hepatic metabolism and consequently increased plasma levels of the active compound.[3,50]

Apixaban

This drug also directly inhibits factor Xa by acting on free and prothrombinase complex factor Xa. Similar to rivaroxaban, apixaban has high oral bioavailability (50%). The peak plasma level of apixaban occurs within 3 to 4 hours after oral ingestion and the half-life is in the range of 8 to 15 hours in healthy volunteers. Apixaban is metabolized in the liver and elimination occurs primarily by hepatobiliary (75%) followed by renal (25%) pathway.[49] The dose of 5 mg twice a day used for stroke prophylaxis in patients with AF should be reduced by half if patients have 2 of the following charac-teristics: age ≥80 years, body weight ≤60 kg, or serum creatinine ≥1.5 mg/dL. This recommendation originated from the Aristotle trial when apixaban was compared with warfarin in patients with AF.[2] Apixaban is however contraindicated in patients with severe liver disease.

Edoxaban

Edoxaban is also an oral direct factor Xa inhibitor, similar to rivaroxaban and apixaban. The drug is predominantly and rapidly absorbed in the upper gastrointestinal tract leading to bioavailability of approximately 60%. Absorption is not influenced by food. Peak plasma levels are attained after only 1 to 2 hours of administration, and its half-life averages 10 hours allowing daily administration of the drug.[29,50,51]

Monitoring Direct Oral Anticoagulants

Given its predictable pharmacokinetics, the DOACs can be administered in fixed doses and do not require routine monitoring of their anticoagulant activity. Assays that quantify the concentration of the agent or its activity might be rather helpful in situations in which there is concern for nonadherence, decreased absorption, drug-drug interaction, life-threatening bleeding, overdose, or accumulation of the drug due to renal insufficiency. This information can be particularly important if the pa-tient needs urgent surgery or systemic thrombolysis for stroke.[50,52]

It has been shown that the DOACs can prolong the results of the global tests pro-thrombin time (PT/INR) and activated partial thromboplastin time (aPTT) depending on the interval after ingestion. This interference, however, does not have a linear rela-tionship with the concentration of the agent but rather to the thromboplastin used in the assay and that is why these global tests cannot be used to monitor activity of these agents.[53] Quantitative tests using high-pressure liquid chromatography were used by manufacturers in the preclinical phases but these are not available in real practice. For that matter, a normal thrombin-time (TT) or a normal anti-Xa chromogenic assay will help exclude dabigatran and factor Xa inhibitors, respectively.[50,53,54]

Management of Bleeding Complications

All randomized controlled trials comparing the DOACs with conventional therapy have documented a decrease in the incidence of fatal bleeding. Nevertheless, intracranial hemorrhage and major gastrointestinal bleed still poses a risk to the life of patients tak-ing these medications. The limited availability of specific antidotes and guidelines in how to manage patients with DOACs-related life-threatening bleeding has made physicians hesitant to prescribe it.[32,55]

Patients who present with bleeding should receive usual supportive measures, mechanical compression, surgery, and endoscopic therapy when appropriate. Different from the factor Xa inhibitors, the thrombin inhibitor dabigatran can be partially removed by hemodialysis. Use of coagulation factor concentrate such as the activated prothrombin complex concentrate (aPCC) can be considered in potentially life-threatening bleeding complications, although current data are limited regarding its clinical efficacy in this setting and potential for recurrent thromboembolism.[56]

Highly specific reversal agents for the direct thrombin inhibitor dabigatran (eg, idarucizumab) and factor Xa inhibitors (eg, andexanet alpha, aripazine) have been under clinical investigation.[1,56] The dabigatran antidote idarucizumab (Praxbind) was approved in the United States in October 2015 for use in adult pa-tients who require rapid reversal of its anticoagulant effect for emergency surgery, urgent procedures, or life-threatening bleeding.[57]

Drug-Drug Interactions

The DOACs have minimal drug-drug interactions when compared with warfarin; however, they can be significant and physicians should be aware of possible mechanisms, as the list will probably grow if there is more frequent use of the new agents.

Dabigatran and edoxaban metabolism is dependent on P-glycoprotein (P-gp) transporters and therefore, concomitant use P-gp inhibitors or inducers should be avoided or dose adjustment should be considered. Apixaban and rivaroxaban are affected by both cytochrome P450 (CYP) 3A4 and P-gp strong inhibitors (eg, azoles, human immunodeficiency virus protease inhibitors) leading to increased plasma concentrations of the DOACs and higher bleeding risk. On the other hand, inducers of CYP3A4 and P-gp (eg, rifampin, St John's wort) can lead to a reduction of rivaroxaban plasma levels.[1,50,58]

It is important to remember that the antiplatelet agents and NSAIDs have pharmacodynamic interactions with the DOACs, leading to increased bleeding risk. Concomitant use of these drugs should be avoided unless specifically recommended (acute coronary syndrome or coronary stenting).[50]

PARENTERAL ANTICOAGULANTS

The parenteral anticoagulants can be divided into 2 subgroups based on their mechanism of action. The indirect parenteral anticoagulants have activity mediated by plasma cofactors and include UFH, LMWH, fondaparinux, and danaparoid. The direct parenteral anticoagulants specifically target the coagulation factor thrombin and include the hirudins, bivalirudin, and argatroban. This section focuses on the pharmacology of UFH and LMWH as those are more commonly used in the internal medicine practice.

Pharmacology

UFH anticoagulant effect is achieved by enhancing the activity of the natural anticoagulant antithrombin (AT) to inactivate both thrombin (factor IIa) and factor Xa.[59] The LMWHs also act via antithrombin to inactivate factor Xa; however, the anti-IIa activity is lower, as this requires a longer saccharide chain length.[60]

Both UFH and LMWHs are given either by intravenous or subcutaneous injection. Metabolism occurs by saturable and nonsaturable mechanisms. The first involves binding to endothelial cells and clearance by the reticuloendothelial system, and the second is obtained by renal clearance. Both mechanisms are important for UFH, but renal clearance predominates for LMWHs. This is clinically important as accumulation of LMWHs may occur, with increased bleeding risk, in renal failure.[60] Intravenous heparin has immediate action, whereas the bioavailability of subcutaneous (SC) injections is less than 50%. The LMWH bioavailability after SC injection averages 90% to 100%. The half-life of intravenous UFH is approximately 45 to 60 minutes whereas the SC LMWH reaches approximately 4 hours.

Dosage

The dose of both UFH and LMWH will vary depending on its indication, especially whether it is being used for prophylactic or therapeutic purposes. The use of intravenous UFH doses based on a patient's weight and adjusted by institutional algorithms has shown to provide faster effect based on achievement of aPTT goal within 24 hours and to decrease recurrence of VTE. The most commonly used doses for UFH and LMWH are summarized on **Table 9**.

Table 9
Commonly used doses of unfractionated heparin and low molecular weight heparins in the management of VTE

Heparin	Prophylactic Dose	Therapeutic Dose
Unfractionated heparin	5.000 U SC every 8 or 12 h	IV CI 80 U/kg initial bolus followed by 18 U/kg/h[a]
Low molecular weight heparin[b]		
Enoxaparin	40 mg SC daily	1 mg/kg/dose SC every 12 h
Dalteparin	5000 U SC daily	200 U/kg SC daily

Abbreviations: CI, continuous infusion; IV, intravenous; SC, subcutaneous; U, units.
[a] Dose will then be adjusted by institutional algorithm based on goal aPTT (~1.5 to 2.5 times the mean of control value).
[b] LMWH doses should be adjusted for older age, obesity and renal failure.
Data from Garcia DA, Baglin TP, Weitz JI, et al. Parenteral anticoagulants: antithrombotic therapy and prevention of thrombosis, 9th ed: American College of Chest Physicians evidence-based clinical practice guidelines. Chest 2012;141(2 Suppl):e24S–43S; and Baglin T, Barrowcliffe TW, Cohen A, et al. Guidelines on the use and monitoring of heparin. Br J Haematol 2006;133(1):19–34.

Monitoring

Before initiation of therapy with heparin, baseline laboratory tests (coagulation, complete blood count, and renal function) should be done to determine dosing and best monitoring strategy. It is also important to assess risk of bleeding to define appropriate intensity of anticoagulation.

- Monitoring of UFH is usually performed using the aPTT.[61] A target ratio versus midpoint of normal range of 1.5 to 2.5 is used.
- The activated clotting time is used to monitor the higher heparin doses given to patients undergoing percutaneous coronary interventions or cardiopulmonary bypass surgery.
- The anti–factor Xa activity assay is available in some institutions to assess heparin activity in situations in which the aPTT might not be reliable: patients with baseline prolonged aPTT (eg, lupus anticoagulant), assessment of LMWH activity in patients with renal failure, and in cases of heparin resistance.[59,61]

Adverse Events

- Osteoporosis: In addition to its anticoagulant effects, heparin also inhibits osteoblast formation and osteoclast activation, which can promote bone loss. The incidence of vertebral fracture has been reported to be as high as 15% in patients receiving UFH. The frequency, however, is lower with LMWHs and so this form is preferred for long-term use.[59,62]
- HIT is a potentially life-threatening prothrombotic complication caused by exposure to UFH and less commonly to LMWH. The development of antibodies directed against complexes formed by a platelet protein, platelet factor 4, and heparin can lead to progressive platelet count decline starting on day 5 to 14 after exposure and in some cases the thrombocytopenia is associated with new arterial and venous thrombosis. Diagnosis is made by clinical risk assessment (4T score) and laboratory evaluation (immunoassays and functional assays).[63] Once HIT is recognized, an alternative anticoagulant (direct thrombin inhibitor or fondaparinux) should be initiated to prevent further complications.[64,65]
- Bleeding complications: severity and location of bleeding are variable, so management should be based on urgency and coagulation parameters. Heparin

administered by intravenous infusion has a fast half-life of 45 to 60 minutes. If there is severe bleeding and urgent reversal is necessary, protamine sulfate can be given by slow infusion to neutralize its effects. Protamine sulfate also can be used for reversal of LMWH, although it might not neutralize it completely.

SUMMARY AND FUTURE DIRECTIONS

The anticoagulation therapy horizon has expanded significantly in recent years with the development of new target-specific oral anticoagulants as an alternative for the widely used VKAs and heparin. The DOACs have been shown to be as effective as the older drugs with associated decreased risk of intracranial bleeding in many of the clinical indications. New ongoing trials will help answer whether the DOACs are also safe and effective in special populations, such as APS, HIT, or CAT. The growing use in clinical practice will also increase the knowledge about its possible drug-drug interactions and tolerability. Finally, the future development of new target-specific agents and respective antidotes is expected to broaden the options and improve the quality of life of patients in need of anticoagulation.

REFERENCES

1. Gomez-Outes A, Suarez-Gea ML, Lecumberri R, et al. Direct-acting oral antico-agulants: pharmacology, indications, management, and future perspectives. Eur J Haematol 2015;95(5):389–404.
2. Mega JL, Simon T. Pharmacology of antithrombotic drugs: an assessment of oral antiplatelet and anticoagulant treatments. Lancet 2015;386(9990):281–91.
3. Bauer KA. Pros and cons of new oral anticoagulants. Hematology Am Soc Hematol Educ Program 2013;2013:464–70.
4. Asmis LM. Direct oral anticoagulants (DOACs) versus "new" oral anticoagulants (NOACs)? Semin Hematol 2014;51(2):87–8.
5. Arepally GM, Ortel TL. Changing practice of anticoagulation: will target-specific anticoagulants replace warfarin? Annu Rev Med 2015;66:241–53.
6. January CT, Wann LS, Alpert JS, et al. 2014 AHA/ACC/HRS guideline for the management of patients with atrial fibrillation: a report of the American College of Cardiology/American Heart Association Task Force on practice guidelines and the Heart Rhythm Society. Circulation 2014;130(23):e199–267.
7. Coppens M, Eikelboom JW, Hart RG, et al. The CHA2DS2-VASc score identifies those patients with atrial fibrillation and a CHADS2 score of 1 who are unlikely to benefit from oral anticoagulant therapy. Eur Heart J 2013;34(3):170–6.
8. van der Hulle T, Dronkers CEA, Huisman MV, et al. Current standings in diagnostic management of acute venous thromboembolism: still rough around the edges. Blood Rev 2016;30(1):21–6.
9. Kearon C, Akl EA, Comerota AJ, et al. Antithrombotic therapy for VTE disease: antithrombotic therapy and prevention of thrombosis, 9th ed: American College of chest physicians evidence-based clinical practice guidelines. Chest 2012; 141(2 Suppl):e419S–494.
10. Kearon C, Akl EA, Ornelas J, et al. Antithrombotic therapy for VTE Disease: CHEST guideline and expert panel report. Chest 2016;149(2):315–52.
11. Alberio L. The new direct oral anticoagulants in special indications: rationale and preliminary data in cancer, mechanical heart valves, anti-phospholipid syndrome, and heparin-induced thrombocytopenia and beyond. Semin Hematol 2014;51(2): 152–6.

12. Lyman GH, Khorana AA, Kuderer NM, et al. Venous thromboembolism prophy-laxis and treatment in patients with cancer: American Society of Clinical Oncology clinical practice guideline update. J Clin Oncol 2013;31(17):2189–204.
13. Lyman GH, Bohlke K, Falanga A. Venous thromboembolism prophylaxis and treatment in patients with cancer: American Society of Clinical Oncology clinical practice guideline update. J Oncol Pract 2015;11(3):e442–4.
14. Prandoni P. The treatment of cancer-associated venous thromboembolism in the era of the novel oral anticoagulants. Expert Opin Pharmacother 2015;16(16): 2391–4.
15. Lee AY, Levine MN, Baker RI, et al. Low-molecular-weight heparin versus a coumarin for the prevention of recurrent venous thromboembolism in patients with cancer. N Engl J Med 2003;349(2):146–53.
16. Spencer FA, Emery C, Reed G, et al. Venous thromboembolism in the outpatient setting. Arch Intern Med 2007;167(14):1471–5.
17. Falck-Ytter Y, Francis CW, Johanson NA, et al. Prevention of VTE in orthopedic surgery patients: antithrombotic therapy and prevention of thrombosis, 9th ed: American College of chest physicians evidence-based clinical practice guide-lines. Chest 2012;141(2 Suppl):e278S–325S.
18. Kahn SR, Lim W, Dunn AS, et al. Prevention of VTE in nonsurgical patients: antith-rombotic therapy and prevention of thrombosis, 9th ed: American College of chest physicians evidence-based clinical practice guidelines. Chest 2012; 141(2 Suppl):e195S–226S.
19. Goldhaber SZ, Leizorovicz A, Kakkar AK, et al. Apixaban versus enoxaparin for thromboprophylaxis in medically ill patients. N Engl J Med 2011;365(23): 2167–77.
20. Cohen AT, Spiro TE, Buller HR, et al. Rivaroxaban for thromboprophylaxis in acutely ill medical patients. N Engl J Med 2013;368(6):513–23.
21. Prandoni P, Temraz S, Taher A. Direct oral anticoagulants in the prevention of venous thromboembolism: evidence from major clinical trials. Semin Hematol 2014;51(2):121–30.
22. Kakkar AK, Brenner B, Dahl OE, et al. Extended duration rivaroxaban versus short-term enoxaparin for the prevention of venous thromboembolism after total hip arthroplasty: a double-blind, randomised controlled trial. Lancet 2008; 372(9632):31–9.
23. Muntz JE, Michota FA. Prevention and management of venous thromboembolism in the surgical patient: options by surgery type and individual patient risk factors. Am J Surg 2010;199(1 Suppl):S11–20.
24. Gould MK, Garcia DA, Wren SM, et al. Prevention of VTE in nonorthopedic surgical patients: antithrombotic therapy and prevention of thrombosis, 9th ed: American College of chest physicians evidence-based clinical practice guidelines. Chest 2012;141(2 Suppl):e227S–77S.
25. Daniels PR. Peri-procedural management of patients taking oral anticoagulants. BMJ 2015;351:h2391.
26. Douketis JD, Spyropoulos AC, Spencer FA, et al. Perioperative management of antithrombotic therapy: antithrombotic therapy and prevention of thrombosis, 9th ed: American College of chest physicians evidence-based clinical practice guidelines. Chest 2012;141(2 Suppl):e326S–50S.
27. Douketis JD, Spyropoulos AC, Kaatz S, et al. Perioperative bridging anticoagula-tion in patients with atrial fibrillation. N Engl J Med 2015;373(9):823–33.
28. Mar PL, Familtsev D, Ezekowitz MD, et al. Periprocedural management of antico-agulation in patients taking novel oral anticoagulants: review of the literature and

recommendations for specific populations and procedures. Int J Cardiol 2016; 202:578–85.

29. Ferns SJ, Naccarelli GV. New oral anticoagulants: their role in stroke prevention in high-risk patients with atrial fibrillation. Med Clin North Am 2015;99(4):759–80.

30. Weitz JI, Gross PL. New oral anticoagulants: which one should my patient use? Hematology Am Soc Hematol Educ Program 2012;2012:536–40.

31. Connolly SJ, Ezekowitz MD, Yusuf S, et al. Dabigatran versus warfarin in patients with atrial fibrillation. N Engl J Med 2009;361(12):1139–51.

32. Garcia DA. The target-specific oral anticoagulants: practical considerations. Hematology 2014;2014(1):510–3.

33. Granziera S, Hasan A, Cohen AA. Direct oral anticoagulants and their use in treatment and secondary prevention of acute symptomatic venous thromboembolism. Clin Appl Thromb Hemost 2016;22(3):209–21.

34. Dobesh PP, Fanikos J. Direct oral anticoagulants for the prevention of stroke in patients with nonvalvular atrial fibrillation: understanding differences and similarities. Drugs 2015;75(14):1627–44.

35. Ansell J, Hirsh J, Hylek E, et al. Pharmacology and management of the vitamin K antagonists: American College of chest physicians evidence-based clinical practice guidelines (8th edition). Chest 2008;133(6 Suppl):160S–98S.

36. Gaertner S, Cordeanu EM, Mirea C, et al. Prothrombotic risk of vitamin K antagonists during the first days of treatment: one more reason to use new oral anticoagulants. Int J Cardiol 2015;186:141–2.

37. Ageno W, Gallus AS, Wittkowsky A, et al. Oral anticoagulant therapy: antithrombotic therapy and prevention of thrombosis, 9th ed: American College of Chest Physicians evidence-based clinical practice guidelines. Chest 2012; 141(2 Suppl):e44S–88S.

38. Keeling D, Baglin T, Tait C, et al. Guidelines on oral anticoagulation with warfarin - fourth edition. Br J Haematol 2011;154(3):311–24.

39. Holbrook A, Schulman S, Witt DM, et al. Evidence-based management of anticoagulant therapy: antithrombotic therapy and prevention of thrombosis, 9th ed: American College of chest physicians evidence-based clinical practice guidelines. Chest 2012;141(2 Suppl):e152S–84S.

40. Shaw K, Amstutz U, Kim RB, et al. Clinical practice recommendations on genetic testing of CYP2C9 and VKORC1 variants in warfarin therapy. Ther Drug Monit 2015;37(4):428–36.

41. Kimmel SE, French B, Kasner SE, et al. A pharmacogenetic versus a clinical algorithm for warfarin dosing. N Engl J Med 2013;369(24):2283–93.

42. Barta AL, Nutescu EA, Thompson PA, et al. Relationship between time spent at extreme international normalized ratios and time in therapeutic range with bleeding and thrombosis in warfarin-treated patients. Am J Health Syst Pharm 2015;72(14):1188–94.

43. Pokorney SD, Simon DN, Thomas L, et al. Patients' time in therapeutic range on warfarin among US patients with atrial fibrillation: results from ORBIT-AF registry. Am Heart J 2015;170(1):141–8, 148.e1.

44. Pisters R, Lane DA, Nieuwlaat R, et al. A novel user-friendly score (HAS-BLED) to assess 1-year risk of major bleeding in patients with atrial fibrillation: the Euro Heart Survey. Chest 2010;138(5):1093–100.

45. Lip GY. Assessing bleeding risk with the HAS-BLED score: balancing simplicity, practicality, and predictive value in bleeding-risk assessment. Clin Cardiol 2015; 38(9):562–4.

46. Zhu W, He W, Guo L, et al. The HAS-BLED score for predicting major bleeding risk in anticoagulated patients with atrial fibrillation: a systematic review and meta-analysis. Clin Cardiol 2015;38(9):555–61.
47. Goldstein JN, Refaai MA, Milling TJ, et al. Four-factor prothrombin complex concentrate versus plasma for rapid vitamin K antagonist reversal in patients needing urgent surgical or invasive interventions: a phase 3b, open-label, non-inferiority, randomised trial. Lancet 2015;385(9982):2077–87.
48. Coumadin FDA. Approval. Available at: http://www.accessdata.fda.gov/drugsatfda_docs/label/2011/009218s107lbl.pdf.
49. Garcia D, Libby E, Crowther MA. The new oral anticoagulants. Blood 2010; 115(1):15–20.
50. Dempfle CE. Direct oral anticoagulants–pharmacology, drug interactions, and side effects. Semin Hematol 2014;51(2):89–97.
51. Parasrampuria DA, Truitt KE. Pharmacokinetics and pharmacodynamics of edoxaban, a Non-Vitamin K antagonist oral anticoagulant that inhibits clotting factor Xa. Clin Pharmacokinet 2015. [Epub ahead of print].
52. Konkle BA. Monitoring target-specific oral anticoagulants. Hematology Am Soc Hematol Educ Program 2014;2014(1):329–33.
53. Tsakiris DA. Direct oral anticoagulants–interference with laboratory tests and mechanism of action. Semin Hematol 2014;51(2):98–101.
54. Kozek-Langenecker SA. Perioperative management issues of direct oral anticoagulants. Semin Hematol 2014;51(2):112–20.
55. Palareti G. Direct oral anticoagulants and bleeding risk (in comparison to vitamin K antagonists and heparins), and the treatment of bleeding. Semin Hematol 2014;51(2):102–11.
56. Husted S, Verheugt FW, Comuth WJ. Reversal strategies for NOACs: state of development, possible clinical applications and future perspectives. Drug Saf 2016;39(1):5–13.
57. Burness CB. Idarucizumab: first global approval. Drugs 2015;75(18):2155–61.
58. Peacock WF, Levy PD, Gonzalez MG, et al. Target-specific oral anticoagulants in the emergency department. J Emerg Med 2016;50(2):246–57.
59. Garcia DA, Baglin TP, Weitz JI, et al. Parenteral anticoagulants: antithrombotic therapy and prevention of thrombosis, 9th ed: American College of chest physicians evidence-based clinical practice guidelines. Chest 2012;141(2 Suppl): e24S–43S.
60. Baglin T, Barrowcliffe TW, Cohen A, et al. Guidelines on the use and monitoring of heparin. Br J Haematol 2006;133(1):19–34.
61. Uprichard J, Manning RA, Laffan MA. Monitoring heparin anticoagulation in the acute phase response. Br J Haematol 2010;149(4):613–9.
62. Mazziotti G, Canalis E, Giustina A. Drug-induced osteoporosis: mechanisms and clinical implications. Am J Med 2010;123(10):877–84.
63. Lee GM, Arepally GM. Heparin-induced thrombocytopenia. Hematology Am Soc Hematol Educ Program 2013;2013:668–74.
64. Lee GM, Arepally GM. Diagnosis and management of heparin-induced thrombocytopenia. Hematol Oncol Clin North Am 2013;27(3):541–63.
65. Linkins LA, Dans AL, Moores LK, et al. Treatment and prevention of heparin-induced thrombocytopenia: antithrombotic therapy and prevention of thrombosis, 9th ed: American College of chest physicians evidence-based clinical practice guidelines. Chest 2012;141(2 Suppl):e495S–530S.
66. Patel MR, Mahaffey KW, Garg J, et al. Rivaroxaban versus warfarin in nonvalvular atrial fibrillation. The New England journal of medicine 2011;365(10):883–91.

67. Investigators E, Bauersachs R, Berkowitz SD, et al. Oral rivaroxaban for symptomatic venous thromboembolism. The New England journal of medicine 2010; 363(26):2499–510.

68. Schulman S, Kearon C, Kakkar AK, et al. Dabigatran versus warfarin in the treatment of acute venous thromboembolism. The New England journal of medicine 2009;361(24):2342–52.

69. Granger CB, Alexander JH, McMurray JJ, et al. Apixaban versus warfarin in patients with atrial fibrillation. The New England journal of medicine 2011;365(11): 981–92.

70. Agnelli G, Buller HR, Cohen A, et al. Oral apixaban for the treatment of acute venous thromboembolism. The New England journal of medicine 2013;369(9): 799–808.

71. Giugliano RP, Ruff CT, Braunwald E, et al. Edoxaban versus warfarin in patients with atrial fibrillation. The New England journal of medicine 2013;369(22): 2093–104.

Pharmacologic Therapies for Rheumatologic and Autoimmune Conditions

 CrossMark

Alison M. Bays, MD, MPH&TM[a],*, Gregory Gardner, MD[b]

KEYWORDS

- Rheumatology • Autoimmune • Immunosuppression • Gout
- Disease-modifying antirheumatic drugs (DMARDs) • Biologic agents

KEY POINTS

- Steroids should be used at the lowest effective dose, for the least amount of time.
- Colchicine is used as a prophylactic agent for gout or pseudogout at a dosage of 0.6 mg twice per day in those with normal renal function.
- Allopurinol should be started at 100 mg per day, 50 mg per day with existing renal disease.
- All tumor necrosis factor agents have a potential increased risk of tuberculosis and hepatitis B reactivation, and these must be tested for before starting the medications.

NONSTEROIDAL ANTI-INFLAMMATORY DRUGS

Nonsteroidal anti-inflammatory medications (NSAIDs) are used often in rheumatology in conjunction with other medications or as monotherapy for acute gout or the sero-negative spondyloarthropathies.[1,2] NSAIDs act by inhibition of cyclooxygenase, decreasing prostaglandin E_2 and prostacyclin, and have anti-inflammatory properties in addition to some antiplatelet activities. There is not one NSAID medication or dose recommended over other medications, but care should be taken when assessing the patient's comorbidities, such as hypertension, renal insufficiency, gastrointestinal (GI) ulcers, and cardiovascular risk. Studies have shown no difference in selective as compared with nonselective NSAIDs in the treatment of osteoarthritis.[1]

Major side effects include GI bleeding and increased cardiovascular disease risk. NSAIDs should be avoided in patients with known cardiovascular disease, because there is an increased risk for heart failure exacerbations and coronary events in this

Conflict of Interest Disclosures: None.
Role in Authorship: All authors had access to data and a role in writing and revising the article.
[a] Division of Rheumatology, Department of Internal Medicine, Harborview Medical Center, 325 9th Avenue, Box 356428, Seattle, WA 98104, USA; [b] Division of Rheumatology, Department of Internal Medicine, University of Washington, Box 356428, 1959 Pacific Street, Seattle, WA 98195, USA
* Corresponding author.
E-mail address: alisonmb@uw.edu

Med Clin N Am 100 (2016) 719–731
http://dx.doi.org/10.1016/j.mcna.2016.03.001
medical.theclinics.com

population. Care should be taken when prescribing both NSAIDs and steroids, because this has been shown to increase the risk of GI bleeding. Testing and eradication of *Helicobacter pylori* is recommended.[3] A proton pump inhibitor may be considered as well.

Other important side effects include nephrotoxicity, photosensitivity, aseptic meningitis, antiplatelet activity, hepatotoxicity, and, rarely, Stevens-Johnson syndrome.[1]

CORTICOSTEROIDS

Steroids are used commonly in rheumatology for many conditions, such as gout, polymyalgia rheumatica, rheumatoid arthritis (RA), vasculitis, and lupus (**Table 1**). Glucocorticoids act through the cytosolic steroid hormone receptor, resulting in increased expression of anti-inflammatory proteins and decreased production of proinflammatory proteins.[4]

There are a few diseases for which glucocorticoids are used alone, such as with polymyalgia rheumatica. In patients with polymyalgia rheumatica and without concomitant giant cell arteritis, oral prednisone dosages are recommended from

Table 1
Steroids are generally not recommended in spondyloarthropathies[2] and are relatively contraindicated in scleroderma because it may precipitate a scleroderma renal crisis (especially with RNA polymerase III antibodies); also they are relatively contraindicated in psoriatic arthritis due to flares of psoriasis with tapering

Disease	Situation	Initial Prednisone Dosing
ANCA-associated small vessel vasculitis[32]	Biopsy-proven organ threatening disease (diffuse alveolar hemorrhage, glomerulonephritis)	500 mg–1 g methylprednisolone daily for 3 d, then 60 mg daily with taper over months while starting rituximab or oral cyclophosphamide
Giant cell arteritis[33]	Suspected or biopsy-proven without vision changes	Prednisone 40–60 mg with taper started after 2–4 wk while monitoring symptoms and inflammatory markers
	Vision loss	500 mg–1 g methylprednisolone daily for 3 d, then prednisone 60 mg daily with taper
Gout[6]	Prophylaxis	<10 mg/d (generally 5 mg)
	Flare	0.5 mg/kg/d for 5–10 d, then stop or for 2–5 d, then taper for the next 7–10 d
Polymyalgia rheumatica[5]	No evidence of giant cell arteritis	12.5–25 mg prednisone daily as initial dose
Rheumatoid arthritis[29]	Long-term maintenance	5 mg or less in combination with DMARDs or biologics
	Flare	Preferably 10 mg and less, joint injections, increasing DMARD/biologic therapy
SLE[34]	Maintenance	5 mg or less in combination with other therapies is sometimes used.
	Organ-threatening flare (glomerulonephritis)	500 mg–1 g methylprednisolone daily for 3 d, then 0.5–1 mg/kg daily with taper and initiation DMARD therapy

Data from Ward MM, Deodhar A, Akl EA, et al. American College of Rheumatology/Spondylitis Association of America/Spondyloarthritis Research and Treatment Network 2015 recommendations for the treatment of ankylosing spondylitis and nonradiographic axial spondyloarthritis. Arthritis Rheumatol 2016;68(2):282–98.

12.5 to 25 mg per day, using the minimum effective dosage. Initial tapering should involve getting the patient down to 10 mg within 4 to 8 weeks, and if the patient relapses, increasing prednisone to the dosage before relapse and reattempting a slow taper. Once remission is achieved, taper from 10 mg by 1 mg every 4 weeks. In patients who relapse or have high risk of glucocorticoid complications, methotrexate should be considered and used early.[5]

For acute flares of crystalline disease, such as gout or pseudogout, short courses of higher doses of steroids are recommended (for example, 0.5 mg/kg/d and then stop after 5 days or for 2 to 5 days with a taper over 7 to 10 days).[6] If a patient has a gout or pseudogout flare with few joints involved and is amenable to injection, a local joint injection can be performed. Generally, a large joint is injected with 40 mg of triamcinolone, a medium joint with 20 mg triamcinolone, and smaller joints with 5 to 10 mg.

For chronic inflammatory joint pain, such as with RA and systemic lupus erythematosus (SLE), the dosage of glucocorticoids is much lower, generally 5 to 10 mg per day. This dosage should be tapered as other steroid-sparing agents are initiated.

Pulsed steroids are used in rheumatology in organ-threatening conditions, such as with lupus nephritis or with small vessel vasculitis with pulmonary and renal involvement. This dosage is generally 500 mg to 1 g methylprednisolone intravenously daily for 3 days, followed by prednisone at high dosages, 60 mg per day. The high dose steroids are tapered as other immunosuppressive agents are added.

Some consequences of steroid usage include bone loss, hypertension, weight gain, steroid psychosis, impaired glucose tolerance, avascular necrosis, and increased rate of infection. In addition, severe hypokalemia may occur from pulse dose steroids. The underlying principle of all steroid prescriptions is that patients should be on the lowest dose possible for the least amount of time. Important adjunctive therapy includes calcium and vitamin D, and in some situations, prophylactic bisphosphonate therapy and prophylaxis against pneumocystis. Special considerations include patients with high infectious risk, patients with diabetes, and patients with surgical wound healing. In addition, steroid usage may increase the risk of GI bleed in a hospitalized patient setting, and prophylactic proton pump inhibitors should be considered.[7]

COLCHICINE

Colchicine is used for prophylaxis against gout flares while initiating urate-lowering therapy (ULT) and additionally for patients with pseudogout (calcium pyrophosphate deposition disease, CPPD). It is also used for rare diseases, such as familial Mediterranean fever and Behçet's disease, in addition to pericarditis. Colchicine is extracted from the autumn crocus, and the mechanism of action is not fully understood but involves binding to tubulins, preventing the polymerization of microtubules and concentrates in neutrophils, inhibiting chemotaxis.[8]

Prophylaxis against recurrent episodes of gout, with colchicine, NSAIDs, or corticosteroids is recommended when ULT is initiated.[6] The dosage of colchicine recommended is 0.6 mg once or twice per day with dose adjustments with renal impairment.[6] The US Food and Drug Administration recommends close monitoring with creatinine clearance 30 mL/min and above and starting colchicine at 0.3 mg per day if below 30 mL/min or on hemodialysis. In clinical practice, rheumatologists are sometimes more cautious with not using colchicine in hemodialysis patients if possible or dosing at 0.3 mg twice weekly. Prophylaxis should be for 6 months after achieving target serum urate and can be stopped if there have not been gout flares and if there are no tophi present.[9] In addition, colchicine is used as a prophylactic agent for pseudogout (CPPD) at a dosage of 0.6 mg orally once or twice daily.

The major side effect is diarrhea, in which case colchicine should be reduced or stopped. Other warnings include myelosuppression and neuromuscular toxicity, which can occur at treatment doses. In addition, there are many drug interactions, including cyclosporine, clarithromycin, ketoconazole, and some protease inhibitors.[8]

Urate-lowering Therapy

ULT is generally started in patients with tophi present or recurrent attacks of gouty arthritis (traditionally 2 or more) who cannot reduce the serum uric acid (SUA) into the normal range with lifestyle modification (ie, slow weight loss) or medication modifications (ie, stopping diuretics).[9] An SUA level greater than 6.8 mg/dL is considered physiologically abnormal and is the level at which uric acid begins to lose its solubility. It should be noted that the normative range in many laboratories reflects the obesity epidemic, and "normal" levels as high as 8.5 mg/dL are reported.

Like many therapeutic interventions, there is a target level suggested for successful therapy in patients with hyperuricemia. In patients without tophi, the recommended SUA target is between 5 and 6 mg/dL, and for those with tophi, an SUA of less than or equal to 5 mg/dL is suggested.[6]

There are currently 2 xanthine oxidase inhibitors (XOIs) available, one urisosuric agent and a pegylated uricase medication available to treat hyperuricemia. Even though most patients with hyperuricemia are underexcretors of uric acid rather than overproducers, the current recommendation is to start hypouricemic therapy with an XOI rather than a uricosuric agent. ULT can be initiated during a gout attack if an effective anti-inflammatory agent has been initiated.[9]

Allopurinol

Allopurinol is an XOI first synthesized in 1956 as a possible antineoplastic agent and marketed in 1966 for the treatment of gout. It inhibits the conversion of soluble hypoxanthine and then xanthine to the relatively insoluble uric acid in the purine metabolism pathway. Allopurinol is almost completely metabolized to oxypurinol, which is itself an XOI and is eliminated via the kidneys with an elimination half-life of 14 to 29 hours.[6] The approved dosage range is 100 to 800 mg per day. The recent American College of Rheumatology (ACR) guidelines suggest starting at no more than 100 mg once per day in those with no existing renal disease (**Table 2**).[9] Lower starting doses have been shown to reduce early gout flares and decrease the risk of a hypersensitivity reaction.[6] Allopurinol can be increased every 2 to 4 weeks and doses above 300 mg are acceptable, even in renal impairment, to reach the treatment goal but should be accompanied by transaminase and eosinophil monitoring and patient education for signs and symptoms of drug toxicity.[9] Allopurinol does not have an adverse effect on renal function, although patients with decreased renal function can have elevated

Table 2 Allopurinol	
Allopurinol starting dose	100 mg 50 mg/d with CKD stage 4 or worse
Allopurinol up-titration	Every 2–5 wks
Allopurinol laboratory monitoring	Liver function tests Eosinophils
HLA-B5081 testing	Han Chinese patients Thai patients Korean patients with stage 3 CKD

levels of allopurinol in their blood. The initial guidelines for "renal dosing" of allopurinol were developed with the intent of preventing allopurinol hypersensitivity, not because of direct renal toxicity of allopurinol.[10]

Common side effects of allopurinol include rash, diarrhea, and nausea. In addition, lowering SUA can lead to an increased risk of gouty attacks, so most patients should be on prophylaxis (see earlier discussion on colchicine). A rare patient may experience leukopenia or thrombocytopenia. Allopurinol may cause more severe cutaneous disease such as Stevens-Johnson syndrome and toxic epidermal necrolysis. The hypersensitivity syndrome includes fever, rash, hepatitis, acute renal failure, and eosinophilia. The rates of the more severe reactions appear to be decreased with "go low, go slow" implementation.[6] HLA-B*5801 increases the risk of a severe reaction and should be checked before initiation in patients of Han Chinese and Thai descent in addition to Korean patients with stage 3 chronic kidney disease (CKD) or worse.[9] The other factors associated with hypersensitivity syndrome include renal impairment, use of diuretics, and high starting dose of allopurinol. The combination of the HLA-B5801 allele plus renal insufficiency increases the risk of a serious reaction to allopurinol to 18%.[11]

Important drug interactions include significant increase in the blood levels of 6-mercaptopurine, azathioprine, theophylline, and warfarin when taking concomitant allopurinol. These drugs, especially 6-mercaptopurine and azathioprine, should be avoided or have their dosages reduced.[6]

Febuxostat

Febuxostat is a nonpurine agent that also inhibits xanthine oxidase. It was approved in 2009 for use in the treatment of hyperuricemia and gout. It is metabolized almost wholly by the liver with minimal renal elimination, which has made it attractive for those with renal insufficiency. In the trials comparing allopurinol to febuxostat, the latter appeared to be more efficient at meeting target goals, although allopurinol was not dose titrated as it would have been in clinical practice.[12]

Febuxostat is available in the United States in 40-mg and 80-mg dosages with the recommendation to begin at 40 mg and up-titrate in 2 to 4 weeks if the SUA goal is not reached. Doses as high as 120 mg were used in clinical trials but are not approved for use in the United States; they are, however, approved in Europe.[12]

Side effects include nausea and diarrhea, elevation of liver function tests, and rash with very rare severe skin reactions. Monitoring includes intermittent liver enzyme tests. It is recommended to avoid febuxostat in patients with severe renal or hepatic disease. In patients with rash due to allopurinol, no cross-reactivity with febuxostat is recognized. As with allopurinol, febuxostat will increase the risk to gouty attacks, and prophylaxis is recommended, avoiding concomitant use with of 6-mercaptopurine and azathioprine, and use with caution with theophyllines.[11,12] In the Anti-Platelet Trialists collaboration trial, an increase in investigator-reported cardiovascular events was reported compared with the allopurinol group[12]; this was not found in other studies, but the package insert suggests caution in high-risk groups.

The other limitation of febuxostat is cost when compared with allopurinol and will affect its utilization. Thirty tablets of allopurinol 300 mg is around $25.00 compared with $250 for 30 tablets of febuxostat 40 mg at the time of this writing.

Probenecid

Probenecid was synthesized in the late 1940s, and its initial use was in increasing serum concentration of antibiotics, in particular, penicillin. Early studies of probenecid also revealed its uricosuric properties, and it continues today as the only uricosuric on the market in the United States.

Uric acid undergoes a complex back-and-forth dance in the kidney, and its movement is facilitated by a group of proteins known as organic ion transporters. Probenecid inhibits one such transporter, and the end result is the excretion of uric acid into the urine, where it would normally be reabsorbed again.

Probenecid has taken a secondary role in the guidelines for treatment of hyperuricemia and gout but has been shown in combination studies with allopurinol to offer additional benefit over allopurinol alone in helping patients reach SUA target levels.[13] It is also useful for patients who cannot tolerate other forms of ULT but is rarely effective when the GFR is 50 mL/min or less.[13]

Dosage is 250 mg twice a day with dosage increase as guided by SUA target levels to 1000 mg twice daily. It is generally given with meals to take advantage of increased fluid intake and relative alkaline urine, which reduces the risk of stone formation.

Side effects include the usual GI upset and rash. It impairs the excretion of a host of medications besides antibiotics, and medications added to a regimen that includes probenecid should be reviewed for interaction. Because probenecid increases the amount of uric acid passed into the urinary collection system, it may lead to stone formation. It should be used with caution in a patient suspected of being an overproducer of uric acid (approximately 5% of gouty patients) for this reason.

Other Agents

Pegloticase is a polyethylene glycol conjugated with recombinant mammalian enzyme uricase.[14] Just about every other creature on Earth that makes purines has a built-in uricase. Humans, great apes, and for some reason Dalmatian dogs, do not. Pegloticase is given intravenously in a dosage of 8 mg every 2 weeks and can dramatically lower SUA and lead to significant tophi size reduction. It is recommended in patients with severe gout disease burden and lack of response or intolerance to other ULT.[9] Because uricase is not a protein normally found in humans, it can engender an immune response. Thus, side effects include infusion reactions and anaphylaxis.[14] There is, as with all ULT, an increased risk of gouty flares. Patients need a glucose-6-phosphate dehydrogenase deficiency (G6PD) level measured before treatment due to risk of hemolysis in deficient patients. If this medication is considered, it should be administered by someone with experience in its use.

Losartan is an angiotensin II receptor antagonist agent that has modest uricosuric properties due to its ability to inhibit organic ion transport proteins in the kidney.[13] Fenofibrate also has similar qualities, and these medications can be added to the regimen of patients with hyperuricemia and gout who have comorbid conditions for which such therapy might be useful.

DISEASE-MODIFYING ANTIRHEUMATIC MEDICATIONS

A variety of nonbiologic and biologic agents are available for the treatment of inflammatory arthritis by both rheumatologists and primary care physicians. Because of a relative insufficiency of rheumatologists in the United States and the importance of early diagnosis and treatment of patients with diseases such as RA, it is important for the primary care physician to be familiar and comfortable prescribing and monitoring the "anchor drugs" and also be familiar with the potential side effects of the DMARDs typically prescribed by rheumatologists. **Table 3** describes the use of DMARDs in pregnancy.

Table 3
Disease-modifying antirheumatic medications and pregnancy

Medication	Comments
Avoid	
Methotrexate	Teratogen and abortifactant; off 3 mo before conception
Leflunomide	Teratogen; off 3.5 mo before conception
Mycophenolate	Teratogen and abortifactant
Use with caution	
TNF inhibitors	Stop unless necessary, avoid especially in third trimester to improve efficacy of infant immunization
Generally safe	
Hydroxychloroquine	Generally safe in pregnancy; may be beneficial in SLE pregnancy
Sulfasalazine	Generally safe in pregnancy; folate supplementation recommended
Azathioprine	Generally safe during pregnancy; azathioprine is a prodrug not activated by the fetal liver
Calcineurin inhibitors	Generally safe during pregnancy
Unknown	
Other DMARDs	Not sufficient data to recommend continuation during pregnancy

Data from Leroy C, Rigot JM, Leroy M, et al. Immunosuppressive drugs and fertility. Orphanet J Rare Dis 2015;10:136–51.

Anchor Disease-modifying Antirheumatic Medications

Methotrexate

Methotrexate inhibits dihydrofolate reductase and is commonly used by rheumatologists, in much lower doses than used by oncologists, for the treatment of RA and as a steroid-sparing agent in many other conditions. Current uses include most forms of peripheral inflammatory arthritis, in particular RA and psoriatic arthritis. It is not useful for the axial disease of spondyloarthropathies, such as ankylosing spondylitis. It is typically started as a single agent, and other DMARDs can be added as required to reach a target of low disease activity or remission on clinical disease activity measures. Approximately 50% of patients treated with methotrexate will achieve this level of control, but it must be gradually increased to levels of 15 to 20 mg/wk to achieve these results.

Methotrexate dosing is once weekly, and 1 mg of folic acid is generally prescribed daily along with methotrexate to help with potential side effects without reducing effectiveness.[15] It generally takes 4 to 8 weeks to begin to see clinical efficacy.

Common side effects include liver enzyme elevations and nausea and vomiting. Bone marrow suppression and elevation of liver function tests can also occur. Rare cases of hypersensitivity pneumonitis have been reported with methotrexate. To reduce side effects and increase absorption, patients can split their dose on the same day (half of the pills in the morning and half of the pills at night) especially as the dosage is increased from 7.5 to 10 mg/wk to higher dosages (up to 25 mg/wk). It can also be administered subcutaneously, which may result in higher concentrations of the drug and decreased GI side effects.

Before the start of methotrexate, the ACR recommends getting a complete blood count, liver transaminases level tested, and a creatinine level checked in addition to testing for hepatitis B and C.[16] Complete blood counts, transaminase levels, and serum creatinine levels are recommended every 2 to 4 weeks in the first 3 months of starting therapy and every 8 to 12 weeks during months 3 to 6 and every 12 weeks once the patient has been taking methotrexate for more than 6 months.[10] Women should be prescribed methotrexate with caution, and discussion due to its teratogenic and abortifactant effects and the drug should be completely stopped 3 months before planned conception.

Hydroxychloroquine

Hydroxychloroquine is a derivative of quinine, which was originally derived from the bark of the cinchona tree from South America. The mechanism of action is related to its ability to gently interfere with the way antigen is processed by antigen-presenting cells and by affecting the activity of the innate immune system by inhibiting Toll-like receptors. The latter has a downstream effect of decreasing production of type 1 interferons, which are important in the pathogenesis of autoimmune disease.[17] Hydroxychloroquine was first developed just as WWII was ending and has been used to treat inflammatory arthritis since the 1950s. It has relatively low toxicity but also relatively low potency.

Uses for hydroxychloroquine include an inflammatory arthritis, in particular, RA and SLE. It is useful in the treatment of joint, skin, and systemic involvement in these conditions. In RA, it is often used in so-called triple therapy (methotrexate, sulfasalazine, and hydroxychloroquine) as a DMARD combination regimen.

Hydroxychloroquine is dosed at 6.5 mg/kg/day or less, which is typically 300 to 400 mg per day for the normal sized adult. Onset of action may take 4 to 12 weeks. Side effects can include rash, nausea, vomiting, diarrhea, and hemolysis in patients who are G6PD-deficient. Rare but serious side effects include a neuromyopathy that can affect the heart, and retinopathy. Monitoring for retinopathy includes a baseline examination, to include optical coherence tomography, repeated at 5 years and then every year following.[18] This rare event that can be vision threatening and is generally seen after 10 years or more of use.[19] Of interest, hydroxychloroquine has also been shown to lower low-density lipoprotein and raise high-density lipoprotein levels, has modest antithrombotic qualities, and may reduce the risk of diabetes and cancer in patients with inflammatory diseases.[17]

Other Nonbiologic Disease-modifying Antirheumatic Medications

Sulfasalazine

Sulfasalazine was developed in the 1930s and is a combination of sulfapyridine and 5-aminosalicylic acid (5-ASA). Sulfasalazine is cleaved by gut bacteria into sulfapyridine, which is absorbed, and the 5-ASA molecule that stays in the gut. It is used for RA as a single agent or in combination and the peripheral arthritis/enthesitis of the spondyloarthropathies. It is dosed 500 to 1000 mg twice a day with a maximum dosage of 1500 mg twice a day. Sulfasalazine is most often used as part of triple therapy in RA (methotrexate, sulfasalazine, hydroxychloroquine).[20] Onset of action is 4 to 8 weeks. The most frequent adverse effects are GI side effects, but myelosuppression can also occur. Azospermia has been reported but is reversible.[21]

Leflunomide

Leflunomide was approved for use in RA in 1998. It is a prodrug, and its metabolite inhibits pyrimidine synthesis and is used alone or in combination. Dosing is 10 to 20 mg once per day in an oral pill. Onset of action is 4 to 12 weeks in part due to its long half-life of the metabolite of 15 to 18 days.[22]

The side effects of leflunomide include nausea, vomiting, and diarrhea, and up to 17% of patients experience weight loss. As with methotrexate, leflunomide is a teratogen. If a patient plans pregnancy or becomes pregnant, a cholestyramine washout is recommended at 8 g three times per day for 11 days.[22,23]

Azathioprine

Azathioprine is a prodrug that is converted to 6-mercaptopurine, which inhibits purine synthesis especially in rapid turnover cell populations such as lymphocytes. It is metabolized by the liver and excreted in the urine. Azathioprine is used less for RA than in previous years but is still used in SLE, myositis, and various forms of vasculitis. Side effects include the usual GI distress, bone marrow suppression, drug fever, and a rare but concerning risk of hematologic malignancy. It can be used in pregnancy because even though it crosses the placental barrier, the fetal liver lacks an enzyme to convert azathioprine into 6-mercaptopurine.[23] Patients who are deficient in the enzyme thiopurine methyltransferase are at an increased risk of hematologic side effects and enzyme levels should be checked before initiating therapy.[24]

Mycophenolate

Mycophenolate mofetil is a selective, noncompetitive, and reversible inhibitor of inosine monophosphate dehydrogenase via its active metabolite, mycophenolic acid, which results in the inhibition of the de novo synthesis pathway of purines. T- and B-lymphocyte proliferation depends on the de novo synthesis of purines, while other cell types can use the salvage pathways. Elimination is 93% via kidney and 6% via feces. The elimination half-life is approximately 17 hours. It is used in extensively in SLE and also in vasculitis and for treatment of autoimmune forms of interstitial lung disease.[25]

Side effects include GI upset, bone marrow suppression, and infection; it is a teratogen and leads to miscarriage and a higher rate of congenital malformation. Female patients should be counseled about the risks prior to initiation of therapy. The US Food and Drug Administration approved a risk evaluation and mitigation strategy for mycophenolate prescribers to help inform patients of the risks of exposure to mycophenolate. The information is available online at mycophenolaterems.com.[23]

Calcineurin inhibitors

Cyclosporine and tacrolimus have limited use in rheumatology and are generally used as third-line agents for SLE or other autoimmune disease. They are typically used in transplantation. They inhibit T-cell elaboration of cytokines, in particular interleukin-2 (IL-2). Concerning side effects include hypertension and renal injury, and of interest to rheumatologists, hyperuricemia. Gout is a too-frequent side effect of being on these agents. One advantage is that they are safe to use in pregnancy.[23]

Apremilast

Apremilast is a new agent (2014) approved for the treatment of psoriasis and psoriatic arthritis. It is a phosphodiesterase 4 inhibitor, which has effects on tumor necrosis factor (TNF) production. Dosage is a slow up-titration to 30 mg twice a day. Side effects include GI symptoms and infection but also depression and weight loss.

Biologic Disease-modifying Antirheumatic Medications

All but two of the current biologic agents are proteins with human or human/murine constructs that are directed against inflammatory cytokine activity or against cells that participate in the inflammatory process. They are administered either intravenously or subcutaneously. Many of the cytokines inhibited by these molecules, such as IL-1 or TNF, contribute to disease activity but are also important in other activities, such as response to infection or tumor suppression. Recently, the first of what may be many small molecule agents, a Janus kinase (JAK) inhibitor, has been approved for use in RA and is administered orally.

The biologics, with one exception, are approved for inflammatory arthritis, such as RA, or the spondyloarthropathies. Many are also approved for the treatment of psoriasis. Rituximab is approved for RA and antineutrophil cytoplasmic antibody (ANCA)-associated vasculitis, while belimumab is approved for treatment of SLE.

The strategies for using these agents are beyond the scope of this article. The most commonly used biologic DMARDs are the TNF inhibitors for the treatment of RA or psoriatic arthritis, and it is possible that a primary care physician may institute these agents so these will be discussed. **Table 4** lists all the biologic DMARDs, schedule, initial laboratory testing, and important side effects.[26]

There are currently are five anti-TNF agents. The first agent to be approved was etanercept, a fusion protein combining two TNF p75 receptors with an immunoglobulin G1 (IgG1) Fc region. The circulating half-life of etanercept is 3.5 to 5.5 days, the shortest of all the TNF agents. Infliximab, a chimeric monoclonal antibody against TNF with a half-life of 9.5 days, is generally infused every 6 to 8 weeks for maintenance therapy. Adalimumab is a fully humanized monoclonal antibody against tumor necrosis factor-alpha (TNF-a) and has the longest half-life of the TNF agents of 10 to 20 days, and is generally dosed every 2 weeks via subcutaneous injection. Golimumab is a fully humanized monoclonal antibody with a half-life of 14 days and is dosed once a month by subcutaneous injection or intravenously every 8 weeks. Finally, certolizumab is a Fab' fragment against TNF combined with polyethylene glycol. The half-life is also 14 days with dosing every 2 weeks subcutaneously.

The TNF agents combined with methotrexate have been shown to be very potent inhibitors of disease progression in RA by inhibiting bone and cartilage damage.

All TNF agents have a potential increased risk of tuberculosis (TB) and hepatitis B reactivation, and these must be tested for upfront. Important side effects include infection, including TB and fungal, and drug-induced syndromes, including cutaneous vasculitis, psoriasis, lupus, peripheral neuropathy, and sarcoidosis-like disease.

Table 4
Current biologic disease-modifying antirheumatic medications

Biologic DMARD	Mechanism of Action	Initial Laboratory Testing	Primary Care Concerns
Etanercept	TNF inhibitor	TB, hepatitis B	Infection or drug-induced disease for all TNF
Adalimumab	TNF inhibitor	TB, hepatitis B	agents (see text)
Certolizumab	TNF inhibitor	TB, hepatitis B	
Golimumab	TNF inhibitor	TB, hepatitis B	
Infliximab	TNF inhibitor	TB, hepatitis B	
Rituximab	Anti-CD20 B cell depleter	Hepatitis B	Viral infections, progressive multifocal leukoencephalopathy
Abatacept	CTLA4 Ig T-cell inhibitor	TB	Infection especially in patients with chronic obstructive pulmonary disease
Ustekinumab	IL-12, IL-23 inhibitor	TB	Infection
Tocilizumab	IL-6 inhibitor	TB	Infection, GI perforation, liver enzyme elevation
Tofacitinib	Janus kinase inhibitor	TB	Infection, GI perforation, liver enzyme elevations, cytopenias

Vaccination Recommendations

One of the most important undertakings before initiating patients on DMARD or biologic therapy is vaccination because patients with autoimmune diseases such as RA and SLE are at high risk of pneumococcal disease, likely due to the disease as well as therapies.[27] Before initiating therapy with any agent, including DMARD monotherapy or combination DMARD therapy, anti-TNF biologics or abatacept, rituximab, or tocilizumab, recommendations include immunizing with pneumococcal vaccination and influenza in addition to hepatitis B, human papillomavirus, and herpes zoster, if indicated.[28,29] However, if a patient is taking anti-TNF biologic agents or abatacept, rituximab, or tocilizumab, they should not receive any live-attenuated vaccines such as herpes zoster.[28,29] If the patient is immunized before starting therapy, they should have at least a 2-week waiting period following zoster vaccination before starting biologic agents.[29]

In terms of pneumococcal vaccinations, the Advisory Committee on Immunization Practices, Centers for Disease Control and Prevention, and the ACR are now recommending vaccination with both PPSV23 (pneumovax) and PCV13 (prevnar) in immunosuppressed patients 19 years of age and older, including those patients who are taking immunosuppressive agents.[30,31]

REFERENCES

1. American College of Rheumatology Ad Hoc Group on Use of Selective and Nonselective Nonsteroidal Antiinflammatory Drugs. Recommendations for use of selective and nonselective nonsteroidal antiinflammatory drugs: an American College of Rheumatology white paper. Arthritis Rheum 2008;59: 1058–73.

2. Ward MM, Deodhar A, Akl EA, et al. American College of Rheumatology/Spondylitis Association of America/Spondyloarthritis Research and Treatment Network 2015 recommendations for the treatment of ankylosing spondylitis and nonradiographic axial spondyloarthritis. Arthritis Rheumatol 2016;68(2):282–98.

3. Scarpignato C, Lanas A, Blandizzi C, et al. Safe prescribing of non-steroidal anti-inflammatory drugs in patients with osteoarthritis–an expert consensus addressing benefits as well as gastrointestinal and cardiovascular risks. BMC Med 2015;13:55.

4. Stahn C, Buttgereit F. Genomic and nongenomic effects of glucocorticoids. Nat Clin Pract Rheumatol 2008;4:525–33.

5. Dejaco C, Singh YP, Perel P, et al. 2015 recommendations for the management of polymyalgia rheumatica: a European League Against Rheumatism/American College of Rheumatology Collaborative Initiative. Arthritis Rheumatol 2015;67:2569–80.

6. Khanna D, Khanna PP, Fitzgerald JD, et al. 2012 American College of Rheumatology guidelines for management of gout. Part 2: therapy and antiinflammatory prophylaxis of acute gouty arthritis. Arthritis Care Res (Hoboken) 2012;64:1447–61.

7. Narum S, Westergren T, Klemp M. Corticosteroids and risk of gastrointestinal bleeding: a systematic review and meta-analysis. BMJ Open 2014;4:e004587.

8. Leung YY, Li L, Hui Y, et al. Colchicine—update on mechanisms of action and therapeutic uses. Semin Arthritis Rheum 2015;45:341–50.

9. Khanna D, Fitzgerald JD, Khanna PP, et al. 2012 American College of Rheumatology guidelines for management of gout. Part 1: systematic nonpharmacologic and pharmacologic therapeutic approaches to hyperuricemia. Arthritis Care Res 2012;64:1431–46.

10. Singh JA, Saag KG, Bridges SL Jr, et al. 2015 American College of Rheumatology guideline for the treatment of rheumatoid arthritis. Arthritis Rheumatol 2015;68(1):1–26.
11. Stamp LK, Day RO. Yun J. Allopurinol hypersensitivity: investigating the cause and minimizing the risk. Nat. Rev. Rheumatol. Online Publication September 29, 2015. http://dx.doi.org/10.1038/nrrheum.2015.132.
12. Ernst ME, Fravel MA. Febuxostat: a selective xanthine-oxidase/xanthine dehydrogenase inhibitor for the management of hyperuricemia in adults with gout. Clinical Therapeutics 2009;31(11):2503–18. http://dx.doi.org/10.1016/j.clinthera.2009.11.033.
13. Bach MH, Simkin PA. Uricosuric drugs: the once and future therapy for hyperuricemia? Curr. Opin. Rheumatol 2014;26:169–75. http://dx.doi.org/10.1097/BOR.0000000000000035.
14. Lyseng-Williamson KA. Pegloticase in treatment-refractory chronic gout. Drugs 2011;71(16):2179–92.
15. Schmajuk G, Miao Y, Yazdany J, et al. Identification of risk factors for elevated transaminases in methotrexate users through an electronic health record. Arthritis Care Res (Hoboken) 2014;66(8):1159–66.
16. Saag KG, Gim GT, Patkar NM, et al. American College of Rheumatology 2008 recommendations for the use of nonbiologic and biologic disease-modifying antirheumatic drugs in rheumatoid arthritis. Arthritis Care Res 2008;59(6):762–84.
17. Costedoat-Chalumeau N, Dunogue B, Morel N, et al. Hydroxychloroquine: a multifaceted treatment for lupus. Presse Med 2014;43:167–80.
18. Marmor MF, Kellner U, Lai TY, et al. Revised recommendations on screening for chloroquine and hydroxychloroquine retinopathy. Ophthalmology 2011;118:415–22.
19. Wolfe F, Marmor MF. Rates and predictors of hydroxychloroquine retinal toxicity in patients with rheumatoid arthritis and systemic lupus erythematous. Arthritis Care Res 2010;62:775–84.
20. Moreland LW, O'Dell JR, Paulus HE, et al. A randomized comparative effectiveness study of oral triple therapy versus etanercept plus methotrexate in early aggressive rheumatoid arthritis. Arthritis Rheum 2012;64:2824–35.
21. Plasker GL, Croom KF. Sulfasalazine: a review of its use in the management of rheumatoid arthritis. Drugs 2005;66:1825–49.
22. Ranganath VK, Furst DE. Disease-modifying antirheumatic drug use in the elderly rheumatoid arthritis patient. Rheum Dis Clin North Am 2007;33:197–217.
23. Leroy C, Rigot JM, Leroy M, et al. Immunosuppressive drugs and fertility. Orphanet J Rare Dis 2015;10:136–51.
24. Clunie GP, Lennard L. Relevance of thiopurine methyltransferase status in rheumatology patients receiving azathioprine. Rheumatology (Oxford) 2004;43:13–8.
25. Ginzler EM, Dooley MA, Arnow C, et al. Mycophenolate mofetil or intravenous cyclophosphamide for lupus nephritis. N Engl J Med 2013;353:2219–28.
26. Zampeli E, Panayiotis GV, Athanasios GT. Treatment of rheumatoid arthritis: unraveling the conundrum. J Autoimmun 2015;65:1–18.
27. Shea KM, Edelsberg J, Weycker D, et al. Rates of pneumococcal disease in adults with chronic medical conditions. Open Forum Infect Dis 2014;1(1):ofu024.
28. Singh J, Furst D, Bharat A, et al. 2012 update of the 2008 American College of Rheumatology recommendations for the use of disease-modifying antirheumatic drugs and biologic agents in the treatment of rheumatoid arthritis. Arthritis Care Res 2012;64(5):625–39.
29. Singh JA, Saag KG, Bridges SL Jr, et al. 2015 American College of Rheumatology guideline for the treatment of rheumatoid arthritis. Arthritis Rheumatol 2016;68:1–26.

30. Tomczyk S, Bennett N, Stooecker C, et al. Use of 13-valent pneumococcal conjugate vaccine and 23-valent pneumococcal polysaccharide vaccine among adults aged ≥65 years: recommendations of the advisory committee on immunization practices (ACIP). MMWR Morb Mortal Wkly Rep 2014;63(37):822–5.
31. Kim DK, Bridges CB, Harriman KH, Centers for Disease Control and Prevention (CDC), Advisory Committee on Immunization Practices (ACIP); ACIP Adult Immunization Work Group. Advisory committee on immunization practices recommended immunization schedule for adults aged 19 years or older–United States, 2015. MMWR Morb Mortal Wkly Rep 2015;64(4):91–2.
32. Specks U, Merkel PA, Seo P, et al. Efficacy of remission-induction regimens for ANCA-associated vasculitis. N Engl J Med 2013;369:417–27.
33. González-Gay MA, Pina T. Giant cell arteritis and polymyalgia rheumatica: an update. Curr Rheumatol Rep 2015;17(2):6.
34. Hahn BH, McMahon MA, Wilkinson A, et al. American College of Rheumatology guidelines for screening, treatment, and management of lupus nephritis. Arthritis Care Res (Hoboken) 2012;64(6):797–808.

Movement Disorders
A Brief Guide in Medication Management

Anthony Julius, MD[a], Katelan Longfellow, MD[b],*

KEYWORDS

- Movement disorders • Parkinson's disease • Nonmotor symptoms
- Essential tremor • Restless leg syndrome

KEY POINTS

- A concise overview of medication for management of Parkinson disease addressed primary motor manifestations, nonmotor symptoms, and rapid eye movement sleep behavior disorder.
- A review of helpful medications in essential tremor with some detail regarding ranges where medications are more likely to have clinical efficacy.
- An overview of some effective medications for restless leg syndrome divided into primary and secondary restless leg syndrome to guide treatment.

MOVEMENT DISORDERS: PART I
Parkinson's Disease

Parkinson's disease is a neurodegenerative disorder of the nigrostriatal pathway caused by loss of dopaminergic neurons in the substantia nigra pars compacta.[1] It is the second most common neurodegenerative condition after Alzheimer's disease, affecting 1% of those over 65 years old, more than 1 million people in North America, and more than 7.5 million worldwide.[2,3] The cardinal features include resting tremor, cogwheel rigidity, bradykinesia, and postural instability.[4] Treatment is focused on augmentation of the dopaminergic pathway (**Fig. 1**) through dopamine repletion, dopamine receptor stimulation, and inhibition of enzymes responsible for dopamine metabolism: monoamine oxidase (MAO) type-B and catechol O-methyltransferase.

The goal of therapy is to replete dopamine levels and alleviate motor symptoms (referred to as medication "on" time), increasing medication dose and/or dosing frequency when therapeutic effect is insufficient (medication "off" time), and also monitoring for hyperkinetic involuntary movements known as dyskinesias (medication

Disclosure Statement: The authors have nothing to disclose.
[a] VA Puget Sound, University of Washington Medical Center, 1660 South Columbian Way, Seattle, WA 98108, USA; [b] VA Puget Sound, University of Washington Medical Center, 1660 South Columbian Way, Seattle, WA 98108, USA
* Corresponding author.
E-mail address: katelanlongfellow@catholichealth.net

Med Clin N Am 100 (2016) 733–761
http://dx.doi.org/10.1016/j.mcna.2016.03.002
0025-7125/16/$ – see front matter © 2016 Elsevier Inc. All rights reserved.

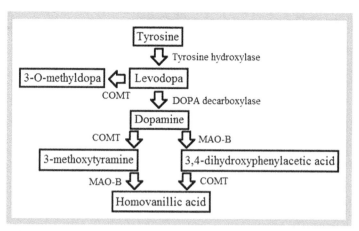

Fig. 1. Metabolic pathway of dopamine. COMT, catechol O-methyltransferase; DOPA, dihydroxyphenylalanine; MAO, monoamine oxidase.

"on-time with dyskinesias"). Treatment is initiated when motor symptoms (tremor, rigidity, bradykinesia) begin to have an impact on quality of life. This can include mobility, stiffness, fine motor control, dexterity, and detriment on activities of daily living (eg, eating, grooming, bathing, dressing). Freezing of gait and postural instability, however, are features of Parkinson's disease that are least likely to respond to pharmacologic treatment.

Levodopa

Levodopa was the first drug available to treat Parkinson's disease, in clinical use since the 1960s. It remains the most potent and effective pharmacologic treatment for parkinsonism.[3] The addition of peripheral dihydroxyphenylalanine (DOPA) decarboxylase inhibitor (carbidopa, or benserazide outside United States), which does not cross the blood–brain barrier, allows conversion of levodopa into dopamine only within the central nervous system, thus reducing side effects of levodopa (eg, nausea, constipation, orthostasis).[5,6]

Carbidopa/levodopa (C/L) is available in immediate release (IR) tablets of several strengths: 25/100, 10/100, and 25/250. Sustained action (SA) tablets are available in 25/100 and 50/200. The first number refers to mg carbidopa; the latter number refers to mg levodopa. Bioavailability of levodopa in SA tablets is approximately 70% compared with IR, which should be considered when adjusting dose.[7,8] Orally disintegrating tablets are also available in the same strengths as IR. A novel formulation of C/L, combining immediate and extended-release beads, recently became available; it reportedly improves "on" time without dyskinesias, reduces "off" time, and allows for less frequent dosing.[9,10] There are no strict rules when starting levodopa therapy, but generally an IR formulation is used, because it is easier to assess for symptomatic improvement. Begin one-half tablet of 25/100 IR 3 times per day, increasing by one half tablet every 1 to 2 weeks as tolerated until taking total of 6 tablets per day (divided TID). Nausea is often the limiting factor when initiating levodopa therapy. For very sensitive patients, additional stand-alone carbidopa can be useful when initiating therapy, as can the antiemetic trimethobenzamide. Over time, C/L doses may start to wear off earlier, requiring increasingly frequent dosing. For some patients, the SA formulation may be more convenient, and a portion of their total levodopa dosage can be converted to this. The levodopa bioavailability is 70% in SA tablets, compared with IR, which should be kept in mind when making dose conversions (**Box 1**).

Box 1
Case 1

A 58-year-old gentleman returns to clinic with 6 to 9 months of unilateral resting tremor, cogwheel rigidity, and bradykinesia. Suspecting Parkinson's disease, you prescribe a trial of carbidopa/levodopa 25/100 IR, half-tablet 3×/d, with goal to titrate up by half-tablet each week until taking 2 tablets 3×/d. You counsel him that the levodopa is absorbed best on an empty stomach (1 hour before or 2 hours after food) because it interacts with protein.

He calls, stating he has had difficulty increasing the dose beyond the 1/2 tablet owing to persistent nausea. You recommend additional carbidopa (Lodosyn) 25 mg tablets with each dose, to help mitigate the side effects of levodopa while he is building up the dose. You also prescribe trimethobenzamide (Tigan) 300 mg PRN if the additional carbidopa is not sufficient, because it has no dopaminergic blockade.

He returns in 3 months, having titrated C/L up to 25/100 IR, 2 tabs 3×/d. He no longer has nausea, so you have him stop the trimethobenzamide and stand-alone carbdidopa. His parkinsonian symptoms respond extremely well to the levodopa, solidifying your diagnosis of Parkinson's disease.

Levodopa is absorbed via amino acid transporters in proximal small intestine, and dietary protein actively competes with it for absorption.[11] Levodopa ingested while there is protein in the gut is significantly less well-absorbed. Taking doses away from food (1 hour before or 2 hours after meals) maximizes bioavailability. Patients who cannot take levodopa on an empty stomach owing to excessive nausea can take with a carbohydrate snack. Ginger ale and ginger candies can be helpful in alleviating levodopa-induced nausea. Ondansetron can be used, but has serotonergic drug–drug interactions with other medications that Parkinson's patients often take (eg, selective serotonin reuptake inhibitors [SSRIs], monoamine oxide B inhibitors), increasing the risk of serotonin syndrome. Trimethobenzamide is the only antiemetic reported not to have any dopaminergic blockade, and is recommended as the pharmacologic agent of choice in Parkinson's patients with severe nausea.[12] Avoid metoclopramide, promethazine, and prochlorperazine owing to dopaminergic blockade. Delayed medication onset can be improved by chewing IR tablets and taking with carbonated beverage to accelerate the onset of action. SA tablets have slower onset of action; patients taking purely the SA formulation frequently develop dose stacking with dyskinesias later in day.[13] Dyskinesias are hyperkinetic involuntary movements that become more prevalent the longer one has been taking levodopa. If dose stacking occurs on SA formulation, it is suggested to convert a portion of each dose to the IR formulation (**Box 2**).

Box 2
Case 2

A 71-year-old gentleman with Parkinson's disease, onset at age 62. He establishes care with you and is complaining of severe dyskinesias later in the day. His symptoms are reasonably well-controlled in the morning and early afternoon, but he complains of severe dyskinesias and mild visual hallucinations later in the afternoon and evening. He is taking carbidopa/levodopa 50/200 SA, 2.5 tabs 4×/d.

Because he is taking purely sustained-action formulation, you suspect he is having dose-stacking side effects owing to the delayed release effects. You decide to convert approx. 50% of his total levodopa to IR formulation. His daily levodopa intake is 1400 mg/d (accounting for 70% SA bioavailability). You reduce his C/L 50/200 SA to 1.5 tab 4×/d, and add C/L 25/100 IR 1 tab 4×/d. His total levodopa intake is now 1240 mg/d.

Despite the slight reduction in total levodopa dose, he feels much better, with only slight residual dyskinesias and resolution of hallucinations.

Carbidopa

Peripheral DOPA decarboxylase is not saturated fully until carbidopa intake reaches approximately 75 mg/d.[14] Patients taking low doses of C/L may not receive adequate carbidopa to block peripheral DOPA decarboxylase, leading to excessive side effects (especially nausea). Additional carbidopa can be given (stand-alone carbidopa) in 25-mg tablets with each dose. For those taking high doses of C/L, where total carbidopa exceeds 300 to 400 mg/d, it has been postulated that some carbidopa may cross the blood–brain barrier and impair central conversion of levodopa to dopamine.[15,16] For those taking high doses, it is suggested to limit total daily carbidopa to less than 400 mg/d by using a 1:10 ratio C/L (10/100 or 25/250, available in IR only; **Box 3**).[17]

Dopamine Agonists

Dopamine agonists directly stimulate dopamine receptors. They can be used as initial treatment of Parkinson's disease, particularly in younger patients, which can delay the need to initiate levodopa for a few years and delay onset of levodopa-induced dyskinesias.[4] Potential psychiatric side effects include hallucinations, psychosis, and impulse control disorder (hypersexuality, compulsive spending, and pathologic gambling). Other adverse effects are lower extremity edema, orthostasis, and sleep attacks.[18–21]

There is no specific age cutoff, but many providers consider avoiding dopamine agonist in those older than 60 given higher incidence of psychiatric side effects in elderly. Dopamine agonists should not be discontinued abruptly, but rather tapered, particularly if at higher doses. Risk of dopamine agonist withdrawal syndrome, characterized by dysphoria, depression, panic, anxiety, diaphoresis, orthostasis, and cravings to resume the dopamine agonist, which occurs in 15% to 20% of patients.[22–24]

Start dopamine agonists gently to maximize tolerability:

- Ropinirole: start 0.25 mg 3 times per day, increase weekly up to maximum of 24 mg/d.
- Pramipexole: start 0.125 mg 3 times per day, increase weekly up to maximum of 4.5 mg/d.
- Rotigotine: transdermal patch provides 24-hour coverage; start 1 to 2 mg per 24 hours, increase to maximum of 8 mg per 24 hours.

Box 3
Case 3

An 83-year-old lady with Parkinson's disease, onset at age 67. She is taking C/L 25/100 IR, 2 tabs 4×/d, plus 50/200 SA, 1 tab 4×/d. Doses are effective, but wear off an hour early, so you decide to increase dosing to 5×/d. This eliminates her early wearing off. However, she feels that each dose is somewhat less effective that previously.

The recent dose increase had the following effects: Her total daily levodopa intake went from 1360 to 1700 mg/d (accounting for the 70% bioavailability of SA levodopa), and total daily carbidopa intake went from 340 to 425 mg/d (also similar reduction in bioavailability). This high level of carbidopa could be crossing the blood–brain barrier, inhibiting central DOPA decarboxylase and conversion of levodopa to dopamine in the brain, thereby reducing efficacy of each dose.

You decide to switch her IR carbidopa/levodopa to 1:10 ratio 10/100. You prescribe 2 tabs of C/L 10/100 IR 5×/d, plus 1 tab of 50/200 SA 5×/d. Total levodopa dose remains unchanged, but carbidopa is reduced from 425 to 275 mg/d. She has some slight nausea for the first few days which then goes away, but the doses regain their prior effectiveness.

- o Some patients obtain smoother symptom control by applying 2 separate patches, changing one in the morning and one in the evening.
- o Application site should be varied to minimize skin irritation.
- Apomorphine: subcutaneous injection used as rescue treatment for severe motor fluctuations ("off episodes").
  - o Initiating therapy is complex; requires 3 days of antiemetic pretreatment with trimethobenzamide (ondansetron must not be used with apomorphine owing to the risk of severe hypotension).[25]
  - o A 2-mg test dose of apomorphine injected under supervision, monitoring supine and standing blood pressure immediately before and after, and at 20, 40, and 60 minutes.
  - o If clinical improvement not observed, incrementally higher doses of 4 to 6 mg can be used after a 2-hour waiting period, but only if blood pressure stable (**Box 4**).[26]

Monoamine Oxidase-B Inhibitors

Dopamine is metabolized predominantly by MAO type-B and catechol O-methyltransferase.[27] Nonselective MAO inhibitors have been around for decades (primarily used for depression), but use complicated by dietary and drug–drug interactions (hypertensive crisis, tyramine reaction).[28] Catecholamines, serotonin, and dietary tyramine are metabolized by MAO-A, whereas dopamine is metabolized by MAO-B.[29,30] Selective MAO-B inhibition allows for augmentation of dopamine levels within nigrostriatal pathway in patients with Parkinson's disease.

Two MAO-B inhibitors are selegiline and rasagiline. They can be used as monotherapy in early Parkinson's disease, but have a modest effect by themselves.[31,32] They are particularly helpful in reducing end-of-dose wearing off and motor fluctuations in patients taking levodopa.

Selegiline

Selegiline is available in 5-mg oral tablets, dosed twice daily (morning and noon) owing to amphetamine metabolite that can cause insomnia if taken later in day.[33] Metabolite can also exacerbate tremor. It is also available in orally dissolving tablet for those with dysphagia, dosed 1.25 mg/d (can increase to 2.5 mg/d after 4–6 weeks). A transdermal selegiline patch delivers higher doses and causes nonselective MAO inhibition; it is intended for psychiatric conditions (namely depression), not Parkinson's disease.

Box 4
Case 4

A 49-year-old woman has recently been diagnosed with levodopa-responsive Parkinson's disease. However, owing to her young age, you suggest that she may benefit from being on a dopamine agonist, rather than carbidopa/levodopa, for the first several years. This will delay her exposure to levodopa, and reduce her development of levodopa-induced dyskinesias in the years to come. She has no psychiatric comorbidities to contraindicate a trial of a dopamine agonist.

She agrees, and you begin a trial of pramipexole. However, at doses sufficient to treat her Parkinson's, she develops orthostasis and sleep attacks. She tolerates a trial of ropinirole better, and is able to titrate to an effective dose without side effects. You counsel her to monitor for impulse-control problems such as spending, gambling, or hypersexuality.

Rasagiline

Rasagiline is available in 0.5- and 1-mg oral tablets; start 0.5 mg/d if taking levodopa, or 1 mg/d (daily maximum) for monotherapy. In 1 trial (A Randomized Placebo Controlled Study to Show That Rasagiline May Slow Disease Progression for Parkinson's Disease [ADAGIO]), rasagiline seemed to confer some protective benefits at 1 mg/d, but findings were not observed at higher dose (2 mg/d), leaving the question of neuroprotective benefits inconclusive.[34]

Both MAO-B inhibitors can trigger dyskinesias and neuropsychiatric side effects in patients taking levodopa. At higher doses, they become nonselective MAO inhibitors, so adhering to dosing guidelines is important. Based on known drug–drug interaction between nonselective MAO inhibitors and other reuptake inhibitors (tricyclic antidepressants, SSRIs, selective norepinephrine reuptake inhibitors), there is theoretical potential for serotonin syndrome and noradrenergic crisis. However, use of selective MAO-B inhibitors with a variety of antidepressants is well-tolerated by most patients.[35–37] Advising patients of risks and teaching them to monitor for symptoms of serotonin syndrome, which can include flushing, fever, diarrhea, tremulousness, agitation, confusion, heart palpitations, or seizures is important.

Catechol O-Methyltransferase Inhibitors

Dopamine is predominantly metabolized by MAO type-B and catechol O-methyltransferase.[27] Two catechol O-methyltransferase inhibitors are entacapone and tolcapone. They are not effective as monotherapy and most useful for patients taking levodopa with motor fluctuations (early wearing off).[38–40] Similar to MAO-B inhibitors, they may worsen dyskinesias or the neuropsychiatric side effects of levodopa.[41] They also cause harmless dark orange discoloration of urine.

Entacapone

Entacapone is available in 200-mg oral tablets, taken with each dose of levodopa (short half-life), maximum of 1600 mg/d.[42] A combined tablet of C/L/entacapone in various strengths between 50 and 200 mg of levodopa is also available.[43,44]

Tolcapone

Tolcapone is available in 100 mg oral tablets, taken 3 times per day (maximum 600 mg/d divided TID). Owing to rare but potentially fatal hepatotoxicity, its use is restricted to select patients with severe motor fluctuations who do not respond to entacapone, cannot tolerate other adjunctive therapies, and can comprehend and accept risks and monitoring required with treatment. Monitor liver enzymes (aspartate aminotransferase, alanine aminotransferase) at baseline, every 2 to 4 weeks for 6 months, and then periodically. If no symptomatic improvement within 3 weeks, or if liver enzymes increases to greater than 2 times the upper limit of normal, discontinue treatment.[45,46]

Amantadine

Amantadine was originally an influenza antiviral. It also has anticholinergic action, N-methyl-D-aspartate receptor antagonism, and dopamine receptor agonism and reuptake inhibition.[47] It has modest antiparkinsonian efficacy by itself, but is useful in decreasing levodopa-induced dyskinesias, which can adversely affect dexterity and fine motor control, and contribute to falls by destabilizing center of gravity. Amantadine is noted to be helpful in patients suffering from levodopa side effects as far back as the 1970s.[48]

Dosing is 100 mg 2 to 4 times per day, except in renal disease (excreted by kidney with minimal metabolism). Amantadine is generally well-tolerated, but potential side effects include lower extremity edema, livedo reticularis, hallucinations, and in toxicity, seizures.[49]

Anticholinergic Agents

Anticholinergic agents have no direct effect on dopamine receptors or metabolism, but can treat parkinsonian tremor by reducing cholinergic activity in striatum, which is thought to contribute to tremor.[50] There is conflicting evidence as to whether anticholinergic agents improve symptoms beyond tremor.[51] Use cautiously; anticholinergic agents have a high side effect profile, especially in older patients. They are most useful in young, tremor-predominant patients.[2]

Trihexyphenidyl is most commonly used for Parkinson's disease. It is available in 2- and 5-mg oral tablets. Start gently to minimize side effects: 1 mg/d, increase every few days as tolerated (maximum 15 mg/d, divided 3 to 4 times per day). It has typical anticholinergic side effects (confusion, memory impairment, dry mouth, constipation, urinary retention, glaucoma exacerbation; **Box 5**).[52]

Nonmotor Symptoms

Nonmotor symptoms are increasingly recognized as having major impact on quality of life.[53–56] A detailed assessment of each symptom is beyond the scope of this section, but key points are addressed.

Drooling

Drooling is common in Parkinson's disease, caused by decreased swallowing frequency and salivary overflow.[57] Ophthalmic atropine drops and inhaled ipratropium spray can be applied sublingually throughout day.[58,59] Glycopyrrolate can also be used, 1 mg 3 times per day, and is reported to work well without adverse effects.[60] Botulinum toxin injection is highly effective. Onabotulinum A, abobotulinum A, and rimabotulinumtoxin B have been used with good results. Injections performed in bilateral parotid and submandibular glands, with effect lasting up to 4 months.[61–63]

Box 5
Case 5

A 78-year-old gentleman with Parkinson's disease for more than 15 years comes to clinic with complaints of motor fluctuations. His carbidopa/levodopa is effective, but rapidly wears off before the next dose despite frequent Q2H dosing.

You discuss the options of catechol O-methyltransferase and monoamine oxide B inhibitors. He has insomnia and mild anxiety, so you chose to avoid selegiline (given the amphetamine metabolite). You opt to try entacapone with each dose of C/L, but this causes an intolerable increase in dyskinesias. He decides he would like to try rasagiline, so you prescribe a low dose (0.5 mg/d), which improves his motor fluctuations with minimal change in his dyskinesias.

He also enquires about a medication that his friend is taking for tremor, called Artane (trihexyphenidyl). You advise that this class of medication (anticholinergic agents) is not advised in patients over 65 owing to detrimental effects on cognition, balance, bowel, bladder, heart rhythm, eye pressure, and so on.

The same 78-year-old gentleman returns to clinic 6 months later, and his dyskinesias have worsened. He is reluctant to reduce his levodopa dose or stop rasagiline, because both help to maintain his mobility. Although you caution him about the incidence of side effects, you agree to a careful trial of amantadine to see if it will alleviate his levodopa-induced dyskinesias. He fortunately tolerates it well, with moderate reduction in the severity of dyskinesias.

Constipation

Constipation can precede motor symptoms by several years.[64] It is exacerbated by medications (including levodopa), physical inactivity, and inadequate hydration. Treatments include increased fluid intake, physical mobilization, a high-fiber diet (eg, vegetables, grains, whole grain pasta, bran), fiber supplements, stool softeners (docusate), and when necessary, laxatives and enemas.[65,66]

Orthostatic hypotension

Orthostatic hypotension is the manifestation of autonomic dysfunction, occurring in more than one-half of patients.[67] It is exacerbated by dopaminergic medications such as levodopa and (especially) dopamine agonists.[68] Orthostatic hypotension treatments include:

- Increased fluid and salt intake, including 1 g sodium chloride tablets.[69,70]
- Compression stockings: loss of peripheral vasospasm reflex causes orthostatic hypotension. Thigh-high or waist-high compression stockings are very helpful.[71]
- Fludrocortisone: if fluid, salt, and compression stockings inadequate.
  - Start 0.1 mg/d, increase weekly as needed to maximum of 0.5 mg/d.[72]
  - Causes fluid retention; use with caution if congestive heart failure is present.
- Midodrine: if above plus fludrocortisone inadequate, peripheral alpha-1-agonist can be added.[73]
  - Start 2.5 mg 3 times per day, cautiously increase up to 10 mg 3 times per day if needed.
  - Causes supine hypertension; monitor carefully. Patient is advised to sleep with the head of bed elevated 20° to 30° and avoid taking third dose within 4 hours of laying down.[74]
- Droxidopa: recently approved for neurogenic orthostatic hypotension.[75,76]
  - Start 100 mg 3 times per day, cautiously increase by 300 mg/d every few days as needed (may 1800 mg/d).
  - Same issues with supine hypertension as midodrine; monitor carefully.

Dementia

Progression from mild cognitive impairment to dementia occurs later in course of Parkinson's (average 14 years after diagnosis), in up to 80% of patients.[77] Rivastigmine (oral and transdermal) is approved by the US Food and Drug Administration for Parkinson's disease dementia. Donepezil, galantamine, and memantine are also used off label.

Hallucinations and psychosis

- Visual hallucinations most common. They are exacerbated by dopaminergic and anticholinergic medications. Reducing the offending medication alleviates symptoms.
- Quetiapine and clozapine are helpful without worsening parkinsonism.[78–81]
  - Quetiapine is easier to use (no need for blood monitoring); start at 12.5 to 25 mg per dose, and titrate individually.

Depression

There is a high prevalence of depression in Parkinson's patients, up to 50%, because the disease significantly impacts motor symptoms and quality of life.[82,83] It is important to diagnose and treat. There are no contraindications to using common antidepressant agents in Parkinson's disease patients on any dopaminergic agents (including MAO-B inhibitors).

Rapid eye movement sleep behavior disorder

Excessive movement during rapid eye movement sleep, when muscle tone should be at minimum. Up to 46% of Parkinson's patients exhibit symptoms.[84] This can be worsened by SSRIs, selective norepinephrine reuptake inhibitors, and tricyclic antidepressants.[85]

- Melatonin
  - Reduces night-time motor activity; requires higher doses than used for insomnia, but has a benign side effect profile.[86,87]
  - Start 6 mg at night; increase to maximum 18 mg at night as needed.
- Clonazepam
  - Also effective, but has a less benign side effect profile. Use if there is no or an inadequate response to melatonin.[88]
  - Start low, depending on patient 0.125 to 0.5 mg at night; maximum 1 mg at night.

The treatment of Parkinson's disease requires a complex, multifaceted approach, incorporating both medication management and nonpharmacologic approaches. It requires a targeted, individualized strategy, based on the specific needs of the patient, balancing demographic factors such as age, gender, and preexisting conditions and comorbidities, as well as recognizing the other medications that each individual may be taking, and taking into account potential side effects and drug–drug interactions of the medicines available for treatment of their Parkinson's disease. This basic principle applies to all of medicine, but the unique aspect of caring for patients with Parkinson's disease is the incredibly broad spectrum that is involved in their care. Although the complexity of interweaving the motor and nonmotor symptoms of Parkinson's disease may seem daunting, the first step is simply to remember to address both aspects of this care (**Tables 1** and **2**).

MOVEMENT DISORDERS: PART II
Essential Tremors

Essential tremors are characterized as action and postural tremors that can vary in amplitude, but maintain a relatively consistent frequency around 8 to 12 Hz.[89] Tremors most commonly involve the bilateral upper extremities in a symmetric manner. As the disease progresses, it may also involve the legs, head, voice, and tongue. Essential tremor is one of the most common types of tremor, with a 4.6% prevalence in populations greater than 65 years of age, approaching 20% in those greater than 95 years of age.[90] Although often termed "benign," the impact of quality of life can be significant. Social stigmatization, limitation in hobbies, impairment in job performance, and even the ability to feed and dress oneself may be impaired. The pathophysiology remains cryptic. The main theories include cerebellothalamic pathway dysfunction.[91,92] Treatments focus on improving quality of life with an emphasis on avoiding medications or supplements that enhance the adrenergic system. Avoidance of caffeine, nicotine, valproic acid, lithium, tricyclic antidepressants, SSRIs, steroids, and bronchodilators are encouraged because they can cause or enhance tremors. Although there is no cure, the goal of treatment is to decrease the amplitude of tremor enough to improve function, but it is not likely to change frequency, which is thought to be a central generator (**Fig. 2**).[93]

Beta Blockers

These antiarrhythmic agents work to decrease adrenergic activity.[94] Propranolol hydrochloride[94] is a nonselective beta blocker (B1 and B2) favored by neurologists owing

Table 1
Medications for motor symptoms in Parkinson's disease

Drug (Generic)	Drug (Brand)	Monotherapy	Side Effects	Clinical Pearls
Carbidopa/ levodopa	Sinemet, Parcopa, Rytary, Stalevo[a]	Yes	Nausea, constipation, fatigue, dyskinesias, hallucinations	Immediate release: protein inhibits absorption; take on empty stomach (1 h before food); chew tablets to accelerate onset; use 1:10 ratio carbidopa/levodopa to keep carbidopa dose <400 mg/d. Sustained action: reduced bioavailability (70%) compared with immediate release; dose stacking can occur later in the day
Carbidopa	Lodosyn	No	None significant	Useful to prevent nausea when starting levodopa therapy, especially when carbidopa dose <75 mg/d
Pramipexole	Mirapex	Yes	Orthostatic hypotension, peripheral edema, sleep attacks, hallucinations, impulse control dysregulation, nausea, constipation, dyskinesias	All dopamine agonists: increased risk of neuropsychiatric side effects (especially hallucinations, impulse control disorder) in patients with preexisting symptoms, and those >65 y old Rotigotine: vary application site to minimize skin irritation Apomorphine: useful for rescue therapy for severe off periods refractory to oral medications; careful initiation regimen required
Ropinirole	Requip	Yes		
Rotigotine	Neupro	Yes		
Apomorphine	Apokyn	No		
Selegiline	Eldepryl, Zelapar	Yes[b]	Amphetamine metabolite (can exacerbate action tremor, insomnia, anxiety)	Has amphetamine metabolite; give second dose no later than noon to avoid insomnia
Rasagiline	Azilect	Yes[b]	Dyskinesias, hallucinations	Both monoamine oxide B inhibitors have theoretical risk of serotonin syndrome with concomitant SSRI/SNRI use, although in clinical practice have been used safely; counsel patients on risk if applicable. Primary use is extending levodopa half-life, reducing motor-fluctuations

Entacapone	Comtan	No	Dyskinesias, hallucinations, orange discoloration of urine	Primary use is extending levodopa half-life, reducing motor fluctuations; harmless orange discoloration of urine
Tolcapone	Tasmar	No	Dyskinesias, hallucinations, orange discoloration of urine, fulminant hepatotoxicity (rare)	Strict monitoring of liver enzymes required; not recommended for general practitioner use
Amantadine	Symmetrel	No	Confusion, hallucinations, livedo reticularis, peripheral edema, constipation, seizures	Primary use is levodopa-induced dyskinesias; multiple mechanisms of action incur variety of side effects, which may limit use
Trihexyphenidyl	Artane	Yes	Confusion, hallucinations, delirium, glaucoma exacerbation, constipation, urinary retention, cardiac arrhythmia	Useful for tremor, but not for rigidity or bradykinesia; owing to high incidence of side effects, advise against use in patients >65 y or those with preexisting cognitive impairment

Abbreviations: MAOI, monoamine oxidase inhibitor; SNRI, selective norepinephrine reuptake inhibitor; SSRI, selective serotonin reuptake inhibitor.
a In combination with entacapone.
b Much more useful in combination with carbidopa/levodopa that monotherapy.

Table 2
Medications for nonmotor symptoms in Parkinson's disease

Symptom	Drug (Generic)	Drug (Brand)	Side Effects	Clinical Pearls
Nausea	Carbidopa	Lodosyn	None significant	Useful to prevent nausea when starting levodopa therapy, especially when carbidopa dose <75 mg/d
	Trimethobenzamide	Tigan	Blurred vision, diarrhea	Generally well-tolerated, reputed to be the best antiemetic agent for Parkinson's patients, with no dopamine-blocking capacity, and no serotonergic properties
Constipation	Docusate Sennosides Fiber supplement	—	None significant	Adequate hydration is also key to helping stool softeners and fiber supplements work adequately; these methods are gentler on the bowel than stimulants like polyethylene glycol
Sialorrhea	Glycopyrrolate Atropine drops	—	Dry mouth, confusion, urinary retention	Some patients tolerate without cognitive side effects
	Botulinum toxin injection	Botox Dysport Myobloc	Dry mouth, dysphagia, distant toxin spread	Parotid and submandibular toxin injection offers up to 3 mo of symptom alleviation if atropine/glycopyrrolate fail
Orthostatic hypotension	Salt tablets	—	Fluid retention, congestive heart failure	First-line treatment of orthostasis is hydration, thigh-high compression stockings, and increased salt intake (cardiac/renal status permitting)
	Fludrocortisone	Fluorinef	Fluid retention, hypertension	Second-line if above are inadequate
	Midodrine	ProAmatine	Hypertension (especially supine), bradycardia	Third-line; owing to supine hypertension, elevate head of bed and take last dose >4 h before bed
	Droxidopa	Northera	Supine hypertension	Similar to midodrine
Hallucinations	Quetiapine Clozapine	Seroquel Clozaril	Worsening of parkinsonism; agranulocytosis, seizures (clozapine)	Reducing dopaminergic medications (especially dopamine agonists) can often lessen or alleviate hallucinations, but when necessary, these atypical neuroleptics are the agents of choice

			Side effects	Comments
Depression	[a]	[a]	Vary by agent	No specific treatment preference; Parkinson's patients typically do well on many SSRIs/SNRIs, even when taking MAO-B inhibitor; depression common in Parkinson's (<50% prevalence)
Dementia	Rivastigmine Donepezil Galantamine	Excelon Aricept Razadyne	Diarrhea, nausea, hypotension, bradycardia, hallucinations, vivid dreams, seizures	Rivastigmine is FDA approved for Parkinson's disease dementia; others are off label
	Memantine	Namenda	Confusion, dizziness, headache, GI upset	Memantine can be trialed if patient cannot tolerate side effects of acetylcholinesterase inhibitors; also off label
REM sleep behavior disorder	Melatonin	—	None significant	First-line, well-tolerated
	Clonazepam	Klonopin	Confusion, hallucinations, delirium, respiratory depression, paradoxical agitation	Second-line; may try if severe symptoms unresponsive to melatonin; caution advised in older patients or preexisting cognitive impairment

Abbreviations: FDA, US Food and Drug Administration; GI, gastrointestinal; MAO, monoamine oxidase; REM, rapid eye movement; SNRI, selective norepinephrine reuptake inhibitor; SSRI, selective serotonin reuptake inhibitor.
[a] Any SSRI or SNRI can be used.

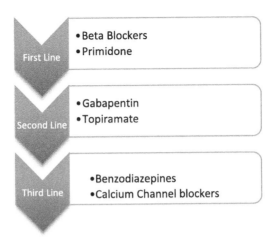

Fig. 2. Essential tremor treatments.

to a higher lipophilic profile. The higher lipophilic profile allows it to freely cross the blood–brain barrier, with greater central effect on tremor.[93] Alternative beta blockers, including nadolol, sotalol, and atenolol, are also effective making the importance of high lipid solubility and central action under question.[95,96] Additionally, based on studies, main action of propranolol is mediated peripherally via B2-adrenergic receptors action.[93] For this reason, if someone is already on a beta blocker for another indication, maximizing the one they are currently on is preferable.

Beta blockers are a preferred first-line agent based on a relatively benign side effect profile. It is preferred in someone who has comorbid hypertension. However, in those with history of severe reactive airway disease such as asthma or chronic obstructive pulmonary disease, beta blockers should not be used based on the risk of bronchospasm.[94] Do not use in people with significantly depressed cardiac function owing to risk of heart failure or who have second-degree atrioventricular block.[93] Additionally, beta blockers should be avoided in those with insulin-dependent diabetes because they can mask symptoms of hypoglycemia.[97] With the use of propranolol you may hope for 30% to 50% amplitude reduction at peak dose.[98] For this reason, twice daily dosing of IR is preferred; however, long-acting, once daily formulations are thought to be equally effective.

Side effects include dizziness, lowered heart rate and blood pressure titration should be gradual as tolerated. Usual dose range is around 60 to 160 mg twice daily in IR formulation (120–320 mg/d).[96] In addition, if someone is only bothered by their tremor in certain situations, giving a presentation, preforming for an event, an as needed option can be very useful. A suggested dose is 20 to 80 mg 2 hours before a specific event (**Fig. 3**).[93]

Primidone

This benzodiazepine was developed originally as an anticonvulsant. Primidone is metabolized hepatically into phenobarbital and phenylethylmalonamide and increases inhibitory gamma-amino butyric acid (GABA)-A activity.[99,100] Primidone is a first line agent and ideal for those who report a strong response to alcohol. Familial autosomal-dominant essential tremor is known for alcohol responsiveness. Additionally, primidone can be synergistic with beta blockers allowing for a lower overall dose to be used. Caution should be taken in those with history of alcoholism owing to

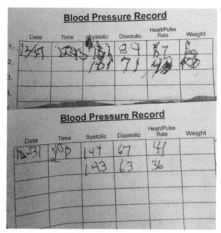

Fig. 3. Essential tremor: demonstration of treatment efficacy with use of propranolol.

combined GABAergic action and sedation. Those on concurrent warfarin require careful monitoring because primidone increases warfarin clearance through P450 activity.[100,101] It absolutely should not be used in pregnant woman, and may reduce the effectiveness of oral contraceptive agents. Primidone can worsen depression, so must be used with extreme caution in those with past history of suicidality. Usual dose range is 25 to 250 mg/d with doses of greater than 250/mg nightly unlikely to provide additional effect.[93,97,102] The main side effects include sedation, gastrointestinal distress, dizziness, and ataxia. These are often limiting factors in dose escalation. A primidone level and phenobarbital metabolite should be measured if toxicity is suspected.

Gabapentin

Originally developed as an antiepileptic agent, gabapentin is now used for a variety of indications including the treatment of neurogenic pain, tremor, and even anxiety. Although the neurochemical action is unknown, it seems that gabapentin binding sites are associated with alpha-2-delta voltage gated calcium channels.[103,104] Although the impact on tremor may not be as reliable as with the first-line agents, gabapentin is a good choice for those who have contraindications to, side effects from, or fail first-line therapies. Additionally, those with comorbid pain (peripheral neuropathy, radiculopathy) or anxiety may have additional benefit. Usual dose range for tremor is around 1200 to 3600 mg/d divided into 3 times daily dosing. Maximum efficacy may be reached at up to 1800 mg in divided doses daily.[105] The main side effects include dizziness, weight gain, and sedation.[103] To prevent these side effects, a slow titration is useful. Gabapentin is excreted through the renal system, so it must be used with caution in those with impaired renal function.

Topiramate

This anticonvulsant can additionally decrease tremor, mainly by enhancing GABA-A activity and antagonistic action via certain glutamate receptors.[106,107] Although this may have a modest impact on tremor, it is an option in those who fail first-line agents. It is sometimes used for mood stabilization and can be helpful for those with a comorbid mood disorder. Additionally, it may be a helpful agent for an obese or overweight patient with the serendipitous side effect of weight loss.[97] Topiramate is contraindicated in those with history of kidney stones or acute angle closure glaucoma.[97] Concurrent use of valproic acid should be used cautiously. The combination increases risk of kidney stones.[97] Women of child bearing age should be counseled about pregnancy prevention owing to increased risk of birth defects. If toxicity is suspected, such as mental status changes or ataxia, consider evaluation of ammonia and for metabolic acidosis.[97] A slow titration is helpful up to 150 mg twice daily as tolerated.[108,109] The average dose in certain trails was around 200 mg/d divided twice daily.[107]

Other Agents

If the therapies discussed are poorly tolerated or contraindicated, benzodiazepines may be considered, with anecdotal preference for clonazepam owing to longer a duration of action, or calcium channel blockers with verapamil as the preferred agent. Discussion about surgical options including deep brain stimulation or gamma knife can be offered.

Although often termed "benign," essential tremor can have a significant impact on quality of life and occupational functioning. Medications are for symptomatic benefit only and do not change the course of disease. The goal of medical therapy is for approximately 50% reduction in tremor amplitude. If this is insufficient, surgical options can be considered in appropriate cases (**Table 3**).

Idiopathic Restless Leg Syndrome

This distressing syndrome is characterized by sensation of discomfort while awake, which causes a desire to move and stretch. Characteristic nocturnal predominance and relief with movement is a key feature. It is a relatively common disorder; 2% to 3% of the population has clinically significant symptoms.[110] In a cross-sectional study by Scholz and colleagues,[111] restless leg syndrome (RLS) causes significant psychological distress. Undertreated patients had increased levels of compulsivity, depression, anxiety, and other forms of psychological unwellness. Although the exact cause of primary RLS is unknown, symptomatic improvement when using dopaminergic therapies makes dopaminergic dysregulation enticing. Additionally, correction

Table 3
Essential Tremor medication quick reference guide

Drug	Drug Type	Dose Range	Preferred Populations	Significant Side Effects	Populations to Avoid
Propranolol	Beta blocker	60–160 mg twice daily	Hypertensive	Bradycardia, hypotension	Severe reactive airway disease, first-degree AV block
Primidone	Benzodiazepine	25–250 mg	Alcohol responsive tremors	Sedation, dizziness	Elderly, alcoholics
Gabapentin	Anticonvulsant	400–1200 mg 3× daily	Concurrent pain, neuropathy	Dizziness, weight gain, lethargy	Renal failure requires reduced dosage
Topirimate	Anticonvulsant	50–100 mg twice daily	Concurrent mood disorder	Weight loss, kidney stones, cognitive blunting	History of kidney stones

Abbreviation: AV, atrioventricular.

of iron deficiency has been shown to improve symptoms. Iron is a cofactor in the production of dopamine.[93,112,113] Initial laboratory evaluation should include serum iron and total iron-binding capacity, ferritin, folate, and magnesium. Ferritin is particularly important. A goal of greater than 75 for those will clinically suspected RLS is advised thought secondary to altered iron metabolism and/or storage in the central nervous system, which is why goal ferritin at this level is suggested.[114,115] Avoid drugs that can exacerbate RLS including alcohol, caffeine, SSRIs, lithium, and antihistamines.[114]

Primary Restless Leg Syndrome

To guide therapy, primary RLS is divided into intermittent, daily/moderate persistent and refractory to determine the best treatment paradigm (**Fig. 4**). This classification is useful to prevent augmentation from therapies over time. Augmentation is defined as earlier symptoms, more severe symptoms, or less response to dopaminergic therapy.[93] This is hypothesized to be related to dopaminergic (D1 receptor) overstimulation.[116]

Intermittent Restless Leg Syndrome: One or Fewer Episodes Weekly

Levodopa

Owing to the risk of augmentation, C/L dose is limited and should be reserved for intermittent symptoms. Levodopa is a decarboxylase inhibitor and also used to treat Parkinson disease.[117] It is thought to be helpful for RLS symptoms based on its dopaminergic effect. Levodopa is prescribed with carbidopa, which prevents decarboxylation of levodopa before passing through the blood-brain barrier to help with nausea.[118] The usual dose of C/L is 25/100 mg tablets, 1 tablet as needed. Avoid greater than 200 mg/d to prevent augmentation.[115] Protein prevents absorption of levodopa centrally, so taking this no sooner than 2 hours after dinner and ideally 30 minutes before the typical onset of symptoms for IR formulations.[119]

Clonazepam

Benzodiazepines that increase GABA activity

- The IR can last 6 to 12 hours.[120,121]
- Initial dose: 0.25 mg nightly.
- Dose range: 0.25 to 2 mg/d.

Considerations that limit use include sedation and the addictive nature of this medication. Avoid in those with concurrent use of other medications that have sedating effects on the central nervous system, or those with impaired kidney or liver function. Owing to risk of respiratory sedation, do not use in those with untreated obstructive sleep apnea.

Daily/Moderate Persistent Restless Leg Syndrome: Two or More Episodes Weekly

For those who experience daily symptoms, the risk of augmentation with the use of levodopa is increased. This is still possible with agonists, but considered less likely. If augmentation develops on 1 dopamine agonist, switch to another. If no other comorbidities are present, dopaminergic therapy may be the primary focus.

Dopamine Agonists

Dopamine agonists are anti-Parkinson agents that include ropinirole and pramipexole. These drugs work primarily via the D2 (dopaminergic) receptor, but can modulate D2 and D3 receptor activity.[93,122]

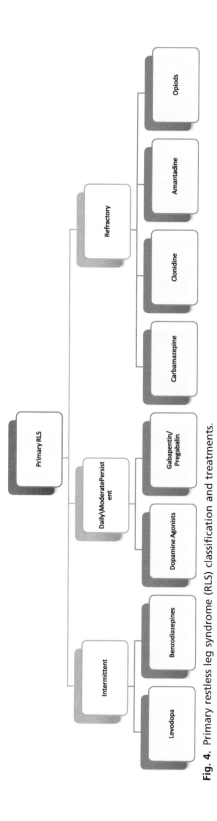

Fig. 4. Primary restless leg syndrome (RLS) classification and treatments.

Ropinirole

- Dose range: Ropinirole: 0.25 to 4 mg at night, approximately 1 hour before typical symptom onset.[113]
- Time to peak concentration: 1 to 2 hours.[123]
- Half-life: approximately 6 hours.[123]

Pramipexole

- Dose range: Pramipexole: 0.125 to 1 mg at night, 1 to 2 hours before typical symptom onset.[113]
- Time to peak concentration: 2 hours.[124]
- Half-life: approximately 8 hours.[124]

There are several difficulties with using dopamine agonists related to physical and behavioral side effects. Dopamine behavioral dysregulation must be discussed before prescribing these medications. This is defined as a potential for uncontrollable urges including pathologic gambling, oversnacking, and sexual disinhibition. A clinician should discuss this before prescribing, and should screen for symptoms on follow-up. It might be important to advise a family member to specifically watch for these behaviors. Similar to levodopa formulations, if taken with protein the onset of action can be delayed by 2.5 hours.[123]

Gabapentin

Gabapentin is an anticonvulsant medication thought to act via alpha-2-delta voltage-gated calcium channels.[104] Gabapentin is a good choice for those with concurrent peripheral neuropathy.

- Onset of action/time to peak dose: 2 to 4 hours.[105]
- Half-life: 5 to 7 hours.[103,125]
- Mean dose for RLS: about 700 mg at night.[113,125]

Pregabalin

Pregabalin is an anticonvusant thought to modulate pain by binding to alpha-2-delta voltage gated calcium channels. This may increase GABA levels.[126]

- Onset of action/time to peak dose: 2 to 4 hours.
- Half-life: approximately 6 hours.[127]
- Doses of greater than 300 mg may not have increased effect. It is given at night.[127,128]

Food can delay absorption and reduce peak potency by 30%.[127]

Refractory Restless Leg Syndrome

Carbamazepine

The mean effective dose for carbamazepine is around 250 mg/d.[129] Owing to side effects of hyponatremia, recommended monitoring tests include sodium and liver function at baseline and annually.[130] Additionally, high-resolution HLA-B*1502 typing in certain Asian populations on other antiseizure drugs may be considered owing to increased risk of Stevens–Johnson syndrome.[131]

Clonidine

Clonidine is an antihypertensive with centrally acting alpha-2-adrenergic agonist activity. It is thought to be helpful in RLS and other pain syndromes via stimulation of alpha-2-adrenoreceptors, potentially effecting spinal pain transmission.[132]

- Onset of action: 30 minutes to 1 hour.
- Half-life: 6 to 12 hours.[133]
- Average effective dose: 0.5 mg.[134]

Amantadine

Amantadine was developed originally as an antiviral agent, but it is used to treat Parkinson disease. It acts as a dopamine agonist and hypothesized effect through N-methyl-D-aspartate activity.[135] Should not be used in people with concurrent dementia or psychosis as can increase confusion and hallucinations.

- Time to peak in plasma: 2 to 4 hours.
- Mean effective dose: around 225 mg/d.[136]

Opioids

May be required if above therapies fail.[110,113]

Secondary Restless Leg Syndrome and Special Populations

Iron deficiency

If iron deficiency is identified, provide an oral iron supplement with 100 to 200 mg of vitamin C to maximize absorption (**Fig. 5**). The target ferritin is greater than 75 mcg/L. Because constipation is a frequent side effect, it is helpful to recommend use of a stool softener and hydration to prevent constipation.[113] Avoid iron overload by rechecking ferritin 3 to 4 months after supplementation.[115]

Pregnancy

RLS is the most common movement disorder in pregnancy in up to 25% to 30% of pregnant women, and is worsened in the third trimester.[137] The hypothesized reason is thought to be related to volume expansion and a decrease in ferritin. Generally, RLS in pregnancy resolves within a few months after delivery.[93] Emphasize nonpharmacologic approaches, including exercise, stretching, and compression stockings. Iron supplementation should be given when indicated.

End-stage renal disease on hemodialysis

RLS is more common in end-stage renal disease. Its incidence ranges from 20% to 60% and symptoms are heightened by peripheral neuropathy. Potential therapies are more frequent dialysis or neuropathic pain medications, such as gabapentin,

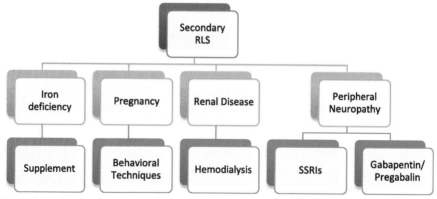

Fig. 5. Secondary restless leg syndrome (RLS) causes and treatments. SSRI, selective serotonin reuptake inhibitor.

Table 4
RLS medication quick reference guide

Drug	Drug Type	Dose Range Nightly	Preferred Populations	Significant Side Effects	Populations to Avoid
Carbidopa/levodopa	Anti-Parkinson agent	<50/200 mg	Intermittent RLS ≤1 episode per week.	Hypotension, nausea	—
Clonazepam	Benzodiazepine	0.25–2 mg nightly	Intermittent RLS	Sedation, respiratory depression	Those with untreated OSA
Ropinirole	Dopamine agonist	0.25–4 mg	Moderate primary RLS ≥2 episodes weekly	Hypotension, sleep attacks, peripheral edema, behavioral dysregulation	Those with underlying psychosis or dementia
Pramipexole	Dopamine agonist	0.125–1 mg	Moderate primary RLS	Hypotension, sleep attacks, peripheral edema, behavioral dysregulation	Those with underlying psychosis or dementia
Gabapentin	Anticonvulsant	About 700 mg	Moderate RLS, chronic pain, neuropathy	Dizziness, weight gain, lethargy	Renal failure requires reduced dosage
Pregabalin	Anticonvulsant	≤300 mg	Moderate RLS chronic pain, neuropathy	Dizziness, weight gain, lethargy	—
Carbamazepine	Anticonvulsant	Around 250 mg	Refractory RLS	Hyponatremia, can affect liver function Monitor Na, CBC, LFTs	Hyponatremia Abnormal liver function
Clonidine	Antihypertensive	Around 0.5 mg	Refractory RLS, hypertension, chronic pain	Hypotension	Hypotensive patients
Amantadine	Antiflu agent Dopamine agonist	Around 225 mg	Refractory RLS	—	Those with underlying psychosis or dementia

Abbreviations: CBC, complete blood count; LFT, liver function test; Na, sodium; OSA, obstructive sleep apnea; RLS, restless leg syndrome.

pregabalin, venlafaxine, or duloxetine. Personally, this author would avoid tricyclic antidepressants specifically for RLS.[138]

Concurrent peripheral neuropathy

These populations may be less responsive to dopaminergic agents. Medications that focus on neuropathic pain treatments should be tried first.

Periodic limb movements of sleep

Periodic limb movements of sleep comprise involuntary triple flexion or jerking motions that occur at night. There are clusters of moments that can last around 30 seconds or brief jerking motions that occur during sleep arousal (stages I and II of sleep). This phenomenon is different than RLS; is it is asymptomatic and not associated with uncomfortable sensations.[93] Although periodic limb movements of sleep are strongly associated with RLS (85% correlation) periodic limb movements of sleep can be associated with any systemic or environmental factors that disrupt sleep and cause frequent arousals. In fact, Baran and colleagues[139] found a positive association with periodic limb movements of sleep and the effectiveness of continuous positive airway pressure therapy and severity of periodic limb movements of sleep. Controlling sleep apnea can improve symptoms. Additionally, clonazepam is a known effective treatment.

RLS is often underrecognized and can have a significant impact on a person's physical and emotional well-being. In evaluation, it is important to classify RLS as primary or secondary. The former is more likely to respond to dopaminergic agents, whereas the latter may respond better to treatment of underlying iron deficiency, peripheral neuropathy, renal disease. Although sometimes associated with periodic limb movements of sleep, periodic limb movements of sleep can be from any process that disrupts quality of sleep (**Table 4**).

REFERENCES

1. Fearnley JM, Lees AJ. Ageing and Parkinson's disease: substantia nigra regional selectivity. Brain 1991;114:2283–301.
2. Clarke CE. Neuroprotection and pharmacotherapy for motor symptoms in Parkinson's disease. Lancet Neurol 2004;3:466–74.
3. Pringsheim T, Jette N, Frolkis A, et al. The prevalence of Parkinson's disease: a systematic review and meta-analysis. Mov Disord 2014;29:1583–90.
4. Connolly BS, Lang AE. Pharmacological treatment of Parkinson disease: a review. JAMA 2014;311:1670–83.
5. Ferreira JJ, Katzenschlager R, Bloem BR, et al. Summary of the recommendations of the EFNS/MDS-ES review on therapeutic management of Parkinson's disease. Eur J Neurol 2013;20:5–15.
6. Huebert ND, Palfreyman MG, Haegele KD. A comparison of the effects of reversible and irreversible inhibitors of aromatic L-amino acid decarboxylase on the half-life and other pharmacokinetic parameters of oral L-3,4-dihydroxyphenylalanine. Drug Metab Dispos 1983;11:195.
7. Yeh K, August T, Bush D, et al. Pharmacokinetics and bioavailability of Sinemet CR: a summary of human studies. Neurology 1989;39:25.
8. Sage JI, Mark MH. Pharmacokinetics of continuous-release carbidopa/levodopa. Clin Neuropharmacol 1994;17:S1.
9. Pahwa R, Lyons KE, Hauser RA, et al. Randomized trial of IPX066, carbidopa/levodopa extended release, in early Parkinson's disease. Parkinsonism Relat Disord 2014;20:142.

10. Nausieda PA, Hsu A, Elmer L, et al. Conversion to IPX066 from standard levo-dopa formulations in advanced Parkinson's disease: experience in clinical trials. J Parkinsons Dis 2015;5(4):837–45.

11. Salat D, Tolosa E. Levodopa in the treatment of Parkinson's disease: current status and new developments. J Parkinsons Dis 2013;3:255.

12. Hauser RA, Isaacson S, Clinch T. Randomized, placebo-controlled trial of trime-thobenzamide to control nausea and vomiting during initiation and continued treatment with subcutaneous apomorphine injection. Parkinsonism Relat Disord 2014;20:1171.

13. Gauthier S, Amyot D. Sustained release antiparkinson agents: controlled release levodopa. Can J Neurol Sci 1992;19:153.

14. Hoehn MM. Increased dosage of carbidopa in patients with Parkinson's disease receiving low doses of levodopa. A pilot study. Arch Neurol 1980;37:146.

15. Jonkers N, Sarre S, Ebinger G, et al. Benserazide decreases central AADC activity, extracellular dopamine levels and levodopa decarboxylation in striatum of the rat. J Neural Transm 2001;108:559.

16. Carvey PM, Zhao CH, Hendey B, et al. 6-Hydroxydopamine-induced alterations in blood-brain barrier permeability. Eur J Neurosci 2005;22:1158.

17. Brod L, Alfred J, Nutt J. Are high doses of carbidopa a concern? A randomized clinical trial in Parkinson's disease. Mov Disord 2012;27:750.

18. Warren Olanow C, Kieburtz K, Rascol O, et al. Factors predictive of the devel-opment of levodopa-induced dyskinesia and wearing-off in Parkinson's disease. Mov Disord 2013;28:1064.

19. Marras C, Lang A. Invited article: changing concepts in Parkinson disease: moving beyond the decade of the brain. Neurology 2008;70(21):1996.

20. Pontone G, Williams JR, Bassett SS, et al. Clinical features associated with impulse control disorders in Parkinson disease. Neurology 2006;67:1258.

21. Stowe RL, Ives NJ, Clarke C, et al. Dopamine agonist therapy in early Parkin-son's disease. Cochrane Database Syst Rev 2008;(2):CD006564.

22. Pondal M, Marras C, Miyasaki J, et al. Clinical features of dopamine agonist withdrawal syndrome in a movement disorders clinic. J Neurol Neurosurg Psy-chiatr 2013;84:130.

23. Rabinak CA, Nirenberg MJ. Dopamine agonist withdrawal syndrome in Parkin-son disease. Arch Neurol 2010;67:58.

24. Nirenberg MJ. Dopamine agonist withdrawal syndrome: implications for patient care. Drugs Aging 2013;30:587.

25. Apomorphine (Apokyn) for advanced Parkinson's Disease. Med Lett Drugs Ther 2005;47:7.

26. Apokyn(R) [prescribing information]. Louisville (KY): Brittania Pharmaceuticals Limited; 2014. Available at: http://www.apokyn.com/assets/APOKYN_PI.pdf. Accessed November 24, 2015.

27. Meiser J, Weindl D, Hiller K. Complexity of dopamine metabolism. Cell Commun Signal 2013;11:34.

28. Grady M, Stahl S. Practical guide for prescribing MAOIs: debunking myths and removing barriers. CNS Spectr 2012;17:2.

29. Wimbiscus M, Kostenko O, Malone D. MAO inhibitors: risks, benefits, and lore. Cleve Clin J Med 2010;77:859.

30. Youdim MB, Weinstock M. Therapeutic applications of selective and non-selective inhibitors of monoamine oxidase A and B that do not cause significant tyramine potentiation. Neurotoxicology 2004;25:243.

31. Ives NJ, Stowe RL, Marro J, et al. Monoamine oxidase type B inhibitors in early Parkinson's disease: meta-analysis of 17 randomised trials involving 3525 patients. BMJ 2004;329:593.

32. Turnbull K, Caslake R, Macleod A, et al. Monoamine oxidase B inhibitors for early Parkinson's disease. Cochrane Database Syst Rev 2012;(3):CD004898.

33. Horn S, Stern MB. The comparative effects of medical therapies for Parkinson's disease. Neurol 2004;63:S7.

34. Olanow CW, Rascol O, Hauser R, et al, for the ADAGIO Study Investigators. A double-blind, delayed-start trial of rasagiline in Parkinson's disease. N Engl J Med 2009;361:13.

35. Waters CH. Fluoxetine and selegiline–lack of significant interaction. Can J Neurol Sci 1994;21:259.

36. Toyama SC, Iacono RP. Is it safe to combine a selective serotonin reuptake inhibitor with selegiline? Ann Pharmacother 1994;28:405.

37. Richard IH, Kurlan R, Tanner C, et al. Serotonin syndrome and the combined use of deprenyl and an antidepressant in Parkinson's disease. Neurology 1997;48: 1070.

38. Olanow CW, Kieburtz K, Stern M, et al. Double-blind, placebo-controlled study of entacapone in levodopa-treated patients with stable Parkinson disease. Arch Neurol 2004;61:1563.

39. Nutt JG. Catechol-O-methyltransferase inhibitors for treatment of Parkinson's disease. Lancet 1998;351:1221.

40. Brooks DJ, Sagar H, UK-Irish Entacapone Study Group. Entacapone is beneficial in both fluctuating and non-fluctuating patients with Parkinson's disease: a randomised, placebo controlled, double blind, six month study. J Neurol Neurosurg Psychiatry 2003;74:1071.

41. Stocchi F, Rascol O, Kieburtz K, et al. Initiating levodopa/carbidopa therapy with and without entacapone in early Parkinson disease: the STRIDE-PD study. Ann Neurol 2010;68:18.

42. Comtan(R) [prescribing information]. Espoo (Finland): Orion Pharma; 2014. Marketed by Novartis Pharmaceuticals Corporation. East Hanover (NJ). Available at: https://www.pharma.us.novartis.com/product/pi/pdf/comtan.pdf. Accessed November 25, 2015.

43. Solla P, Cannas A, Marrosu F, et al. Therapeutic interventions and adjustments in the management of Parkinson disease: role of combined carbidopa/levodopa/ entacapone (Stalevo). Neuropsychiatr Dis Treat 2010;6:483.

44. Stalevo(R) (carbidopa, levodopa, and entacapone) [prescribing information]. Espoo (Finland): Orion Pharma; 2014. Marketed by Novartis Pharmaceuticals Corporation. East Hanover (NJ). Available at: https://www.pharma.us.novartis. com/product/pi/pdf/stalevo.pdf. Accessed November 26, 2015.

45. Olanow CW. Tolcapone and hepatotoxic effects. Tasmar advisory panel. Arch Neurol 2000;57:263.

46. Tasmar(R) [prescribing information]. Bridgewater (NJ): Valeant Pharmaceuticals North America LLC; 2013. Available at: http://www.accessdata.fda.gov/ drugsatfda_docs/label/2013/020697s004lbl.pdf. Accessed November 25, 2015.

47. Amantadine and other antiglutamate agents: management of Parkinson's disease. Mov Disord 2002;17:S13.

48. Godwin-Austen RB, Frears CC, Bergmann S, et al. Combined treatment of parkinsonism with L-dopa and amantadine. Lancet 1970;2:383.

49. Symmetrel(R) (amantadine hydrochloride) [prescribing information]. Chadds Ford (PA): Endo Pharmaceuticals Inc; 2009. Available at: http://www.accessdata. fda.gov/drugsatfda_docs/label/2009/016023s041,018101s016lbl.pdf. Accessed November 25, 2015.

50. Duvoisin RC. Cholinergic-anticholinergic antagonism in parkinsonism. Arch Neurol 1967;17:124.

51. Katzenschlager R, Sampaio C, Costa J, et al. Anticholinergics for symptomatic management of Parkinson's disease. Cochrane Database Syst Rev 2003;(2): CD003735.

52. Artane(R) (trihexyphenidyl) [prescribing information]. Philadelphia: Wyeth Pharmaceuticals Inc; 2003. Available at: http://www.accessdata.fda.gov/ drugsatfda_docs/nda/2003/006773_s036_artane.pdf. Accessed November 25, 2015.

53. Barone P, Antonini A, Colosimo C, et al. The PRIAMO study: a multicenter assessment of nonmotor symptoms and their impact on quality of life in Parkinson's disease. Mov Disord 2009;24:1641.

54. Goetz CG, Wuu J, Curgian LM, et al. Hallucinations and sleep disorders in PD: six-year prospective longitudinal study. Neurology 2005;64:81.

55. Lee AH, Weintraub D. Psychosis in Parkinson's disease without dementia: common and comorbid with other non-motor symptoms. Mov Disord 2012;27:858.

56. Fasano A, Visanji NP, Liu LW, et al. Gastrointestinal dysfunction in Parkinson's disease. Lancet Neurol 2015;14:625.

57. Srivanitchapoom P, Pandey S, Hallett M. Drooling in Parkinson's disease: a review. Parkinsonism Relat Disord 2014;20:1109.

58. Thomsen TR, Galpern WR, Asante A, et al. Ipratropium bromide spray as treatment for sialorrhea in Parkinson's disease. Mov Disord 2007;22:2268.

59. Hyson HC, Johnson AM, Jog MS. Sublingual atropine for sialorrhea secondary to parkinsonism: a pilot study. Mov Disord 2002;17:1318.

60. Arbouw ME, Movig KL, Koopmann M, et al. Glycopyrrolate for sialorrhea in Parkinson disease: a randomized, double-blind, crossover trial. Neurology 2010;74:1203.

61. Lagalla G, Millevolte M, Capecci M, et al. Botulinum toxin type A for drooling in Parkinson's disease: a double-blind, randomized, placebo-controlled study. Mov Disord 2006;21:704.

62. Mancini F, Zangaglia R, Cristina S, et al. Double-blind, placebo-controlled study to evaluate the efficacy and safety of botulinum toxin type A in the treatment of drooling in parkinsonism. Mov Disord 2003;18:685.

63. Chinnapongse R, Gullo K, Nemeth P, et al. Safety and efficacy of botulinum toxin type B for treatment of sialorrhea in Parkinson's disease: a prospective double-blind trial. Mov Disord 2012;27:219.

64. Edwards LL, Quigley EM, Pfeiffer RF. Gastrointestinal dysfunction in Parkinson's disease: frequency and pathophysiology. Neurology 1992;42:726.

65. Zesiewicz TA, Sullivan KL, Arnulf I, et al. Practice parameter: treatment of nonmotor symptoms of Parkinson disease: report of the Quality Standards Subcommittee of the American Academy of Neurology. Neurology 2010;74:924.

66. Okun M. Parkinson's treatment tips for constipation. 2011. Available at: http://movementdisorders.ufhealth.org/2011/09/12/parkinsons-treatment-tips-for-constipation. Accessed November 26, 2015.

67. Asahina M, Vichayanrat E, Low DA, et al. Autonomic dysfunction in parkinsonian disorders: assessment and pathophysiology. J Neurol Neurosurg Psychiatry 2013;84:674.

68. Senard JM, Raï S, Lapeyre-Mestre M, et al. Prevalence of orthostatic hypotension in Parkinson's disease. J Neurol Neurosurg Psychiatry 1997;63:584.
69. Shannon JR, Diedrich A, Biaggioni I, et al. Water drinking as a treatment for orthostatic syndromes. Am J Med 2002;112:355.
70. Young TM, Mathias CJ. The effects of water ingestion on orthostatic hypotension in two groups of chronic autonomic failure: multiple system atrophy and pure autonomic failure. J Neurol Neurosurg Psychiatry 2004;75:1737.
71. Henry R, Rowe J, O'Mahony D. Haemodynamic analysis of efficacy of compression hosiery in elderly fallers with orthostatic hypotension. Lancet 1999;354:45.
72. Hussain RM, McIntosh SJ, Lawson J, et al. Fludrocortisone in the treatment of hypotensive disorders in the elderly. Heart 1996;76:507.
73. Low PA, Gilden JL, Freeman R, et al. Efficacy of midodrine vs placebo in neurogenic orthostatic hypotension. A randomized, double-blind multicenter study. Midodrine Study Group. JAMA 1997;277:1046.
74. Raj SR, Coffin ST. Medical therapy and physical maneuvers in the treatment of the vasovagal syncope and orthostatic hypotension. Prog Cardiovasc Dis 2013; 55:425.
75. Kaufmann H, Norcliffe-Kaufmann L, Palma JA. Droxidopa in neurogenic orthostatic hypotension. Expert Rev Cardiovasc Ther 2015;13:875.
76. Zhao S, Cheng R, Zheng J, et al. A randomized, double-blind, controlled trial of add-on therapy in moderate-to-severe Parkinson's disease. Parkinsonism Relat Disord 2015;21:1214.
77. Aarsland D, Andersen K, Larsen JP, et al. Prevalence and characteristics of dementia in Parkinson disease: an 8-year prospective study. Arch Neurol 2003;60:387.
78. Forsaa EB, Larsen JP, Wentzel-Larsen T, et al. A 12-year population-based study of psychosis in Parkinson disease. Arch Neurol 2010;67:996.
79. Fernandez HH, Friedman JH, Jacques C, et al. Quetiapine for the treatment of drug-induced psychosis in Parkinson's disease. Mov Disord 1999;14:484.
80. Morgante L, Epifanio A, Spina E, et al. Quetiapine versus clozapine: a preliminary report of comparative effects on dopaminergic psychosis in patients with Parkinson's disease. Neurol Sci 2002;23(Suppl 2):S89.
81. Juncos JL, Roberts VJ, Evatt ML, et al. Quetiapine improves psychotic symptoms and cognition in Parkinson's disease. Mov Disord 2004;19:29.
82. Aarsland D, Larsen JP, Lim NG, et al. Range of neuropsychiatric disturbances in patients with Parkinson's disease. J Neurol Neurosurg Psychiatry 1999;67:492.
83. Tandberg E, Larsen JP, Aarsland D, et al. The occurrence of depression in Parkinson's disease. A community-based study. Arch Neurol 1996;53:175.
84. Sixel-Döring F, Trautmann E, Mollenhauer B, et al. Associated factors for REM sleep behavior disorder in Parkinson disease. Neurology 2011;77:1048.
85. Schenck CH, Mahowald MW. Rapid eye movement sleep parasomnias. Neurol Clin 2005;23:1107.
86. Kunz D, Mahlberg R. A two-part, double-blind, placebo-controlled trial of exogenous melatonin in REM sleep behaviour disorder. J Sleep Res 2010;19:591.
87. Boeve BF, Silber MH, Ferman TJ. Melatonin for treatment of REM sleep behavior disorder in neurologic disorders: results in 14 patients. Sleep Med 2003;4:281.
88. Olson EJ, Boeve BF, Silber MH. Rapid eye movement sleep behaviour disorder: demographic, clinical and laboratory findings in 93 cases. Brain 2000; 123(Pt 2):331.
89. Elble RJ. Tremor: clinical features, pathophysiology, and treatment. Neurol Clin 2009;27:679–95.

90. Louis ED, Ferreira JJ. How common is the most common adult movement disorder? Update on the worldwide prevalence of essential tremor. Mov Disord 2010; 25(5):534–41.

91. Deuschl G, Wenzelburger F, Loffler K, et al. Essential tremor and cerebellar dysfunction. Clinical and kinematic analysis of intention tremor. Brain 2000; 123:1568–80.

92. Jenkins IH, Bain PG, Colebatch JG, et al. A positron emission tomography study of essential tremor: evidence for overactivity of cerebellar connections. Ann Neurol 1993;34:82–90.

93. Fahn S, Jankovic J, Hallett M. Principles and practice of movement disorders. 2nd edition. Philadelphia: Elsevier Saunders; 2011.

94. Ayerst Laboratories Inc. Inderal (propranolol hydrochloride) tablets prescribing information. Philadelphia: Ayerst Laboratories Inc; 2002.

95. Leigh PN, Jefferson D, Twomey A, et al. Beta-adrenoreceptor mechanisms in essential tremor; a double-blind placebo controlled trial of metoprolol, sotalol and atenolol. J Neurol Neurosurg Psychiatry 1983;46(8):710–5.

96. Koller WC. Dose-response relationship of propranolol in the treatment of essential tremor. Arch Neurol 1986;43(1):42–3.

97. Hedera P, Cibulčík F, Davis TL. Pharmacotherapy of essential tremor. J Cent Nerv Syst Dis 2013;5:43–55.

98. Koller WC, Royse VL. Time course of a single oral dose of propranolol in essential tremor. Neurology 1985;35(10):1494–8.

99. Baumel IP, Gallagher BB, Mattson RH. Phenylethylmalonamide (PEMA). An important metabolite of primidone. Arch Neurol 1972;27(1):34–41.

100. Mysoline (primidone, USP) [packageinsert]. Aliso Viejo (CA): Valeant Pharmaceuticals NA; 2009. Available at: http://www.accessdata.fda.gov/drugsatfda_docs/label/2009/009170s036lbl.pdf.

101. AHFS drug information 2007. In: McEvoy GK, editor. Primidone. Bethesda (MD): American Society of Health-System Pharmacists; 2008.

102. Zesiewicz TA, Elble R, Louis ED, et al. Practice parameter: therapies for essential tremor: report of the Quality Standards Subcommittee of the American Academy of Neurology. Neurology 2005;64(12):2008–20.

103. Parke-Davis. Neurontin (gabapentin) capsules prescribing information. New York: Parke-Davis; 2005.

104. Hendrich J, Van Minh AT, Heblich F, et al. Pharmacological disruption of calcium channel trafficking by the alpha2delta ligand gabapentin. Proc Natl Acad Sci U S A 2008;105(9):3628–33.

105. Ondo W, Hunter C, Vuong KD, et al. Gabapentin for essential tremor: a multiple-dose, double-blind, placebo-controlled trial. Mov Disord 2000;15(4):678–82.

106. Ortho-McNeil. Topamax (topiramate) tablets and capsules prescribing information. Raritan (NJ): Ortho-McNeil; 2004.

107. Connor GS, Edwards K, Tarsy D. Topiramate in essential tremor: findings from double-blind, placebo-controlled, crossover trials. Clin Neuropharmacol 2008; 31(2):97–103.

108. Johannessen SI. Pharmacokinetics and interaction profile of topiramate: review and comparison with other newer antiepileptic drugs. Epilepsia 1997; 38(Suppl 1):S18–23.

109. Jankovic J, Ondo WG, Stacy MA, et al. Multi-center, double-blind, placebo-controlled trial of topiramate in essential tremor. Mov Disord 2004;19(Suppl 9): S448–9.

110. Walters AS, Wagner ML, Hening WA, et al. Successful treatment of the idiopathic restless legs syndrome in a randomized double-blind trial of oxycodone versus placebo. Sleep 1993;16:327.

111. Scholz H, Benes H, Happe S, et al. Psychological distress of patients suffering from restless legs syndrome: a cross-sectional study. Health Qual Life Outcomes 2011;9:73–9.

112. Linke R, Eisensehr I, Wetter T-C, et al. Presynaptic dopaminergic function in patients with restless legs syndrome: are there common features with early Parkinson's disease? Mov Disord 2004;19:1158–62.

113. Comella CL. Treatment of restless leg syndrome. Neurotherapeutics 2014;11: 177–87.

114. American Academy of Neurology. https://www.aan.com.

115. Trotti LM, Bhadriraju S, Becker LA. Iron for restless legs syndrome. Cochrane Database Syst Rev 2012;(5):CD007834.

116. Paulus W, Trenkwalder C. Less is more: pathophysiology of dopaminergic-therapy-related augmentation in restless legs syndrome. Lancet Neurol 2006; 5(10):878–86.

117. Available at: Rxlist.com.

118. Azur Pharma. Parcopa (carbidopa-levodopa) orally disintegrating tablets prescribing information. Philadelphia: Azur Pharma; 2009.

119. Nutt JG, Fellman JH. Pharmacokinetics of levodopa. Clin Neuropharmacol 1984; 7:35–49.

120. Hanson RA, Menkes JH. A new anticonvulsant in the management of minor motor seizures. Dev Med Child Neurol 1972;14(1):3–14.

121. Roche Laboratories Inc. Klonopin (clonazepam) tablets prescribing information. Nutley (NJ): Roche Laboratories Inc; 1997.

122. Perachon S, Schwartz JC, Sokoloff P. Functional potencies of new antiparkinsonian drugs at recombinant human dopamine D-1, D-2 and D-3 receptors. Eur J Pharmacol 1999;366:293–300.

123. GlaxoSmithKline. Requip (ropinirole hydrochloride) tablets prescribing information. Research Triangle Park (NC): GlaxoSmithKline; 2005.

124. Boehringer Ingelheim. Mirapex (pramipexole dihydrochloride) tablets prescribing information. Ridgefield (CT): Boehringer Ingelheim; 2011.

125. Happe S, Klösch G, Saletu B, et al. Treatment of idiopathic restless legs syndrome (RLS) with gabapentin. Neurology 2001;57:1717.

126. Pfizer, Inc. Lyrica(pregabalin) capsules prescribing information. New York: Pfizer, Inc; 2007.

127. Taylor CP, Angelotti T, Fauman E. Pharmacology and mechanism of action of pregabalin: the calcium channel alpha2-delta (alpha2-delta) subunit as a target for antiepileptic drug discovery. Epilepsy Res 2007;73(2):137–50.

128. Garcia-Borreguero D, Kohnen R, Silber MH, et al. The long-term treatment of restless legs syndrome/Willis-Ekbom disease: evidence-based guidelines and clinical consensus best practice guidance: a report from the International Restless Legs Syndrome Study Group. Sleep Med 2013;14:675–84.

129. Novartis Pharmaceuticals. Tegretol (carbamazepine) chewable tablets, tablets, and suspension and Tegretol XR (carbamazepine) extended-release tablets prescribing information. East Hanover (NJ): Novartis Pharmaceuticals; 2003.

130. Telstad W, Sørensen O, Larsen S, et al. Treatment of the restless legs syndrome with carbamazepine: a double blind study. Br Med J (Clin Res Ed) 1984; 288(6415):444–6.

131. US Food and Drug Administration. Public health advisory: Information for health-care professionals: carbamazepine (marketed as Carbatrol, Equetro, Tegretol, and generics). Rockville (MD): US Food and Drug Administration; 2007. https://www.FDA.gov.

132. Sierralta F, Naquira D, Pinardi G, et al. alpha-Adrenoceptor and opioid receptor modulation of clonidine-induced antinociception. Br J Pharmacol 1996;119(3): 551–4.

133. Boehringer Ingelheim Pharmaceuticals, Inc. Catapres-TTS (clonidine) Trans-dermal Therapeutic System prescribing information. Ridgefield (CT): Boeh-ringer Ingelheim Pharmaceuticals, Inc; 2004.

134. Wagner ML, Walters AS, Coleman RG, et al. Randomized, double-blind, placebo-controlled study of clonidine in restless legs syndrome. Sleep 1996;19(1):52–8.

135. Endo Laboratories. Symmetrel (amantadine hydrochloride) tablets and syrup prescribing information. Chadds Ford (PA): Endo Laboratories; 2009.

136. Evidente VG, Adler CH, Caviness JN, et al. Amantadine is beneficial in restless legs syndrome. Mov Disord 2000;15:324.

137. Hensley JG. Leg cramps and restless legs syndrome during pregnancy. J Midwifery Womens Health 2009;54:211–8.

138. Gigli GL, Adorati M, Dolso P, et al. Restless legs syndrome in end-stage renal disease. Sleep Med 2004;5:309–15.

139. Baran AS, Richert AC, Douglass AB, et al. Change in periodic limb movement index during treatment of obstructive sleep apnea with continuous positive airway pressure. Sleep 2003;26(6):717–20.

Pharmacologic Therapies in Women's Health

Contraception and Menopause Treatment

Caitlin Allen, MD[a],*, Ginger Evans, MD[b], Eliza L. Sutton, MD[c]

KEYWORDS

- Long-acting reversible contraception • Combined hormonal contraception
- Emergency contraception • Menopause transition
- Genitourinary syndrome of menopause • Estrogen therapy

KEY POINTS

- Estrogens and progestogens may be prescribed in a variety of forms and doses for contraception and for relief from menopausal symptoms.
- Long-acting reversible contraception is recommended as first-line contraception for nearly all women due to ease of use, high efficacy, safety, and relatively limited contraindications.
- Emergency contraception to prevent unintended pregnancy should be administered as soon as possible after unprotected intercourse.
- Vasomotor symptoms in the menopause transition can be treated with hormonal, nonhormonal, or nonpharmaceutical approaches.
- Menopausal symptoms respond well to estrogen administered locally for genitourinary symptoms or systemically for vasomotor symptoms; systemic use warrants consideration of risks, alternative approaches, and endometrial protection.

INTRODUCTION

Women's health can refer to aspects of health and disease that are unique to women, are more common in women, manifest differently in women, and/or are treated differently in women. Women's health and its pharmacotherapy are not synonymous with female sex steroids; however, female hormones do play a significant role in the etiology and treatment of commonly encountered women's health conditions.

The authors have nothing to disclose.
[a] Department of Medicine, University of Wisconsin School of Medicine and Public Health, 5120 MFCB, 1685 Highland Avenue, Madison, WI 53705, USA; [b] Department of Medicine, VA Puget Sound Health Care System, University of Washington, 1660 South Columbian Way, S-123-PCC, Seattle, WA 98108, USA; [c] Department of Medicine, Women's Health Care Center, University of Washington, 4245 Roosevelt Way Northeast, Box 354765, Seattle, WA 98105, USA
* Corresponding author.
E-mail address: callen@uwhealth.org

Med Clin N Am 100 (2016) 763–789
http://dx.doi.org/10.1016/j.mcna.2016.03.008
0025-7125/16/$ – see front matter
medical.theclinics.com

This article will focus on hormonal therapy for routine and emergency female contraception and control of menopausal symptoms, since these are common; additionally, the myriad of available pharmacotherapeutic regimens can be confusing and difficult to remember, as can the safety considerations around prescribing.

Estrogen is a steroid hormone that binds to estrogen receptors α and β; 17β-estradiol is the main endogenous female sex hormone. Progestogens are steroid hormones that bind to progesterone receptors α and β; the major endogenous progestogen is progesterone, and synthetic progestogens are called progestins.

Pharmacologic therapies that bind estrogen receptors and progesterone receptors are listed in **Table 1**. This article will address the most commonly used therapies for the following indications.

- Hormonal contraception
- Control of hormone-responsive symptoms between puberty and menopause, for example acne and irregular or heavy menses (typically off-label)

Table 1
Pharmacologic therapies that bind estrogen receptors and/or progesterone receptors

	Reproductive Use	Menopausal Use	Other Uses
Estrogens	Hormonal contraception (with a progestogen): ethinyl estradiol, estradiol hemihydrate, mestranol	Reduction in vasomotor and/or GSM; bone preservation: estradiol, conjugated estrogens, esterified estrogens	Prostate cancer Transgender women Turner syndrome Hypothalamic amenorrhea Osteoporosis prevention Treatment of arteriovenous malformations[1]
Progestogens	Hormonal contraception, progestin with an estrogen: see combined hormonal contraception **(Table 2)**; Hormonal contraception, progestin without an estrogen: etonogestrel levonorgestrel (LNG), medroxyprogesterone acetate (MPA), norethindrone	Endometrial protection: LNG, micronized progesterone, MPA, norethindrone	Palliative treatment of advanced breast or endometrial carcinoma; Appetite stimulation: megestrol acetate Respiratory stimulation: MPA
SERMs	Ovulation induction: clomiphene	Protection of endometrium during estrogen use; bone preservation: bazedoxifene Treatment of GSM: ospemifene	Prevention or treatment of breast cancer: raloxifene, tamoxifen, toremifene
Selective Progesterone Receptor Modulators (SPRMs)	Emergency contraception: ulipristal Abortifacient: mifepristone	—	—

- Control of menopause-related symptoms (vasomotor symptoms [VMS]) and/or genitourinary syndrome of menopause (GSM)

Uses of pharmacotherapeutics binding female sex steroid receptors in certain other situations will not be covered in this article but include.

- Breast cancer prevention (primary prevention and prevention of recurrence)
- Osteoporosis prevention and treatment
- Ovulation induction
- Prostate cancer treatment
- Secondary sex characteristic development for transgender women

Sex steroid hormonal therapy poses several class-specific risks. Estrogens and partial-agonist selective estrogen receptor modulators (SERMs) can increase the risk of venous thromboembolic disease (VTE) and cardiovascular events (heart attack and stroke). Hormonal therapies can also promote or retard the growth of hormone-dependent cells, including tumors. Specific risks are discussed for hormonal contraception and for menopausal hormone therapy.

Hormonal contraception and hormonal treatment of menopausal symptoms share several features. Treatment is with estrogen and/or a progestogen; treatment can be delivered by different routes (**Box 1**), and nonhormonal treatment approaches exist.

Differences include purpose, predominant hormone, dosage, and user characteristics such as age. Hormonal contraception aims to prevent unintended pregnancy primarily through the action of a *progestin* in suppressing ovulation by suppressing

---

Box 1
Routes for administration of therapeutics

Contraception:

- Oral
- Transdermal
- Transmucosal/vaginal
- Parenteral
- Intrauterine

Emergency contraception:

- Oral (hormones)
- Intrauterine (copper)

Menopause transition (systemic effect):

- Oral
- Transdermal
- Transmucosal/vaginal
- Injection (rarely used)

Menopause transition or postmenopause (local effect):

- Topical/vaginal
- Intrauterine LNG (off-label for endometrial protection with estrogen use)
- Oral (ospemifene)

the hypothalamic–pituitary–gonadal axis, thickening cervical mucus as a barrier, and preventing buildup of the endometrium. Estrogen, included in some forms of oral hormonal contraception, reduces irregular bleeding and increases efficacy of oral hormonal contraception. Hormonal contraception is also used (largely off-label) for a control of a number of other conditions including acne, hirsutism, irregular and/or heavy periods, dysmenorrhea, and pain from endometriosis.

Noncontraceptive hormonal treatment in and after the menopause transition, on the other hand, relies on *estrogen* to suppress vasomotor symptoms and/or to address GSM and/or to prevent bone loss. Menopause-related symptoms respond to much lower doses of estrogen than the doses used in combined hormonal contraception, with 10 µg ethinyl estradiol (EE) equivalent to 1.25 µg conjugated equine estrogen[2] (see **Table 5**). GSM responds to even lower doses when applied topically. The lowest-dose options for each use are referred to as ultralow-dose estrogen.

In allopathic hormonal treatment of menopause-related symptoms, a progestogen is only used in women with a uterus who are taking estrogen at doses used for systemic effect, in which case the progestogen's purpose is to oppose the effect of estrogen on the endometrium, reducing the risk of endometrial hyperplasia and cancer.

CONTRACEPTION
Effectiveness of Different Contraceptive Methods

Fortunately, there are many effective methods of contraception available. With perfect use, many of the methods would be extremely effective, resulting in less than 1% of women using any one of them becoming pregnant per year. However, in practice, the forgettable contraception[3] methods (implants or intrauterine devices [IUDs]) strongly outperform other options. For example, in actual use, an implant or IUD results in less than 1% of users experiencing unintended pregnancies in each year of use. The pill, patch, and ring each result in approximately a 9% annual rate of unintended pregnancies in actual use.[4] **Fig. 1** from the US Centers for Disease Control and Prevention (CDC) highlights the performance of each of these methods.

Emergency contraception (EC) can also decrease the risk of pregnancy after a single episode of unprotected sexual intercourse from 3% to 10%[5–7] (depending on which day in the fertile window this occurs) to about 0.1% with the copper IUD[8–10] or about 2% with oral hormonal methods.[7,11]

Long-acting Reversible Contraception

Long-acting reversible contraceptives (LARCs, **Box 2**) achieve high efficacy by gradually releasing an active ingredient from an implanted device, bypassing reliance on daily adherence. LARCs have higher continuation rates at 2 years than other forms of hormonal contraception.[12] LARCs are recommended as first-line contraception options for women who want or need highly effective contraception, women who have contraindications to estrogen, and/or women who have comorbid medical conditions for which pregnancy should be avoided or carefully planned.[13] Current LARCs are safe and effective in adolescents[14] and in nulliparous women, as well as parous women.[13] Duration of effectiveness varies from 3 years for progestin subdermal implants, 3 to 7 years for the progestin IUDs, to 10 to 12 years for copper IUDs. Choosing an IUD depends on the individual; at this time there is limited evidence to support 1 progestin LARC over the other, and the choice should between patient and provider preference and could be based on desired years of contraception, parous status, and cost. LARCs have fewer contraindications than do combined hormonal contraceptives (**Table 2** shows contraindications for hormone use). No LARC contains latex.

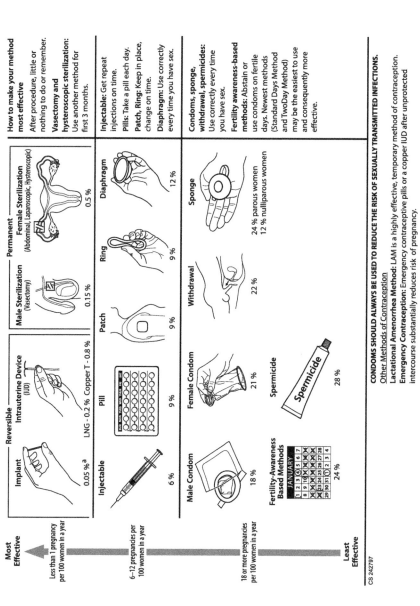

Fig. 1. Effectiveness of contraceptive methods. [a] The percentages indicate the number out of every 100 women who experienced an unintended pregnancy within the first year of typical use of each contraceptive method. (*From* Centers for Disease Control and Prevention. Effectiveness of contraceptive methods. Available at: http://www.cdc.gov/reproductivehealth/unintendedpregnancy/pdf/contraceptive_methods_508.pdf. Accessed February 7, 2016.)

Box 2
Long-acting reversible contraceptives

Subdermal implant (progestin)

- Nexplanon (etonogestrel 68 mg, single rod implant)
  Effective for 3 years
  Insertion is easier than Implanon, and rod is radio-opaque

- Implanon (etonogestrel 68 mg, single rod implant)
  Effective for 3 years

- Norplant (LNG 36 mg × 6 capsules)
  Effective for 5 years
  Not marketed in United States since 2002

Intrauterine device (progestin IUDs)

- Mirena (LNG 52 mg)
  FDA-approved for 5 years, but effective for 7 years[15]

- Skyla (LNG 13.5 mg)
  FDA-approved for 3 years; no evidence of longer duration efficacy[15]

- Liletta (LNG 52 mg)
  FDA-approved for 3 years (may be extended at a later date)

Intrauterine device (copper IUD)

- Paragard T 380A
  FDA-approved for 10 years, but effective for 12 years[15]

Common adverse effects of LARCs include irregular bleeding for progestin-based LARC methods, acne for progestin implants, and heavy menstrual bleeding with the copper IUD.[16] Menstrual irregularity is the main reason for discontinuation of LARCs, plus spontaneous expulsion for IUDs. Routine counseling on expected bleeding pattern can improve likelihood of continuation with the method .[17] Although LARCs have become more widely used in the past 5 years,[18] they remain underutilized.[19]

LARCs can be used shortly after childbirth with several considerations.

- Progestin-only methods and copper IUDs do not affect risk of VTE, unlike estrogen-containing methods.
- IUD insertion poses higher risk of uterine perforation when performed greater than 10 minutes and less than 6 weeks after delivery, and during lactation. In addition, spontaneous expulsion occurs more often after postpartum insertion.
  - Copper IUDs may be inserted immediately after Cesarean section[20]; otherwise "insertion should be delayed to the second postpartum month."[21]
  - Progestin IUD insertion has been shown to be effective and safe (albeit with higher risk of higher expulsion) if performed within 48 hours postpartum,[22] but insertion is recommended later than 6 weeks in prescribing information.[23]
- Progestin implant may be inserted between 3 and 4 weeks after delivery in women who are not breast feeding, but it is not recommended before 4 weeks postpartum in women who are breast feeding.[24] However, studies show no reduction in breast feeding and no impairment in infant weight gain with early implant insertion compared with no contraceptive or delayed initiation of contraceptive.[25]

Fertility returns quickly after removal of a LARC. After IUD removal, the pregnancy rate among women attempting to conceive is similar to that of women discontinuing

Table 2
Key contraindications to hormonal therapies or forms

	Estrogen (Systemic) Menopausal Vasomotor Symptoms[46]	Estrogen (Systemic) Contraception Use	Progestin	Any IUD	Copper IUD
Known allergy to any component	✓	✓	✓	✓	✓[21]
Current pregnancy	✓	✓	✓	4	4 (except may be inserted as EC)
Unexplained vaginal bleeding with potential concerning cause, before evaluation		2	2 for oral 3 for implant or injection	4	4
Hypercoagulable state, current or past VTE or arterial thrombosis	✓	4	2	1	1
Breast cancer (current or past)	✓	4 if current (within 5 y) 3 if disease-free for ≥5 y	4 if current (within 5 y) 3 if disease-free for ≥5 y	LNG IUD: see column to left Copper IUD: see column to right	1
Liver disease	✓	4 for advanced or decompensated cirrhosis, hepatic adenoma, or hepatocellular carcinoma 2 for focal nodular hyperplasia 1 for mild compensated cirrhosis	3 for advanced or decompensated cirrhosis, hepatic adenoma, or hepatocellular carcinoma 2 for focal nodular hyperplasia 1 for mild compensated cirrhosis	LNG IUD: see column to left Copper IUD: see column to right	1

(continued on next page)

Table 2
(continued)

	Estrogen (Systemic) Menopausal Vasomotor Symptoms[46]	Estrogen (Systemic) Contraception Use	Progestin	Any IUD	Copper IUD
Gallbladder disease	✔	3 if symptomatic, with or without medical treatment 2 if asymptomatic or after cholecystectomy	2	LNG IUD: see column to left Copper IUD: see column to right	1
Hyperlipidemia	✔ (relative contraindication for those with triglycerides >400 mg/dL)	2–3 depending on level and other CHD risks, but screening not indicated before initiation of CHC	2	LNG IUD: see column to left Copper IUD: see column to right	1
Hypertension	✔ If uncontrolled	4 if systolic ≥160 or diastolic ≥100 or in presence of vascular disease 3 otherwise in patient with hypertension	3 (for DMPA) or 2 (for other progestin methods) if systolic ≥160 or diastolic ≥100 or in presence of vascular disease 2 (for DMPA) or 1 (for other progestin methods) otherwise in patient with hypertension	LNG IUD: 2 Copper IUD: see column right	1
Gestational trophoblastic disease with persistently elevated HCG	—	1	1	4 for malignant disease or persistently elevated β-HCG level 3 for undetectable or declining β-HCG level	4 for malignant disease or persistently elevated β-HCG level 3 for undetectable or declining β-HCG level

Condition				
Endometrial hyperplasia ✔	✔ for unopposed estrogen / 1 if combined with progestin	1	1 for endometrial hyperplasia / 4 for insertion in setting of endometrial cancer	1 for endometrial hyperplasia / 4 for insertion in setting of endometrial cancer
Current pelvic inflammatory disease or mucopurulent cervicitis	—	1	4 for insertion in setting of active mucopurulent infection / 2 for continuation in setting of active infection	4 for insertion in setting of active mucopurulent infection / 2 for continuation in setting of active infection
Postpregnancy endometritis in past 3 months	—	—	4	4
Known or suspected uterine or cervical malignancy	—	—	4	4
Abnormal anatomy of uterine cavity, or existing IUD	—	—	4	4
Wilson disease	—	—	✔21	—

Category	Description
4	Method contraindicated in this condition; unacceptable health risk
3	Method not recommended; risks may outweigh advantages
2	Advantages outweigh risks for this method in this condition
1	No restriction for this method in this condition

Key: MEC for contraceptive use.[45]
Contraindications are marked by MEC category[45] or by "✔" if not addressed in MEC classification.
Table is not inclusive; check MEC or product insert for additional information.

other methods, with 50% of former IUD-users conceiving by 3 months after removal of that device.[26] Likewise, removal of progestin implant is followed by ovulation within 1 month in 40% of women, and conception within 12 months in 95.8% of patients.[27]

Progestin LARCs offer the noncontraceptive health benefit of reduced menstrual flow and thus reduced likelihood of iron deficiency anemia, and reduction in dysmenorrhea and pain from endometriosis.

Other Progestin-only Contraception

Progestin-only contraception is also available in oral and injection forms as the progestin-only pill (POP or minipill) and depot medroxyprogesterone acetate (DMPA), respectively.

DMPA can be as effective as LARCs[14] with ideal use, but efficacy depends on regular dosing every 12 weeks, and discontinuation rate of DMPA is high.[12] DMPA offers the benefits of efficacy and intermittent dosing without exposure to estrogen, but without the cost or commitment of an IUD or implant. Bleeding is irregular (and often heavy) initially, although with continued use amenorrhea occurs. DMPA has a reputation of causing weight gain, but systematic review has found the mean gain in studies up to 12 months in duration to be less than 2 kg.[28] DMPA has been associated with decline in bone density and increase in fracture risk.[29]

POPs are less effective than other hormonal methods, and regular daily dosing is key to efficacy. Their most common use is in the postpartum period, as POPs may be started at any time after delivery, may be used during breastfeeding, and do not increase the risk of VTE (unlike combined hormonal contraceptives [CHCs]).

Combined Hormonal Contraception: Combined Oral Contraception, the Patch, and the Ring

CHCs contain an estrogen as well as a progestin. The addition of estrogen improves efficacy by improving ovulation suppression, and avoids irregular bleeding by stabilizing the endometrium. However, it also increases the potential risks and contraindications to use.

Currently available delivery mechanisms include: pills, a patch, and a vaginal ring. **Table 3** details the different components of oral formulations of estrogen and progestin, which have been combined in myriad permutations to form the available combination oral contraceptive (COC) regimens. These combinations are available as monophasic regimens or as more complex regimens in which the dose of the progestin and/or estrogen component changes over the month. COCs are most commonly packaged as 21 days of active pills, followed by 7 days of placebo during which a withdrawal bleed is experienced. Extended-cycle formulations are now available, packaged so that a withdrawal bleed is experienced only every 3 months, and a continuous formulation is also available. Any monophasic pill can be used off-label in an extended-cycle or continuous fashion. Although not as extensively investigated, the vaginal ring has also been studied (by changing the ring each month, foregoing a withdrawal bleed for a various number of cycles) and can be used off-label in an extended-cycle manner.[30–32]

Serious risks and contraindications

As mentioned previously, the most important risks of hormonal contraception are VTE and cardiovascular risk (heart attack and stroke). For VTE, the baseline risk in nonusers is 0.19 to 0.37 cases per 1000 person–years. The relative risk is about 2 to 4 times higher in COC users, which still corresponds to a low absolute risk.[33] In a large French

Table 3
Ingredients and formulations of combination hormonal contraceptives available in the United States[a,b]

Estrogens Available forms and doses	Ethinyl estradiol (EE) 10 μg[c] **20 μg** 25 μg **30 μg** 35 μg 40 mcg[d] 50 mcg Estradiol valerate[c,d] (EV) 1, 2, and 3 mg Mestranol (EE pro-drug) 50 μg (equivalent to 35 μg EE)

Progestins	First generation
	  Ethynodiol diacetate
	  Norethindrone
	  Norethindrone acetate
	 Second generation
	  Levonorgestrel
	  Norgestrel
	 Third generation
	  Desogestrel
	  Etonorgestrel[c] (ring, implant)
	  Norelgestromin[c] (patch)
	  Norgestimate
	 Fourth generation
	  Dienogest[c]
	  Drospirenone

Phasing	**Monophasic** (estrogen and progestin dose stable over $\geq$21 d)
	 Multiphasic (progestin dose changes over 21 d)
	  Biphasic
	  Triphasic
	 Estrophasic (estrogen dose changes over 21–91 d)

Cycle length
 Pills per pack
 Active pills per cycle
	21-d pack
	  21 active pills
	 28-d pack
	  21 active pills
	  24 active pills[c]
	  28 active pills
	 91-d pack
	  84 active pills
	  84 active pills + 7 d of 10 μg EE pills

Bold indicates recommended first-line COC.[33]
Italics indicate progestins available only in non-oral contraceptives.
[a] This information is current as of November 2015.
[b] New brands with new synthetic hormones and formulations, and generics of previously approved brands, become available frequently.
[c] As a contraceptive, available only as brand name (as of November 2015).
[d] Available only within an estrophasic formulation (as of November 2015).

study, the overall annual number of VTE events attributable to contraceptive use was 0.56 cases per 1000 person–years.[43]

The cardiovascular risk of CHCs follows a similar pattern, but events are less common than VTE in the CHC-using population by 2 orders of magnitude. The baseline risk in nonusers is 13.2 cases per 100,000 person–years for myocardial infarction (MI) and 24.2 cases per 100,000 person–years for stroke. Current use of COCs with EE doses of 20 to 40 μg has an adjusted relative risk ranging from 0.9 to 2.3. Even assuming the highest risk multiplier, this corresponds to an absolute risk of 32.1 and 52.5 cases per 100,000 person–years for MI and stroke, respectively.[44] Furthermore, any increase in risk does not appear to persist after discontinuation of the method; previous use of CHCs does not confer an increased risk above baseline risk in nonusers.[44]

The absolute risk of cancer in COC users is lower than in non-users. In a general practitioner data set, the absolute risk reduction for ever-use of COCs was 10 per 100,000 person-years.[47] The effect on risk of specific cancers is mixed, with a decrease in the risk of endometrial, ovarian and colorectal cancer but a slight increase in breast and cervical cancer.[34] The risk reduction for endometrial and ovarian cancer appears to persist for decades after use.[47]

In 1996, the World Health Organization (WHO) first developed medical eligibility criteria for contraceptive use (MEC), a system of rating the safety of specific contraceptive methods in different health conditions. The MEC have been updated periodically and have been adapted for use in individual countries. The CDC created the US MEC[45] and from it the US Selected Practice Recommendations for Contraceptive Use,[48] helpful and practical guides to selecting safe contraceptive options for patients. A helpful app, available for iOS and Android users (CDC MEC) contains the same data. In the MEC classification, specific methods are rated from 1 (no contraindication) to 4 (contraindicated) for specific clinical situations. Key contraindications for hormonal contraception and IUDs are shown in **Table 2**, with MEC level. Clinicians should be aware of the MEC and review it when prescribing CHCs; unfortunately, CHCs are still being prescribed for many women with level 3 and 4 contraindications.[49]

The risk of VTE with CHCs concerns many providers and patients but should be put into context. Pregnancy elevates the risk of VTE significantly more than CHC use does. Providers should communicate the risk in terms of absolute risk (which is generally low) and not relative risk, which can be misleading.[50] Counseling regarding CHCs also provides an opportunity to highlight noncontraceptive benefits and common adverse effects. **Box 3** highlights a few key discussion points.

Nonoral combined hormonal contraceptive options: patch and ring

The contraceptive patch (ORTHO EVRA) contains EE and norelgestromin (the active metabolite of norgestimate). The patch delivers 20 μg EE daily, but because the pharmacodynamics differ from oral administration, a user's overall exposure to estrogen is about 60% greater than for a COC containing 35 μg EE. In other words, the daily estrogen exposure from the patch is roughly equivalent to 50 μg EE taken orally.[51] A new patch is applied once weekly for 3 weeks, followed by 1 week off the patch for a withdrawal bleed.

The vaginal ring (NuvaRing) is a soft, flexible polymer ring that is inserted into the vagina for 21 days, followed by removal by the patient for 7 days of withdrawal bleeding. The marketed vaginal ring releases 120 μg of etonogestrel (a third-generation progestin) and 15 μg of EE daily.[52]

The same women who are candidates for COCs are also candidates for the patch or vaginal ring, because the risks and contraindications are similar. These are thoroughly laid out by the WHO and CDC,[45] and common risks and contraindications are highlighted in **Table 2**. In the early postmarketing phase of the patch, concern was raised over a possible increased risk of VTE with the patch over the known risk of VTE with the pill. Subsequent data on this are mixed, with some showing greater risk,[53] from the patch and some showing no difference.[54–56]

Box 3
Combined hormonal contraception: discussion points with patients

Effectiveness for Pregnancy Prevention

- Risk of pregnancy with 1 year of typical use is about 9%[4]
- Long-acting reversible contraceptives are more effective than the pill, patch, or ring[4]

Noncontraceptive Benefits

- Decrease risk of endometrial, ovarian, and colorectal cancer[34]
- Improve acne[35]
- Improve primary dysmenorrhea[36–38]

Common adverse effects

- Bleeding irregularity (12%)[39]
- Nausea (7%)[39]
- Weight gain (5%)[39]; has not been linked to CHC use when studied more rigorously[40]
- Headache (4%); tends to improve or disappear over months of use[39,41]
- Breast tenderness (4%)[39]
- Mood changes (5%)[39,42]

Major adverse effects

- VTE; absolute risk attributable to use about 0.56 per 1000 person–years[43]
- Cardiovascular disease; absolute risk attributable to use about 18.9 cases per 100,000 person–years for myocardial infarction and 28.3 cases per 100,000 person–years for stroke[44]
- Cancer; slight increase in risk of breast cancer (odds ratio [OR] 1.08; confidence interval [CI], 1.00–1.17) and cervical cancer[34]

The patch and ring offer improved ease of administration over COCs, and patch users have reported more consistent use of the method than pill users.[57] However, pregnancy rates between all 3 methods are similar, and discontinuation rates are lowest among pill users.[57] Nonoral options may be preferred in some situations, because they do not undergo first-pass metabolism in the liver. Vaginal ring users report less acne, nausea, and emotional changes, as well as fewer bleeding problems than pill users.[57] On the other hand, compared with pill users, patch users report more breast discomfort, painful menses, nausea, and vomiting. Ring users report more vaginal irritation and discharge.[57]

Choosing between different combined hormonal contraception options
The plethora of CHCs available requires clinicians and patients to select between numerous options. Efficacy is essentially equivalent, thus when choosing between CHC options, clinicians and patients should attempt to optimize all applicable considerations.

- Lowest risk of serious adverse events (VTE or cardiovascular disease)
- Fewest side effects
- Most appropriate noncontraceptive benefit(s)
- Ease and acceptability of dosing and delivery for that patient
- Out-of-pocket costs

Box 4 highlights some tips to consider during shared decision-making.

Box 4

Tips for choosing between different combined hormonal contraceptive options

- Monophasic preparations are recommended over multiphasic preparations[58]
- Of the preparations available, those with the lowest VTE risk are[33]:
  - LNG plus 20 μg EE
  - LNG plus 30 μg EE
- 30 μg EE results in less unscheduled bleeding and lower discontinuation rates than 20 μg EE[59]
- Nonoral options avoid first-pass hepatic metabolism, so could theoretically avoid some drug interactions[51]
- Nonoral options avoid first-pass hepatic metabolism, so are theoretically not as effective against acne[51,60,61]
- Patch users report more breast discomfort, painful menses, nausea, and vomiting than pill users and ring users[57]
- Ring users report fewer bleeding problems and less nausea and emotional changes than pill users, but more vaginal irritation and discharge[57]

Emergency Contraception

The goal of EC is to prevent an undesired pregnancy in the days following an episode of unprotected intercourse (UPI). The 4 main methods of EC are shown in **Table 4**. Because many women are not aware of the proper use of EC[62] and because EC is time-sensitive, advanced provision of medications during a routine

Table 4
Options for emergency contraception

Method	Dosage	Availability and FDA Status	Timing of Use (Maximum Days After Unprotected Intercourse)	Pregnancy Rates After Use[c] (Approximate)
Copper IUD	—	Device placed in office procedure	Up to 5 d	~ 0.1%
Ulipristal	30 mg once	With prescription	Up to 5 d	~ 1.4%
LNG	1.5 mg once	Over the counter No age restrictions	Up to 3 d[a]	~ 2%
LNG	0.75 mg twice taken 12 h apart	Behind the counter Age >17 only Photo identification required	Up to 3 d[a]	~ 2%
Yuzpe method	Various doses (approximately 100 μg EE + 0.5 mg LNG twice, taken 12 h apart)[b]	Not labelled for EC	Up to 3 d[a]	~ 2%

[a] Some benefit demonstrated at 3 to 5 days; all EC should be used as soon as possible after unprotected intercourse.[63,65]
[b] See http://ec.princeton.edu/questions/dose.html#dose for list of specific options.
[c] Baseline risk of pregnancy after one episode of UPI is variably estimated at 3% to 10%.[5–7] General estimates of effectiveness of each method are listed here.[9–11,71,72,75]

family planning visit is recommended by the American Congress of Obstetricians and Gynecologists (ACOG)[63] and the CDC.[64] This practice does not increase risky sexual behavior.[65]

EC should also be provided post-UPI for any woman who desires not to become pregnant, regardless of whether the UPI is thought to have occurred during the fertile window and without delaying for (or requiring) a pregnancy test.[63] There are no contraindications to hormonal EC used in the appropriate timeframe after UPI.[48] Tips for counseling at prescription of EC are included in **Box 5**, and common side effects are found in **Box 6**. When prescribing EC after an episode of UPI, also discuss the patient's options for routine contraception. Hormonal contraception can be started immediately after levonorgestrel (LNG) or Yuzpe method EC without waiting for menses (quick start),[66] but should not be started sooner than 5 days after ulipristal (a selective progesterone receptor modulator or SPRM), in order to maintain the effectiveness (**Box 7**).[67–69] If the copper IUD is chosen, it can remain in place to provide ongoing, continuous, highly effective routine contraception.

Method of action

- The copper IUD works as EC by affecting sperm viability and function; if ovulation has occurred, then it may affect the oocyte and endometrium, inhibiting fertilization and implantation.[70]
- Ulipristal, an SPRM, has a direct inhibitory effect on follicular rupture, even if the luteinizing hormone (LH) surge has begun, and a dominant follicle has been chosen.[70]
- LNG, a progestin, delays or inhibits ovulation prior to the LH surge; it has no effects on the endometrium or on sperm function.[70]

Comparative effectiveness of each method

Table 4 shows the approximate risk of pregnancy with use of the various methods. Baseline risk of pregnancy after a single episode of UPI is approximately 3% to 10%[5–7] (depending on the fertile window). Copper IUD is by far the most effective of the EC methods, nearly eliminating the risk of pregnancy after placement.[8–10] Ulipristal is the second most effective method, with 1.4% of women becoming pregnant.[11] LNG and Yuzpe method have similar efficacy, with an absolute risk of pregnancy about 2%.[7,11,71] Of the hormonal methods, ulipristal has the advantage of equal effectiveness up to 5 days post-UPI until ovulation has occurred,[11] whereas LNG and the Yuzpe method have diminishing effectiveness over the 5 days after UPI.[63,72]

In studies, a higher pregnancy rate has been observed in obese women using hormonal EC.[73,74] The effect seems to be less pronounced for ulipristal than LNG.[74] In obese women, the copper IUD is the most efficacious choice for EC.

Box 5
Common adverse effects of hormonal emergency contraception

- Headache, fatigue, dizziness, back pain (LNG, Ulipristal, Yuzpe method)[63]
- Earlier-onset next menses (LNG)[72]
- Delay of next menses (Ulipristal)[72]
- Nausea and vomiting (Yuzpe method)[63]

Box 6
Tips for prescribing emergency contraception

- EC is appropriately discussed and prescribed in advance[64]
- Copper IUD is the most effective form of EC[9,10,63]
- Ulipristal is more effective than LNG[11]
- Obesity does not affect performance of the copper IUD[74]
- Obesity can decrease effectiveness of all hormonal forms of EC[73,74]
- The Yuzpe method is less favored due to significant nausea[63]

Box 7
When to start routine hormonal contraception after emergency contraception

- Barrier methods should always be used after EC until the next menstrual cycle; conception can occur from a second episode of unprotected intercourse in the same cycle[63]
- Routine contraception can be started or resumed immediately after LNG EC or the Yuzpe method[63]
- Routine hormonal contraception should not be initiated or resumed for at least 5 days after ulipristal, per updated FDA labeling; starting hormonal contraception immediately after ulipristal can interfere with ulipristal's ability to prevent pregnancy[67–69]

MENOPAUSE

By 2025, the number of postmenopausal women is expected to rise to 1.1 billion worldwide.[76] **Box 8** contains definitions of menopause.

The hallmark of the menopause transition is vasomotor symptoms (VMS) otherwise known as hot flashes and/or night sweats. New evidence suggest these symptoms are likely to last up to 7 years or longer for some women, and providers should counsel women about these symptoms.[77] Cigarette smoking, obesity, and increased age also correlate with increased number of VMS.[78] In the years following

---

Box 8
Definitions used in menopause

- Natural menopause: cessation of menses (amenorrhea) for 1 year, a retrospective diagnosis
- Induced menopause: cessation of menstruation after bilateral oophorectomy/iatrogenic ablation of ovarian function (radiation/chemotherapy)
- Menopause transition: course of time leading up the last menses (final menstrual period)
- Primary ovarian insufficiency: transient or permanent loss of ovarian function with amenorrhea in a woman less than 40 years old
- Laboratory: follicle-stimulating hormone (FSH) greater than 30 mIU/mL twice separated by at least 8 weeks

Adapted from Shifren JL, Gass MLS. The North American Menopause Society recommendations for clinical care of midlife women. Menopause 2014;21(10):1040.

Box 9
Common symptoms of menopause transition and post-menopause

- Vasomotor symptoms. Hot flashes and night sweats: sensation of heat, intense sweating and flushing affecting the face and chest lasting 1 to 5 minutes[79]

- GSM. Vulvovaginal atrophy manifesting as vaginal or vulvar dryness, discharge, itching, dyspareunia, vaginal bleeding and easy tearing; urinary symptoms: frequency, urgency and frequent urinary tract infections[80]

- Sleep disruption[81]

- Cognitive and mood changes, difficulty concentrating[81]

- Breast tenderness[81]

- Nonspecific complaints of headache, joint aches/stiffness, back pain[81]

---

menopause, chronic genitourinary symptoms related to low estrogen levels predominate.

Hot flashes are not well understood, but the predominant theory is that the thermoregulatory zone narrows with the decrease in estrogen, increasing the likelihood for the threshold for sweating or chills to be reached. Additionally, as estrogen levels drop, norepinephrine receptors in the brain increase. Noradrenergic and serotonin pathways are upregulated, which is thought to further narrow the thermoregulatory zone. These pathways have been the target for nonhormonal therapies in treatment of menopause symptoms.[79] **Box 9** further describes the symptoms of menopause transition.

Treatment of Menopause Symptoms

Treatment of menopause symptoms focus on the 2 most common concerns: vasomotor and genitourinary symptoms. ACOG, American Association of Clinical Endocrinologists (AACE), and North American Society of Menopause (NAMS) have agreed that the most effective treatment for moderate-to-severe hot flashes (usually >10/d, can be less if disabling to the patient) is hormonal therapy as long as there is not a contraindication.[46,82,83] **Table 2** lists contraindications of hormone therapy. The NAMS recently released a mobile application (MenoPro) available for iOS and Android users that goes through an algorithm to choose the best treatments for patients with vasomotor and/or GSM symptoms.[84] This includes the cardiovascular risk assessment which is important in calculating risk for estrogen therapy. No non-hormonal therapy has been equivalent to estrogen therapy with improving vasomotor symptoms.[85] **Table 5** lists the approximate equivalent doses of estrogen, with **Table 6**

Table 5
Approximate bioavailable equivalent estrogen doses for menopausal hormone therapy

Conjugated equine estrogen (CEE)	0.625 mg
Synthetic conjugated estrogen	0.625 mg
Micronized 17β-estradiol (E2)	1.0 mg
Ethinyl estradiol (commonly used in oral contraceptive pills)	0.005 mg–0.015 mg
Transdermal 17β-estradiol (E2) patch	0.05 mg

Data from Manson JE, Ames JM, Shapiro M, et al. Algorithm and mobile app for menopausal symptom management and hormonal/non-hormonal therapy decision making. Menopause 2015;22(3):252.

Table 6
Commonly prescribed hormonal therapy for vasomotor symptoms available in the United States

	Product	Ultralow Dose	Low Dose	Standard
Estrogen Alone				
Oral	Estrace (E2), Premarin (CEE), Generics available	E2 0.25 mg/d[a]	E2 0.5 mg/d CEE 0.3 mg/d	E2 1.0 mg/d CEE 0.625 mg/d Higher doses available
Transdermal	Various, generics available	E2 0.014md/d[a]	E2 0.025 mg/d	E2 0.0375 mg/d E2 0.05 mg/d
Vaginal Ring	Femring	—	—	E2 0.05–0.10 mg/d for 90 d use
Progestogen Products (added to estrogen to protect endometrium)				Dosing depends on number of days of use (low dose for daily use; higher dose if used for cyclic use: ie 10–14 d of the month)
Oral	Provera MPA (progestin) Prometrium micronized progesterone (in peanut oil) Generics available			2.5 mg, 5 mg, 10 mg 100 mg, 200 mg
Intrauterine system	Mirena[a] Skyla			20 µg/d 5 y use 6 µ/d 3 y use
Combination: Estrogen–Progestogen Products				
Oral Continuous –Cyclic	Premphase CEE + MPA			0.625 E + 5.0 mg P (separate tablets: E alone days 1–14/E + P days 15–28)
Oral Continuous-Combined	Prempro CEE + MPA Activella E2 + norethindrone acetate (P) Angeliq E2 + drospirenone (P) Generics available			0.3 or 0.4 mg E + 1.5 mg P daily 0.5 mg E + 0.1 P daily 1 mg E + 0.5 mg P daily Higher doses available
Oral Intermittent-Combined	Prefest E2 + norgestimate			1 mg E, 1mg E + 0.09 P (E alone for 3d, followed by E + P for 3d, repeated continuously)
Transdermal Combined	CombiPatch E2 + Norethindrone acetate (P) Climara Pro E2 + Levonorgestel (P)			0.05 mg E + 0.14 mg P twice weekly 0.045 mg E + 0.015 P once weekly
Combination: Other Estrogen-SERM Product				
Oral Estrogen + SERM	Duavee CEE + bazedoxifene (SERM)			0.45 E + 20 mg SERM daily

[a] Not FDA approved for the treatment of vasomotor symptoms.

Data from North American Menopause Society. Approved prescription products for menopausal symptoms in the United States and Canada. Available at: http://www.menopause.org/docs/default-source/2014/nams-ht-tables.pdf. Accessed March 4, 2016; with permission.

Box 10
Clinical pearls for treating women during the menopause transition and post-menopause with vasomotor symptoms

- Lifestyle modifications with cooling techniques is a reasonable first-line therapy; however evidence is poor or lacking for the benefit in moderate to severe hot flashes[82]
  - Dressing in layers
  - Keeping a fan and/or ice water handy
  - Avoiding triggers such as alcohol, spicy food, and hot foods or liquids
- Cardiovascular risk assessment (blood pressure and fasting lipid profile)
  - Women with cardiovascular disease risk greater than 10% should not receive hormonal therapy[82]
- Systemic hormone therapy should be not be used in women 10 years or more since menopause onset[82]
- Hormone therapy should be the lowest effective dose for the shortest amount of time
  - Current recommendation: 5 years maximum duration of therapy given increased risk for breast cancer seen in the Women's Health Initiative Trial[83]
- For women with an increased risk for breast cancer, via personal or family history, systemic hormone therapy is not recommended[82]
  - Breast cancer risk can be calculated here: http://www.cancer.gov/bcrisktool.
- For women with intact uterus, progesterone should be used (oral or IUD) to reduce risk of endometrial hyperplasia[86]
- Transdermal estrogen (with progesterone if uterus is present) should be used to reduce hepatic first-pass metabolism and risk for venous thromboembolism.[87]
- Adverse effects of hormonal therapy include breast tenderness, bloating, and uterine bleeding[85]
  - Lower dose may improve these, but reduce the relief of vasomotor symptoms.
- Clinicians can chose to start with standard versus low dosing and titrate to symptom control.[85]
- Monitoring of estrogen levels is not necessary; however, in those not seeing improvement in symptoms with increased doses, measurement of serum estradiol levels can be performed.
  - Serum target range: 40 to 100 pg/mL (from a study using transdermal estradiol).[85]
- Combination conjugated estrogen (CEE)+ bazedoxifene, a SERM (Duavee) has been approved by the FDA for the treatment of moderate-to-severe vasomotor symptoms for women with an intact uterus.
  - Reduced number and severity of hot flashes compared to placebo without an increase in breast density (as often seen with estrogen–progestin therapy), although its risk for breast cancer is unknown[88]
  - Higher rates of amenorrhea and reduced bleeding when compared with traditional hormone therapy[88]
  - Risk of VTE is similar to standard hormonal therapy[88]

---

listing commonly prescribed estrogen and progestin products. **Box 10** highlights clinical pearls for treatment of menopause symptoms. For women with contraindications to hormonal therapy or who wish to avoid hormones for other reasons, **Table 7** lists other pharmaceuticals with potential benefits for treatment of vasomotor symptoms.

Treatment of Genitourinary Syndrome of Menopause

Nonhormonal and hormonal topical treatments are effective for genitourinary symptoms after menopause (**Table 8** lists available treatments and dosages).[93] Mild GSM may respond well to vaginal lubricants or moisturizers, whereas more severe

Table 7
Nonhormonal treatment of vasomotor symptoms

Medication	Dose	Notes
Paroxetine salt (Brisdelle)[a]	7.5 mg/d	Reduction of 33%–67% compared to with placebo[89]
Other SSRI		
Citalopram	10–20 mg/d	Use with caution when also prescribing with tamoxifen therapy[90]; listed are starting doses can increase if effective[91]
Escitalopram	10–20 mg/d	
Fluoxetine	20–30 mg/d	
SNRIs		
Venlafaxine	37.5–150 mg/d	Reduction ranging from 25%–69% in hot flash frequency[90,92]
Desvenlafaxine	100–150 mg/d	
Clonidine	0.1 mg/d	Frequent side effects: dry mouth, constipation, drowsiness; be careful with rebound elevation in blood pressure[90]
Gabapentin	900 mg/d	Start with 300 mg at night, then increase to 600 mg at night, finally add additional separate 300 mg in the morning[90,92]

Abbreviations: SNRI, serotonin–norepinephrine reuptake inhibitors; SSRI, selective serotonin reuptake inhibitor.

[a] Only FDA-approved non-hormonal medication for the treatment of moderate-to-severe hot flashes.

GSM usually necessitates hormonal therapy for significant relief. Vaginal estrogen is the most commonly used hormonal therapy for GSM, but one oral SERM, ospemifene, has also been US Food and Drug Administration (FDA) approved for treatment of moderate-to-severe dyspareunia from menopause.

For women with a history of breast cancer, data are currently insufficient to ascertain the safety of local hormonal therapy for GSM. Use of low-dose vaginal estrogen results in a small rise in serum estradiol levels, more so with vaginal tablets than vaginal ring.[94,95] However, in a case–control trial, vaginal estrogen use was not associated with increased risk of recurrence of breast cancer in women treated with tamoxifen.[96] Ospemifene has not been studied in women with a history of breast cancer, although clinical trials to date in women without breast cancer have not observed adverse breast effects, and animal studies have demonstrated an antagonistic effect on breast cancer cells.[97]

In women without a history of breast cancer, systemic estrogen therapy can also treat GSM; however, it should only be used if moderate-to-severe vasomotor symptoms are also present. Additionally, 10% to 15% of women using systemic hormone therapy will still experience GSM symptoms, in which case Femring (E2 0.05 mg/d or 0.10 mg/d, a systemic dosing of hormone therapy) may improve symptoms of both.[85] Femring should be combined with a progestogen in a women with an intact uterus.

Low-dose vaginal estrogen does not necessitate a progestogen for women with a uterus. A postmenopasual woman with a uterus who experiences vaginal spotting or bleeding should undergo a transvaginal ultrasound and/or endometrial biopsy to evaluate for the possibility of endometrial hyperplasia or carcinoma, regardless of her history of hormone exposure.[93]

Vaginal conjugated equine estrogen (CEE) cream results in higher serum estrogen levels than vaginal estradiol tablets or ring, and may be more likely to cause adverse effects of uterine bleeding, breast pain, and perineal pain, as well as endometrial overstimulation.[94] Women appeared to favor the estradiol-releasing ring for ease of use and comfort.[94]

Table 8
Treatment of genitourinary syndrome of menopause

	Product-Trade Name	Dosage	Notes
OTC water-based vaginal lubricants	Astroglide K-Y Jelly Pre-Seed Slippery Stuff Liquid Silk	Use as needed	Reduces friction during sexual activity
OTC silicone-based vaginal lubricants	Astroglide X K-Y Intrigue Pink Pjur Eros	Use as needed	Reduces friction during sexual activity
Vaginal Moisturizers	Replens Vagisil Feminease K-Y SILK-E	Use as needed or daily	Reduce vaginal pH to premenopausal level if used daily
Vaginal Ring	Estring (17β Estradiol 2 mg total)	Ring releases 7.5 µg/d for 90 d	Also FDA approved for urinary urgency and dysuria (of note: systemic hormone therapy can increase urinary incontinence) Pro: convenience every 3 mo per use Con: placement requires dexterity and flexibility
Vaginal Cream	Estrace (17β Estradiol 0.1 mg active ingredient/gram) Premarin (conjugated estrogen 0.625 mg active ingredient/gram)	Initial: 2–4 g/d for 1–2 wk Maintenance: 1 g/1–3 times/wk For dyspareunia: 0.5 g/d for 21d then off 7d, or twice/wk	Pro: applied intravaginal (plastic applicator) as well as vestibular and vulvar tissue Con: Messy
Vaginal Tablet	Vagifem (10 µg Estradiol hemihydrate)	Initial: 1 tablet/d for 2 wk Maintenance: 1 tablet twice/wk	Pro: less messy then cream
Oral SERM	Osphena (ospemifene)	60 mg/d for the treatment of dyspareunia	Hot flashes increased in treatment group

Abbreviations: OTC, over the counter/nonprescription; VVA, Vulvovaginal atrophy.
Data from Kaunitz AM, Manson JE. Management of Menopausal Symptoms. Obstet Gynecol 2015;126(4):859–76; and Management of symptomatic vulvovaginal atrophy: 2013 position statement of The North American Menopause Society. Menopause 2013;20(9):888–902.

Contraception During the Menopause Transition

Although the absolute risk of pregnancy is lower during the menopause transition, unplanned pregnancy rates are higher and result in higher risk to both the mother and child with complications.[98] Although many women use permanent contraception such as sterilization during this point in their lives, those who do not should be counseled on effective methods. There is no contraception that is restricted solely on age.[45] The authors recommend reviewing the aforementioned contraceptive options and the CDC MEC based with patient's risks. For determining when women can discontinue the use of hormonal contraception, see **Box 11** for guidance.

Box 11
Indications to stop contraception

- IUD users: FSH $\geq$ 30 IU/L on 2 occasions 6 to 8 weeks apart, and amenorrhea

- CHC users age $\geq$50: FSH $\geq$30 IU/L on 2 occasions 6 to 8 weeks apart, checked $\geq$14 days after cessation of CHC while using a backup barrier method

- DMPA users age $\geq$50: FSH $\geq$30 IU/L on 2 occasions 90 days apart, checked on the day of injection

- Age 60, if CHCs still in use (not advised)

Adapted from Baldwin MK, Jensen JT. Contraception during the perimenopause. Maturitas 2013;76(3):240.

SUMMARY

In summary, women's health pharmaceutics focus on contraception and menopause treatment. Understanding the contraindications to hormone therapy in women of all ages, preferred doses and routes, and counseling women on adverse effects are paramount for the prescriber.

REFERENCES

1. Szilagyi A, Ghali MP. Pharmacological therapy of vascular malformations of the gastrointestinal tract. Can J Gastroenterol 2006;20(3):171–80.

2. Mandel FP, Geola FL, Lu JK, et al. Biologic effects of various doses of ethinyl estradiol in postmenopausal women. Obstet Gynecol 1982;59(6):673–9.

3. Grimes DA. Forgettable contraception. Contraception 2009;80(6):497–9.

4. Trussell J. Contraceptive failure in the United States. Contraception 2011;83(5): 397–404.

5. Li D, Wilcox AJ, Dunson DB. Benchmark pregnancy rates and the assessment of post-coital contraceptives: an update. Contraception 2015;91(4):344–9.

6. Wilcox AJ, Dunson DB, Weinberg CR, et al. Likelihood of conception with a single act of intercourse: providing benchmark rates for assessment of post-coital contraceptives. Contraception 2001;63(4):211–5.

7. Leung VWY, Soon JA, Levine M. Measuring and reporting of the treatment effect of hormonal emergency contraceptives. Pharmacotherapy 2012;32(3): 210–21.

8. Zhou L, Xiao B. Emergency contraception with Multiload Cu-375 SL IUD: a multicenter clinical trial. Contraception 2001;64(2):107–12.

9. Cleland K, Zhu H, Goldstuck N, et al. The efficacy of intrauterine devices for emergency contraception: a systematic review of 35 years of experience. Hum Reprod 2012;27(7):1994–2000.

10. Wu S, Godfrey EM, Wojdyla D, et al. Copper T380A intrauterine device for emergency contraception: a prospective, multicentre, cohort clinical trial. BJOG 2010; 117(10):1205–10.

11. Glasier AF, Cameron ST, Fine PM, et al. Ulipristal acetate versus levonorgestrel for emergency contraception: a randomised non-inferiority trial and meta-analysis. Lancet 2010;375(9714):555–62.

12. O'neil-Callahan M, Peipert JF, Zhao Q, et al. Twenty-four-month continuation of reversible contraception. Obstet Gynecol 2013;122(5):1083–91.

13. American College of Obstetricians and Gynecologists. ACOG Practice Bulletin No. 121: Long-acting reversible contraception: Implants and intrauterine devices. Obstet Gynecol 2011;118(1):184–96.

14. Winner B, Peipert JF, Zhao Q, et al. Effectiveness of long-acting reversible contraception. N Engl J Med 2012;366(21):1998–2007.

15. Wu JP, Pickle S. Extended use of the intrauterine device: a literature review and recommendations for clinical practice. Contraception 2014;89(6):495–503.

16. Bahamondes L, Brache V, Meirik O, et al. A 3-year multicentre randomized controlled trial of etonogestrel- and levonorgestrel-releasing contraceptive implants, with non-randomized matched copper-intrauterine device controls. Hum Reprod 2015;30(11):2527–38.

17. Modesto W, Bahamondes MV, Bahamondes L. A randomized clinical trial of the effect of intensive versus non-intensive counselling on discontinuation rates due to bleeding disturbances of three long-acting reversible contraceptives. Hum Reprod 2014;29(7):1393–9.

18. Branum AM, Jones J. Trends in long-acting reversible contraception use among U.S. women aged 15-44. NCHS Data Brief 2015;(188):1–8.

19. Pickle S, Wu J, Burbank-Schmitt E. Prevention of unintended pregnancy: a focus on long-acting reversible contraception. Prim Care 2014;41(2):239–60.

20. Goldstuck ND, Steyn PS. Intrauterine contraception after cesarean section and during lactation: a systematic review. Int J Womens Health 2013;5:811–8.

21. FDA Product. Intrauterine copper contraceptive. Available at: http://www.iodine.com/label/paragard-t-380a. Accessed November 29, 2015.

22. Sonalkar S, Kapp N. Intrauterine device insertion in the postpartum period: A systematic review. Eur J Contracept Reprod Health Care 2015;20(1):4–18.

23. MIRENA. Available at: http://www.accessdata.fda.gov/drugsatfda_docs/label/2008/021225s019lbl.pdf. Accessed November 22, 2015.

24. Nexplanon. Available at: https://www.merck.com/product/usa/pi_circulars/n/nexplanon/nexplanon_pi.pdf. Accessed November 22, 2015.

25. Lopez LM, Grey TW, Stuebe AM, et al. Combined hormonal versus nonhormonal versus progestin-only contraception in lactation. Cochrane Database Syst Rev 2015;(3). CD003988. John Wiley & Sons, Ltd. Available at: http://onlinelibrary.wiley.com/doi/10.1002/14651858.CD003988.pub2/abstract. Accessed November 25, 2015.

26. Stoddard AM, Xu H, Madden T, et al. Fertility after intrauterine device removal: a pilot study. Eur J Contracept Reprod Health Care 2015;20(3):223–30.

27. Bhatia P, Nangia S, Aggarwal S, et al. Implanon: subdermal single rod contraceptive implant. J Obstet Gynaecol India 2011;61(4):422–5.

28. Lopez LM, Edelman A, Chen M, et al. Progestin-only contraceptives: effects on weight. Cochrane Database Syst Rev 2013;(7):CD008815.

29. Lopez LM, Chen M, Mullins Long S, et al. Steroidal contraceptives and bone fractures in women: evidence from observational studies. Cochrane Database Syst Rev 2015;(7). CD009849. John Wiley & Sons, Ltd. Available at: http://onlinelibrary.wiley.com/doi/10.1002/14651858.CD009849.pub3/abstract. Accessed November 25, 2015.

30. Miller L, Verhoeven CHJ, Hout JI. Extended regimens of the contraceptive vaginal ring: a randomized trial. Obstet Gynecol 2005;106(3):473–82.

31. Sulak PJ, Smith V, Coffee A, et al. Frequency and management of breakthrough bleeding with continuous use of the transvaginal contraceptive ring: a randomized controlled trial. Obstet Gynecol 2008;112(3):563–71.

32. Barreiros FA, Guazzelli CAF, Barbosa R, et al. Extended regimens of the combined contraceptive vaginal ring containing etonogestrel and ethinyl estradiol: effects on lipid metabolism. Contraception 2011;84(2):155–9.

33. de Bastos M, Stegeman BH, Rosendaal FR, et al. Combined oral contraceptives: venous thrombosis. Cochrane Database Syst Rev 2014;(3):CD010813.

34. Gierisch JM, Coeytaux RR, Urrutia RP, et al. Oral contraceptive use and risk of breast, cervical, colorectal, and endometrial cancers: a systematic review. Cancer Epidemiol Biomarkers Prev 2013;22(11):1931–43.

35. Arowojolu AO, Gallo MF, Lopez LM, et al. Combined oral contraceptive pills for treatment of acne. Cochrane Database Syst Rev 2012;(7). CD004425. John Wiley & Sons, Ltd. Available at: http://onlinelibrary.wiley.com/doi/10.1002/14651858.CD004425.pub6/abstract. Accessed November 25, 2015.

36. Wong CL, Farquhar C, Roberts H, et al. Oral contraceptive pill as treatment for primary dysmenorrhoea. Cochrane Database Syst Rev 2009;(2):CD002120.

37. Osayande AS, Mehulic S. Diagnosis and initial management of dysmenorrhea. Am Fam Physician 2014;89(5):341–6.

38. Harada T, Momoeda M, Terakawa N, et al. Evaluation of a low-dose oral contraceptive pill for primary dysmenorrhea: a placebo-controlled, double-blind, randomized trial. Fertil Steril 2011;95(6):1928–31.

39. Rosenberg MJ, Waugh MS. Oral contraceptive discontinuation: a prospective evaluation of frequency and reasons. Am J Obstet Gynecol 1998;179(3 Pt 1):577–82.

40. Gallo MF, Lopez LM, Grimes DA, et al. Combination contraceptives: effects on weight. Cochrane Database Syst Rev 2014;(1):CD003987.

41. Loder EW, Buse DC, Golub JR. Headache as a side effect of combination estrogen-progestin oral contraceptives: a systematic review. Am J Obstet Gynecol 2005;193(3 Pt 1):636–49.

42. Shahnazi M, Farshbaf Khalili A, Ranjbar Kochaksaraei F, et al. A comparison of second and third generations combined oral contraceptive pills' effect on mood. Iran Red Crescent Med J 2014;16(8):e13628.

43. Tricotel A, Raguideau F, Collin C, et al. Estimate of venous thromboembolism and related-deaths attributable to the use of combined oral contraceptives in France. PLoS One 2014;9(4):e93792.

44. Lidegaard Ø, Løkkegaard E, Jensen A, et al. Thrombotic Stroke and Myocardial Infarction with Hormonal Contraception. N Engl J Med 2012;366(24):2257–66.

45. Centers for Disease Control and Prevention (CDC). U S. Medical Eligibility Criteria for Contraceptive Use, 2010. MMWR Recomm Rep 2010;59(RR-4):1–86.

46. Goodman N, Cobin R, Ginzburg S, et al. American Association of Clinical Endocrinologists medical guidelines for clinical practice for the diagnosis and treatment of menopause. Endocr Pract 2011;17(Suppl 6):1–25.

47. Hannaford PC, Selvaraj S, Elliott AM, et al. Cancer risk among users of oral contraceptives: cohort data from the Royal College of General Practitioner's oral contraception study. BMJ 2007;335(7621):651.
48. Division of Reproductive Health, National Center for Chronic Disease Prevention and Health Promotion, Centers for Disease Control and Prevention (CDC). U.S. Selected Practice Recommendations for Contraceptive Use, 2013: adapted from the World Health Organization selected practice recommendations for contraceptive use, 2nd edition. MMWR Recomm Rep 2013;62(RR-05):1–60.
49. Yu J, Hu XH. Inappropriate use of combined hormonal contraceptives for birth control among women of reproductive age in the United States. J Womens Health 2013;22(7):595–603.
50. Machado RB, Morimoto M, Santana N, et al. Effect of information on the perception of users and prospective users of combined oral contraceptives regarding the risk of venous thromboembolism. Gynecol Endocrinol 2015;31(1):57–60.
51. Deviveni D, Skee D, Vaccaro N, et al. Pharmacokinetics and pharmacodynamics of a transdermal contraceptive patch and an oral contraceptive. J Clin Pharmacol 2007;47(4):497–509.
52. Ethinylestradiol + etonogestrel contraceptive vaginal ring: new drug. Possibly useful in some situations. Prescrire Int 2006;15(82):50–3.
53. Plu-Bureau G, Maitrot-Mantelet L, Hugon-Rodin J, et al. Hormonal contraceptives and venous thromboembolism: an epidemiological update. Best Pract Res Clin Endocrinol Metab 2013;27(1):25–34.
54. Jick SS, Hagberg KW, Kaye JA. ORTHO EVRA and venous thromboembolism: an update. Contraception 2010;81(5):452–3.
55. Jick SS, Hagberg KW, Hernandez RK, et al. Postmarketing study of ORTHO EVRA and levonorgestrel oral contraceptives containing hormonal contraceptives with 30 μg of ethinyl estradiol in relation to nonfatal venous thromboembolism. Contraception 2010;81(1):16–21.
56. Jick SS, Kaye JA, Russmann S, et al. Risk of nonfatal venous thromboembolism in women using a contraceptive transdermal patch and oral contraceptives containing norgestimate and 35 microg of ethinyl estradiol. Contraception 2006;73(3):223–8.
57. Lopez LM, Grimes DA, Gallo MF, et al. Skin patch and vaginal ring versus combined oral contraceptives for contraception. Cochrane Database Syst Rev 2013;(4):CD003552.
58. Van Vliet HAAM, Grimes DA, Lopez LM, et al. Triphasic versus monophasic oral contraceptives for contraception. Cochrane Database Syst Rev 2011;(11):CD003553.
59. Gallo MF, Nanda K, Grimes DA, et al. 20 μg versus >20 μg estrogen combined oral contraceptives for contraception. Cochrane Database Syst Rev 2013;(8):CD003989.
60. Katsambas AD, Dessinioti C. Hormonal therapy for acne: why not as first line therapy? facts and controversies. Clin Dermatol 2010;28(1):17–23.
61. ACOG Practice Bulletin No. 110: noncontraceptive uses of hormonal contraceptives. Obstet Gynecol 2010;115(1):206–18.
62. Foster DG, Harper CC, Bley JJ, et al. Knowledge of emergency contraception among women aged 18 to 44 in California. Am J Obstet Gynecol 2004;191(1):150–6.
63. Practice Bulletin No. 152: Emergency Contraception. Obstet Gynecol 2015;126(3):e1–11.
64. Gavin L, Moskosky S, Carter M, et al. Providing quality family planning services: Recommendations of CDC and the U.S. Office of Population Affairs. MMWR Recomm Rep 2014;63(RR-04):1–54.

65. Rodriguez MI, Curtis KM, Gaffield ML, et al. Advance supply of emergency contraception: a systematic review. Contraception 2013;87(5):590–601.

66. Westhoff C, Kerns J, Morroni C, et al. Quick start: novel oral contraceptive initiation method. Contraception 2002;66(3):141–5.

67. Brache V, Cochon L, Duijkers IJM, et al. A prospective, randomized, pharmacodynamic study of quick-starting a desogestrel progestin-only pill following ulipristal acetate for emergency contraception. Hum Reprod 2015;30(12):2785–93.

68. Glasier A. Starting hormonal contraception after using emergency contraception: what should we recommend? Hum Reprod 2015;30(12):2708–10.

69. ELLA (Ulipristal tablet). Available at: http://www.accessdata.fda.gov/drugsatfda_docs/label/2015/022474s007lbl.pdf. Accessed November 29, 2015.

70. Gemzell-Danielsson K, Berger C, Lalitkumar PG. Mechanisms of action of oral emergency contraception. Gynecol Endocrinol 2014;30(10):685–7.

71. Trussell J, Rodríguez G, Ellertson C. New estimates of the effectiveness of the Yuzpe regimen of emergency contraception. Contraception 1998;57(6):363–9.

72. Cheng L, Che Y, Gulmezoglu AM. Interventions for emergency contraception. Cochrane Database Syst Rev 2012;(8):CD001324.

73. Kapp N, Abitbol JL, Mathé H, et al. Effect of body weight and BMI on the efficacy of levonorgestrel emergency contraception. Contraception 2015;91(2):97–104.

74. Glasier A, Cameron ST, Blithe D, et al. Can we identify women at risk of pregnancy despite using emergency contraception? Data from randomized trials of ulipristal acetate and levonorgestrel. Contraception 2011;84(4):363–7.

75. American College of Obstetricians and Gynecologists. ACOG Practice Bulletin No. 112: Emergency contraception. Obstet Gynecol 2010;115(5):1100–9.

76. Shifren JL, Gass MLS. The North American Menopause Society Recommendations for Clinical Care of Midlife Women. Menopause 2014;21(10):1038–62.

77. Avis NE, Crawford SL, Greendale G, et al. Duration of Menopausal Vasomotor Symptoms Over the Menopause Transition. JAMA Intern Med 2015;175(4):531–9.

78. Gold EB, Colvin A, Avis N, et al. Longitudinal Analysis of the Association Between Vasomotor Symptoms and Race/Ethnicity Across the Menopausal Transition: Study of Women's Health Across the Nation. Am J Public Health 2006;96(7):1226–35.

79. Morrow PKH, Mattair DN, Hortobagyi GN. Hot flashes: a review of pathophysiology and treatment modalities. Oncologist 2011;16(11):1658–64.

80. Portman DJ, Gass MLS, Vulvovaginal Atrophy Terminology Consensus Conference Panel. Genitourinary syndrome of menopause: new terminology for vulvovaginal atrophy from the International Society for the Study of Women's Sexual Health and the North American Menopause Society. Menopause 2014;21(10):1063–8.

81. Hale GE, Robertson DM, Burger HG. The perimenopausal woman: Endocrinology and management. J Steroid Biochem Mol Biol 2014;142:121–31.

82. North American Menopause Society. The 2012 hormone therapy position statement of: The North American Menopause Society. Menopause 2012;19(3):257–71.

83. ACOG Practice Bulletin No. 141: Management of Menopausal Symptoms. Obstet Gynecol 2014;123(1):202–16.

84. Manson JE, Ames JM, Shapiro M, et al. Algorithm and mobile app for menopausal symptom management and hormonal/non-hormonal therapy decision making: a clinical decision-support tool from The North American Menopause Society. Menopause 2015;22(3):247–53.

85. Kaunitz AM, Manson JE. Management of Menopausal Symptoms. Obstet Gynecol 2015;126(4):859–76.
86. Furness S, Roberts H, Marjoribanks J, et al. Hormone therapy in postmenopausal women and risk of endometrial hyperplasia. Cochrane Database Syst Rev 2012;(8). CD000402. John Wiley & Sons, Ltd. Available at: http://onlinelibrary. wiley.com.ezproxy.library.wisc.edu/doi/10.1002/14651858.CD000402.pub4/abstract. Accessed October 29, 2015.
87. Corbelli J, Shaikh N, Wessel C, et al. Low-dose transdermal estradiol for vasomotor symptoms: a systematic review. Menopause 2015;22(1):114–21.
88. Palacios S, Currie H, Mikkola TS, et al. Perspective on prescribing conjugated estrogens/bazedoxifene for estrogen-deficiency symptoms of menopause: A practical guide. Maturitas 2015;80(4):435–40.
89. Carroll DG, Lisenby KM, Carter TL. Critical appraisal of paroxetine for the treatment of vasomotor symptoms. Int J Womens Health 2015;7:615–24.
90. Nelson HD, Vesco KK, Haney E, et al. Nonhormonal therapies for menopausal hot flashes: systematic review and meta-analysis. JAMA 2006;295(17):2057–71.
91. Krause MS, Nakajima ST. Hormonal and nonhormonal treatment of vasomotor symptoms. Obstet Gynecol Clin North A 2015;42(1):163–79.
92. Nonhormonal management of menopause-associated vasomotor symptoms: 2015 position statement of The North American Menopause Society. Menopause 2015;22(11):1155–74.
93. Management of symptomatic vulvovaginal atrophy: 2013 position statement of The North American Menopause Society. Menopause 2013;20(9):888–902.
94. Suckling JA, Kennedy R, Lethaby A, et al. Local oestrogen for vaginal atrophy in postmenopausal women. Cochrane Database Syst Rev 2006;(4). CD001500. John Wiley & Sons, Ltd. Available at: http://onlinelibrary.wiley.com.ezproxy. library.wisc.edu/doi/10.1002/14651858.CD001500.pub2/abstract.   Accessed October 29, 2015.
95. Simmons CE, Kuchuk I, Freedman OC, et al. Are Estring® and Vagifem® equally effective and safe for the treatment of urogenital atrophy in breast cancer patients on aromatase inhibitor therapy? Clin Oncol (R Coll Radiol) 2012;24(8):e128–9.
96. Le Ray I, Dell'Aniello S, Bonnetain F, et al. Local estrogen therapy and risk of breast cancer recurrence among hormone-treated patients: a nested case-control study. Breast Cancer Res Treat 2012;135(2):603–9.
97. Berga SL. Profile of ospemifene in the breast. Reprod Sci 2013;20(10):1130–6.
98. Baldwin MK, Jensen JT. Contraception during the perimenopause. Maturitas 2013;76(3):235–42.

Pharmacologic Therapy in Men's Health

Hypogonadism, Erectile Dysfunction, and Benign Prostatic Hyperplasia

Kathryn E. Berkseth, MD[a],*, Arthi Thirumalai, MBBS[b],
John K. Amory, MD, MPH[c]

KEYWORDS

- Male hypogonadism • Erectile dysfunction (ED) • Benign prostatic hyperplasia (BPH)
- Pharmacologic treatment

KEY POINTS

- Injectable and transdermal preparations of testosterone are the most widely used in clinical practice. Alternative testosterone preparations, including subcutaneous pellets, buccal, and nasal preparations, can be considered for patients in whom injectable or transdermal preparations are ineffective or poorly tolerated.
- Oral phosphodiesterase inhibitors are initial pharmacotherapy for erectile dysfunction. Intraurethral or intrapenile alprostadil can be used for men who do not have a satisfactory response to oral medications.
- Alpha1-adrenergic antagonists are first-line therapy for benign prostatic hyperplasia. 5-Alpha-reductase inhibitors are useful in men with large prostate glands or those unable to tolerate alpha1-adrenergic antagonists.

INTRODUCTION

Male reproductive, sexual, and urologic health concerns are common presenting complaints in both primary care and subspecialty clinic settings. This article reviews current pharmacologic treatment options for 3 common men's health concerns: hypogonadism, erectile dysfunction (ED), and benign prostatic hyperplasia (BPH).

Disclosure Statement: The authors have nothing to disclose.
[a] Division of Metabolism, Endocrinology and Nutrition, Department of Medicine, University of Washington, 1959 Northeast Pacific Street, Box 356426, Seattle, WA 98195, USA; [b] Division of Metabolism, Endocrinology and Nutrition, Department of Medicine, University of Washington, 1959 Northeast Pacific Street, HSB C-209, UW Box# 357138, Seattle, WA 98195, USA; [c] Department of Medicine, University of Washington, 4245 Roosevelt Way Northeast, Box #354760, Seattle, WA 98105, USA
* Corresponding author.
E-mail address: keberks@uw.edu

Med Clin N Am 100 (2016) 791–805
http://dx.doi.org/10.1016/j.mcna.2016.03.006
0025-7125/16/$ – see front matter © 2016 Elsevier Inc. All rights reserved.
medical.theclinics.com

TESTOSTERONE REPLACEMENT THERAPY IN MALE HYPOGONADISM

Male hypogonadism, defined as signs and symptoms of low testosterone combined with confirmation of low serum testosterone concentration, is estimated to affect 2% to 12.8% of adult men.[1] The prevalence of hypogonadism is higher among certain populations, including the elderly and the obese. It is anticipated that the prevalence of male hypogonadism in the United States will likely increase over the coming years due to a combination of factors, including the aging of the population and increases in co-morbid conditions associated with increased risk of hypogonadism such as obesity and diabetes.[1] The evaluation and diagnosis of male hypogonadism are reviewed elsewhere.[2] Here we will focus treatment using testosterone replacement therapy.

Benefits, Side Effects, and Risks

Among men with symptomatic hypogonadism, the potential clinical benefits of testosterone replacement therapy include increased libido, improved muscle strength, improved body composition (eg, decreased fat mass and increased lean mass), maintenance or improvement in bone mineral density, improved mood and cognition, improved erectile function, and maintenance or improvement in secondary sexual characteristics.[2]

The potential clinical benefits must be carefully weighed against potential risks for each patient. Potential adverse effects of testosterone replacement include erythrocytosis, increases in prostate-specific antigen (PSA), and worsening of prostate disorders (eg, BPH symptoms), worsening of existing obstructive sleep apnea, and dermatologic effects such as acne and skin irritation.[2] Testosterone replacement therapy is not appropriate for hypogonadal men who desire fertility because testosterone suppresses luteinizing hormone production and thus can reduce spermatogenesis by lowering intratesticular testosterone concentration.[3]

In addition, the US Food and Drug Administration (FDA) recently added a warning to all testosterone preparations regarding possible increased risk of cardiovascular disease, including myocardial infarction and stroke in patients taking testosterone. Ongoing studies are attempting to better assess this risk. At this time, clinicians in practice should discuss this warning with all patients when starting or continuing testosterone treatment.[4,5]

Testosterone Preparations

There are a variety of testosterone preparations currently available in the United States (**Table 1**). The choice of preparation should be determined by the clinician in conversation with each individual patient and should take into consideration patient preference as well as cost and convenience. The most widely used testosterone preparations in the United States are transdermal and injectable preparations due to their ease of use (transdermal) and relatively low cost (injectable).

Injectable preparations

Testosterone enanthate and testosterone cypionate are widely used long-acting injectable testosterone preparations.[6,7] Both forms are administered as intramuscular (IM) injections and most patients are able to administer injections independently at home with the help of a partner. These preparations are highly effective in improving symptoms of hypogonadism and maintaining virilization. In addition, the long-acting preparation allows most men to administer IM injections every 2 weeks (instead of the daily application of a transdermal preparation). With long-acting IM preparations, testosterone concentration and clinical effects (eg, impacts on mood and libido) peak around 1 to 2 days after the injection and wane over the subsequent 2 weeks.[8] For

Table 1
Testosterone preparations

Formulation	Preparation (US Tradename)	Dosage Forms	Usual Dosing[a]	Site of Application	Advantages	Disadvantages and Risks	Approximate Cost per Month[b]
Intramuscular							
Long-acting	Testosterone cypionate (Depo-Testosterone)	100 mg/mL or 200 mg/mL	100–200 mg every 2 wk or 50–100 mg every 1 wk	Thigh or buttock	Home IM injection, infrequent treatment, low cost, high efficacy	Peak effects or fluctuating testosterone levels, pain or irritation at injection site	$15–60 (generic) $50–70 (brand)
	Testosterone enanthate (Delatestryl)	200 mg/mL					$15–35 (generic) $45–50 (brand)
Extra–long-acting	Testosterone undecanoate (Aveed)	250 mg/mL	750 mg initially, then 750 mg at 4 wk, then 750 mg every 10 wk ongoing	Buttock	Long-acting	Administered in office or hospital by REMS-certified provider, risk of pulmonary oil microembolism and anaphylaxis	$1050 (plus cost of injection)

(continued on next page)

Table 1
(continued)

Formulation	Preparation (US Tradename)	Dosage Forms	Usual Dosing[a]	Site of Application	Advantages	Disadvantages and Risks	Approximate Cost per Month[b]
Transdermal							
Gels	Androgel (1% gel) Testim (1% gel)	25 mg in 2.5 g packet OR 50 mg in 5 g packet 50 mg in 5 g packet	50–100 mg daily	Dry intact skin or back, abdomen, upper thighs or arm	Steady serum testosterone concentration	Risk of transfer, requires daily application, may not achieve normal testosterone levels in all men, occasional skin irritation	$175–400 (generic) $500–525 (brand) $160–320 (generic) $480–520 (brand)
	Androgel (1.62% gel)	20.25 mg in 1.25 g packet 40.5 mg in 2.5 g packet 20.25 mg per actuation, metered-dose pump	20.25–81 mg daily				$480–550 (brand only)
	Fortesta (2% gel)	10 mg per actuation, metered-dose pump	10–70 mg daily	Dry intact skin of front and inner thighs	Ease of application		$160–400
	Axiron (2% solution)	30 mg per actuation, metered-dose pump	30–120 mg daily	Dry, intact skin of axilla	Ease of application, reduced risk for transfer		$260–1200
Patch	Androderm	2 mg/24 h patch 4 mg/24 h patch	2–6 mg daily	Dry intact skin of arm or torso	Limited risk of transfer, no injection	Skin irritation or rash (about 1/3 of men), daily application	$475–510

Other

Route	Brand	Formulation	Usual dose	Administration	Advantages	Disadvantages	Cost
Implanted Subcutaneous Pellet	Testopel	75 mg pellets	150–450 mg every 3–6 mo	Implanted into subcutaneous fat of buttock, lower abdominal wall or thigh	No risk of transfer, no daily treatment	Extrusion, infection, fibrosis at pellet sites Placed in clinic or hospital by trained provider under sterile conditions	$150–175 (plus cost of pellet placement) cost estimate based on dose 150 mg mg every 3 mo
Nasal	Natesto	5.5 mg per actuation, metered-dose pump applicator	11 mg (2 pumps, 1 in each nostril) 3 times daily	Intranasal	Minimal risk of transfer	Frequent administration, rhinorrhea, epistaxis, sinusitis, nasal scab	$600–700
Buccal	Striant SR	30 mg buccal system	30 mg twice daily	Adhere to depression in the gingiva superior to upper incisors	No injection	Frequent administration, gingival irritation	$550–600
Oral	Generally not recommended						

Abbreviations: IM, intramuscular; REMS, Risk Evaluation and Mitigation Strategy.

ª Usual doses are listed but dosing should be adjusted based on specific patient factors and clinician judgment.

ᵇ Cost data based on average cost purchasing monthly supply, various suppliers as listed on goodrx.com at the time of publication and estimated costs at University of Washington Medical Center for facility administered testosterone undecanoate and Testopel.

some patients, these fluctuations in testosterone effect are particularly bothersome. In these cases, alternate dosing of 100 mg every week or use of an alternate testosterone preparation may be preferred.

An extra–long-acting IM testosterone preparation, testosterone undecanoate, has also recently been approved for use in the United States. This preparation is administered as a deep IM injection at baseline, 4 weeks, and then every 10 weeks. This preparation reduces the frequency of IM injection. However, due to risk of pulmonary oil microembolism and anaphylaxis, the drug is only available through a Risk Evaluation and Mitigation Strategy (REMS) program and must be administered by a trained and registered care provider in an office or hospital setting. Thus, this formulation is not recommended unless patients are unable to tolerate or access other available preparations.

Transdermal preparations
There are several transdermal gels currently available in the United States, including Androgel, Testim, Fortesta, and Axiron. Gels are supplied in packets or tubes or in a metered-dose pump and are applied by hand to dry, intact skin on the arms, torso, or thighs. They should not be applied to the scrotum. Gels are generally well-tolerated. They offer the benefit of minimal fluctuation in testosterone concentration from day to day and may be preferable for patients who struggle with peak effects from IM injections. They are occasionally associated with mild skin irritation. Use of gels is limited by the potential for skin-to-skin transfer to others and patients should be instructed to limit this risk by carefully washing their hands after gel application and avoiding skin-to-skin contact with others (particularly female partners or children) on the gel-treated areas.[9] Additionally, some men do not achieve normal testosterone concentrations due to poor absorption of topical applications and monitoring of serum testosterone concentration is important to confirm adequate dosing with these preparations.

One testosterone patch preparation (Androderm) is currently available in the United States. The patch reduces the risk of skin-to-skin transfer of testosterone and is preferable for some patients. However, up to one-third of men who use the patch may have significant rash or skin irritation preventing its ongoing use. Patches should not be applied to the scrotum. Monitoring of testosterone concentration is also important with transdermal patches because absorption can be variable similarly to gel preparations.

Other available preparations
One preparation of subcutaneous testosterone pellet is currently available (Testopel).[10] Pellets are placed in the subcutaneous fat of the buttock, lower abdomen, or thigh every 3 to 6 months. Pellets are placed in sterile conditions in an office or hospital setting. They are associated with risks, including infection, fibrosis, and pellet extrusion. Benefits include avoiding skin-to-skin transfer, no need for self-injection, and infrequent dosing.

Nasal and buccal testosterone preparations are also available. These preparations are infrequently used due to limitations of nasal, sinus, or gingival irritation. In addition, there are limited published data on use of nasal preparation and animal studies suggest possible increases in central nervous system testosterone levels higher than that expected with other preparations.

Oral preparations of testosterone (eg, methyltestosterone) have been available for many years. However, use of these preparations for treatment of male hypogonadism is not recommended because of concerns about possible lack of efficacy in producing virilization, reports of hepatic toxicity with these drugs,[11] and the wide availability of more preferred preparations.

Monitoring and Dose Adjustment

Patients on testosterone replacement therapy should be followed to assess improvement in hypogonadal symptoms and to achieve serum testosterone concentrations in the normal reference range. Among patients being treated with testosterone cypionate or enanthate IM injection every 2 weeks, the clinician should target testosterone levels in the middle to normal range (400–700 ng/dL) 1 week after the last injection.[2] Generally, patients should be seen back approximately 3 months after starting or changing a testosterone dose for clinical assessment; testosterone serum concentration monitoring; if needed; and monitoring of hematocrit and PSA. Once on stable treatment, continued clinical and laboratory follow-up every 6 to 12 months is recommended.[2]

Various formulations of testosterone are available and choice of treatment formulation should be based on discussion of risks and benefits between the provider and each patient. Injectable and transdermal preparations of testosterone are the most widely used in clinical practice and are generally effective and well-tolerated. Alternative testosterone preparations, including subcutaneous testosterone pellets, buccal, and nasal preparations can be considered for patients in whom injectable or transdermal preparations are ineffective or poorly tolerated.

PHARMACOLOGIC TREATMENT OF ERECTILE DYSFUNCTION
Erectile Dysfunction

ED is defined as the inability to achieve and maintain an erection sufficient for intercourse. ED is a common complaint of sexually active men, with a lifetime prevalence of 70%.[12] ED is commonly associated with systemic disorders such as hypertension, diabetes, coronary artery disease, or harmful behaviors such as tobacco or drug use. Other factors that can cause ED include neurologic diseases, hypogonadism, mood disorders, and medications. In addition, the prevalence of ED increases significantly with age, such that most men in their 80s have ED and require treatment if they wish to remain sexually active.[13] Fortunately, there are many efficacious therapies for the treatment of ED in men. Indeed, with current therapies, most men can be successfully treated for ED using 1 of the following therapies.

Approach to Erectile Dysfunction

Before an ED medication is prescribed, it is useful to review the patient's symptoms, sexual frequency, and erectile function. In particular, low libido may be a sign of underlying hypogonadism, which would trigger a measurement of a morning serum total testosterone concentration and possible treatment with testosterone. In addition, several common medications can adversely affect sexual function, including antihypertensives, antidepressants, antipsychotics, antiandrogens (eg, spironolactone and cimetidine), and opiates. Often, ED can be improved by substitution of 1 of these medications for another that is less likely to interfere with erectile function. For example, selective serotonin reuptake inhibitors commonly impair sexual function, both in terms of ED and anorgasmia. Alternative antidepressants, such as bupropion and venlafaxine are associated with a lower incidence of sexual side effects and may result in improvement in symptoms of ED.[14]

Other important historical clues include prior pelvic surgery or the rapid loss of an erection soon after the initiation of sexual activity, which might suggest either anxiety or a venous leak. On physical examination, evidence of neuropathy or testicular atrophy would suggest systemic disease such as diabetes or hypogonadism. Treating men with low serum testosterone concentrations is likely to improve libido and erectile function, as well as improve muscle and bone density, and is reasonable in patients with truly low serum testosterone. If these approaches to treatment do not result in satisfactory improvement in symptoms, it is reasonable to suggest specific treatment of ED with 1 of the following medications.

Oral Phosphodiesterase Inhibitors

Treatment of ED with as-needed oral phosphodiesterase-5 inhibitors (**Table 2**) is recommended as initial therapy for ED because these agents are relatively safe, easy to administer, and have a high likelihood of greatly improving symptoms of ED in most men. Phosphodiesterase inhibitors improve erectile function by increasing the production of nitric oxide in the corpora cavernosum, resulting in increased penile blood flow and improved erectile function. The 4 currently available phosphodiesterase-5 inhibitors have some minor differences in terms of their half-life and dosing. In particular, tadalafil has the longest half-life and excellent bioavailability. Therefore, tadalafil can be dosed with food in contrast to sildenafil and vardenafil, which require dosing on an empty stomach 30 to 60 minutes before intercourse.[15] Tadalafil can also be dosed daily at lower doses for men who do not respond to as-needed treatment with some improvement in overall efficacy.[16]

Oral phosphodiesterase inhibitors are contraindicated in men taking nitrates, such as nitroglycerin, because severe hypotension can develop. Similarly, caution should be exercised when combining these medications with alpha-adrenergic antagonists, especially older nonselective alpha-antagonists prescribed for the treatment of prostatic hyperplasia. Because of the potential for hypotension from the combination of alpha-adrenergic antagonists and oral phosphodiesterase inhibitors, it is frequently recommended that the initial dose of a phosphodiesterase inhibitor be reduced by half, then the dose increased slowly from there to the minimum required for an erection sufficient for intercourse. In addition, switching from a nonselective alpha antagonist, to an alpha1 selective antagonist (see later discussion) in men receiving both therapies is recommended.[17] Common side effects of these medications include headaches, dyspepsia, diarrhea, epistaxis, and a blue tinge to vision (with sildenafil). In addition, all of these medications are metabolized by CYP3A4, so coadministration of any of the phosphodiesterase-5 inhibitors with a CYP3A4 inhibitor results in increased drug concentrations, which could increase the risk of side effects such as hypotension.

Other Oral Medications for Erectile Dysfunction

The antidepressant trazadone has been reported to benefit some men with ED and is occasionally prescribed in men with mild depression and ED for a double effect. Side effects of this medication include dizziness, sedation, and weight gain. In addition, priapism has been rarely reported with this medication.[18] Therefore, men should be counseled to seek medical attention for erections that last more than 4 hours while taking this medication. Finally, yohimbine is occasionally prescribed for ED in the setting of low libido in men with a normal testosterone, although the data supporting this indication are not strong[19] and this medication is not currently approved by the FDA for the treatment of ED. Side effects with yohimbine are frequent and can include potentially serious increases in blood pressure and heart rate. Yohimbine is a common ingredient in nonprescription dietary supplements marketed for sexual potency, so eliciting a history of supplement use in patients with ED may reveal exposure to this drug.

Intraurethral and Intrapenile Alprostadil

Alprostadil (prostaglandin E1) is a direct vasodilator that relaxes vascular smooth muscle to increase blood flow in the penis and results in an erection sufficient for

Table 2
Medications for the treatment of erectile dysfunction

Drug Name	Tradename	Dose Range	Side Effects	Notes
Oral				
Sildenafil	Viagra	25–100 mg as needed	Headaches, dyspepsia, hypotension, rhinitis, visual disturbance (ie, Viagra)	Avoid coadministration with nitrates & alpha-antagonists
Vardenafil	Levitra	5–20 mg as needed		Use with caution in liver & kidney dysfunction
Tadalafil	Cialis	10–20 mg as needed or 2.5–5 mg daily		Avoid strong CYP3A4 inhibitors
Avanafil	Stendra	50–200 mg as needed		
Trazadone	Desyrel	50–300 mg each night, orally	Sedation, dizziness, weight gain, priapism	Potential for QTc prolongation Less potent than PDE-5 inhibitors
Intraurethral Pellet				
Alprostadil	Muse	125–1000 mcg	Vasodilatation, penile pain, priapism	Can be used twice daily Avoid in hematological disease
Intrapenile Injections				
Alprostadil	Caverject, Edex	5–40 mcg	Injection site pain, priapism	Max use 3 times weekly, and once in 24 h Avoid in anticoagulated patient

Abbreviations: PDE-5, phosphodiesterase type 5; QTc, corrected QT interval.

intercourse in most men. Alprostadil is available in both intraurethral forms (tradename Muse in the United States), and intrapenile injection (tradenames Edex and Caverject). Intraurethral alprostadil is introduced into the urethra by an applicator. The penis is then massaged to allow for absorption of the drug into the corpora cavernosum. With treatment, approximately two-thirds of men will experience an erection sufficient for intercourse.[20] Side effects other than penile pain are uncommon. This medication should not be used in men with Peyronie disease, sickle cell anemia, or myeloproliferative disorders due to the risk of priapism.

Intrapenile alprostadil is appropriate for patients who can be trained to perform self-injections and is an especially good choice for those who perform these injections routinely (eg, diabetics using insulin). The sterile alprostadil solution is reconstituted immediately before use and injected into 1 penile corporeal body. Connected circulation between the 2 corpora then delivers the drug to the uninjected side, allowing for a symmetric erection that may last for more than an hour. Almost 90% of men who use intrapenile injections of alprostadil are satisfied with their erectile function with this technique; however, penile pain is a frequent complaint and may lead to discontinuation.[21] Systemic anticoagulation is a contraindication to the use of these injections. Similarly, either form of alprostadil should not be used in men with a penile implant due to the risk of infecting the implant. Intrapenile alprostadil is occasionally combined with other drugs, such as phentolamine and papaverine, by compounding pharmacies; however, these preparations have not been rigorously tested and safety concerns exist regarding these combination therapies, such as penile nodules, hematoma formation (with papaverine), and hepatitis.[22]

Nonpharmacological Therapy for Erectile Dysfunction

Patients who may not respond to pharmacologic therapies, may experience intolerable side effects, may have contraindications to therapy, or may prefer nonmedical therapy do have options for treating ED. Mechanical vacuum pumps can be used to generate an erection sufficient for intercourse, although the necessary occlusive ring placed at the base of the penis often interferes with ejaculation. Penile prostheses are a highly effective form of treated ED. These devices are usually reserved for men who have failed pharmacotherapy and have no contraindications to surgery. Patient satisfaction with these devices is high.

Oral phosphodiesterase inhibitors are initial pharmacotherapy for ED. Intraurethral or intrapenile alprostadil can be used for men who don't have a satisfactory response to oral medications.

PHARMACOLOGIC TREATMENT OF BENIGN PROSTATIC HYPERPLASIA

BPH is a common cause of morbidity in older men. Autopsy studies have shown that the prevalence of BPH starts increasing from 40% to 50% around age 50 to more than 80% older than age 80 years.[23] Using history and digital rectal examinations, the Baltimore Longitudinal Study of Aging also found similar clinical prevalence rates.[24] Symptoms may include a variety of lower urinary tract symptoms, including urinary frequency, urgency, hesitancy, nocturia, and weak urinary stream. The severity of these symptoms can be variable with an insidious onset and slow progression. A meta-analysis of studies that followed untreated men with BPH for 2.6 to 5 years showed that 16% remained stable and 38% showed improvement in symptoms.[25] Therefore, in most men, the decision to treat is based on how much they are affected by their symptoms. The American Urological Association symptoms index, or the International

Prostate Symptom Score (IPSS),[26] can be a useful tool to assess the severity of a patient's symptoms and help identify men who may warrant therapy.

Medical Management

In men with mild-to-moderate symptoms (IPSS<19), monotherapy with alpha1-adrenergic antagonists can be the starting point. Men with more severe symptoms may need to start with combination therapy.

Alpha1-Adrenergic Antagonists

Alpha1-adrenergic antagonist drugs relax the smooth muscle in the bladder neck, prostate capsule, and prostatic urethra, countering the dynamic component of bladder outlet obstruction. There are 5 FDA-approved agents in the United States: terazosin, doxazosin, tamsulosin, alfuzosin, and silodosin. When compared with 5-alpha-reductase inhibitors, these agents have a faster onset of therapeutic benefits (6–12 months vs 1–2 weeks) and are more effective at improving urinary symptoms in the short and long term.[27] A meta-analysis of placebo-controlled trials and comparative studies among terazosin, doxazosin, tamsulosin, and alfuzosin showed these agents reduced IPSS scores by 30% to 40% and increased urinary flow rates by 16% to 25%.[28] All the drugs were more effective than placebo and similar in efficacy to each other. Therefore, when choosing between them, cost, side-effect profile, and drug interactions should be determining factors in the decision. Common side effects of these medications include nasal congestion, dizziness, and headache. **Table 3** summarizes the different approved agents with their side-effect profiles and costs. The nonuroselective agents, terazosin and doxazosin, need to be initiated at a lower dose and then titrated up over several weeks due to the side effect of hypotension. Taking these medications at bedtime also minimizes the postural lightheadedness that may be seen with initial doses.

5-Alpha-Reductase Inhibitors

5-Alpha-reductase inhibitor medications act by reducing the size of the prostate gland; therefore, therapeutic effects may not be seen until after 6 to 12 months of therapy. This is why these agents are more effective in men with larger prostates. In general, these agents can be used in men who desire medical therapy for BPH but are not able to tolerate alpha1-adrenergic antagonists or for combination therapy in men with

Table 3
Alpha1-adrenergic antagonists with their side-effect profiles and cost

Drug	Uroselective	Hypotension	PDE-5i Worsen Hypotension	Ejaculatory Dysfunction	Cost per Month
Terazosin	No	↑↑↑	Yes	No	$48
Doxazosin	No	↑↑↑	Yes	No	$118 (ER) $43 (IR, generic) $107 (IR, Cardura)
Tamsulosin	Yes	—	No	Yes	$126 (generic) $226 (Flomax)
Alfuzosin	Yes	↑	No	No	$126 (generic) $690 (Uroxatral)
Silodosin	Yes	—	No	Yes	$227

Abbreviations: ER, extended release; IR, immediate release; PDE-5i, phosphodiesterase-5 inhibitors.

severe symptoms (IPSS>20). There are 2 approved agents for use: finasteride and dutasteride. A study of 895 men with BPH treated with finasteride for a year noted increased maximal urinary flow rate, 19% decrease in mean prostate volume, and 23% lowering of obstructive and 18% lowering of nonobstructive symptom scores.[29] A study of more than 3000 men has shown that these benefits are sustained for 4 years[30] and 6 years.[31] Additionally, finasteride therapy may halve the risk of needing prostate surgery and acute urinary retention compared with placebo.[30] Dutasteride seems similar to finasteride on all fronts. A trial comparing finasteride and dutasteride therapy for 12 months showed no differences in reduction of prostate volume, improvement in urinary flow rates, urinary symptoms scores, or adverse-effect profiles.[32] In addition, in patients with gross hematuria secondary to BPH or uncertain cause, finasteride has been shown to reduce the rate of recurrent hematuria as well as the need for surgery.[33]

Side effects of 5-alpha-reductase inhibitors

1. Prostate cancer risk: Two large, randomized controlled trials have shown that in men with BPH, although there is overall lower risk of prostate cancer with 5-alpha-reductase inhibitor therapy, the risk of high-grade prostate cancer (Gleason score>7) is increased.[34,35] This has led to an FDA warning label to ensure men are evaluated for prostate cancer before initiation of therapy. A suggested approach is to perform digital rectal examinations and obtain PSA levels before starting the medication and monitoring these while on treatment. Because these agents can lower PSA by up to 50%, any increase in PSA on therapy warrants further evaluation.
2. Sexual dysfunction: Commonly noted problems include decreased libido, ejaculatory dysfunction, and ED; however, these may only manifest in the first year of therapy.[36]

Anticholinergic Agents

Anticholinergic agents are useful in patients with predominantly irritative urinary symptoms (eg, frequency, urgency, incontinence) either as monotherapy or in combination with alpha1-adrenergic antagonists. Commonly used agents include tolterodine and oxybutynin. Other approved agents are darifenacin, solifenacin, fesoterodine, and trospium. Therapy comes with the side effects of peripheral anticholinergic action, including drowsiness, decreased cognitive function, blurry vision, dry mouth, tachycardia, and constipation.

Phosphodiesterase-5-Inhibitors

Tadalafil is the only approved agent in the phosphodiesterase-5-inhibitor class for use in BPH in the United States. It is worth considering in men with symptomatic BPH and ED. It has been shown to improved urinary flow rate and urinary symptom scores.[37,38]

Herbal Therapies

There is no concrete evidence to support the efficacy of agents such as saw palmetto, beta-sitosterol, cernilton, and pygeum africanum. None of these agents are approved for the treatment of BPH in the United States.

The decision to treat men with BPH is based on severity of symptoms and their impact on a patient's life. Alpha1-adrenergic antagonists are first-line therapy with comparable efficacy of the different agents. Their side-effect profiles and cost may be the determining factors for which agent is chosen for treatment. 5-Alpha-reductase inhibitors are useful in men with large prostates or those unable to tolerate alpha1-adrenergic antagonists.

REFERENCES

1. Zarotsky V, Huang MY, Carman W, et al. Systematic literature review of the risk factors, comorbidities, and consequences of hypogonadism in men. Andrology 2014;2(6):819–34.
2. Bhasin S, Cunningham GR, Hayes FJ, et al. Testosterone therapy in men with androgen deficiency syndromes: an Endocrine Society clinical practice guideline. J Clin Endocrinol Metab 2010;95(6):2536–59.
3. Contraceptive efficacy of testosterone-induced azoospermia in normal men. World Health Organization Task Force on methods for the regulation of male fertility. Lancet 1990;336(8721):955–9.
4. Goodman N, Guay A, Dandona P, et al. American Association of Clinical Endocrinologists and American College of Endocrinology Position Statement on the Association of Testosterone and Cardiovascular Risk. Endocr Pract 2015;21(9):1066–73.
5. Morgentaler A, Miner MM, Caliber M, et al. Testosterone therapy and cardiovascular risk: advances and controversies. Mayo Clin Proc 2015;90(2):224–51.
6. Snyder PJ, Lawrence DA. Treatment of male hypogonadism with testosterone enanthate. J Clin Endocrinol Metab 1980;51(6):1335–9.
7. Sih R, Morley JE, Kaiser FE, et al. Testosterone replacement in older hypogonadal men: a 12-month randomized controlled trial. J Clin Endocrinol Metab 1997;82(6):1661–7.
8. Schurmeyer T, Nieschlag E. Comparative pharmacokinetics of testosterone enanthate and testosterone cyclohexanecarboxylate as assessed by serum and salivary testosterone levels in normal men. Int J Androl 1984;7(3):181–7.
9. Swerdloff RS, Wang C, Cunningham G, et al. Long-term pharmacokinetics of transdermal testosterone gel in hypogonadal men. J Clin Endocrinol Metab 2000;85(12):4500–10.
10. McCullough AR, Khera M, Goldstein I, et al. A multi-institutional observational study of testosterone levels after testosterone pellet (Testopel(®)) insertion. J Sex Med 2012;9(2):594–601.
11. Westaby D, Ogle SJ, Paradinas FJ, et al. Liver damage from long-term methyltestosterone. Lancet 1977;2(8032):262–3.
12. Grant P, Jackson G, Baig I, et al. Erectile dysfunction in general medicine. Clin Med 2013;13(2):136–40.
13. Shamloul R, Ghanem H. Erectile dysfunction. Lancet 2013;381(9861):153–65.
14. Safarinejad MR. The effects of the adjunctive bupropion on male sexual dysfunction induced by a selective serotonin reuptake inhibitor: a double-blind placebo-controlled and randomized study. BJU Int 2010;106(6):840–7.
15. Corbin JD, Francis SH. Pharmacology of phosphodiesterase-5 inhibitors. Int J Clin Pract 2002;56(6):453–9.
16. Shabsigh R, Seftel AD, Kim ED, et al. Efficacy and safety of once-daily tadalafil in men with erectile dysfunction who reported no successful intercourse attempts at baseline. J Sex Med 2013;10(3):844–56.
17. Miller MS. Role of phosphodiesterase type 5 inhibitors for lower urinary tract symptoms. Ann Pharmacother 2013;47(2):278–83.
18. Carson CC 3rd, Mino RD. Priapism associated with trazodone therapy. J Urol 1988;139(2):369–70.

19. Ernst E, Pittler MH. Yohimbine for erectile dysfunction: a systematic review and meta-analysis of randomized clinical trials. J Urol 1998;159(2):433–6.

20. Padma-Nathan H, Hellstrom WJ, Kaiser FE, et al. Treatment of men with erectile dysfunction with transurethral alprostadil. Medicated Urethral System for Erection (MUSE) Study Group. N Engl J Med 1997;336(1):1–7.

21. Linet OI, Ogrinc FG. Efficacy and safety of intracavernosal alprostadil in men with erectile dysfunction. The Alprostadil Study Group. N Engl J Med 1996;334(14): 873–7.

22. Levine SB, Althof SE, Turner LA, et al. Side effects of self-administration of intra-cavernous papaverine and phentolamine for the treatment of impotence. J Urol 1989;141(1):54–7.

23. Berry SJ, Coffey DS, Walsh PC, et al. The development of human benign prostatic hyperplasia with age. J Urol 1984;132(3):474–9.

24. Guess HA, Arrighi HM, Metter EJ, et al. Cumulative prevalence of prostatism matches the autopsy prevalence of benign prostatic hyperplasia. Prostate 1990;17(3):241–6.

25. Isaacs JT. Importance of the natural history of benign prostatic hyperplasia in the evaluation of pharmacologic intervention. Prostate Suppl 1990;3:1–7.

26. Barry MJ, Fowler FJ Jr, O'Leary MP, et al. The American Urological Association symp-tom index for benign prostatic hyperplasia. The Measurement Committee of the American Urological Association. J Urol 1992;148(5):1549–57 [discussion: 1564].

27. Tacklind J, Fink HA, Macdonald R, et al. Finasteride for benign prostatic hyper-plasia. Cochrane Database Syst Rev 2010;(10):CD006015.

28. Djavan B, Marberger M. A meta-analysis on the efficacy and tolerability of alpha1-adrenoceptor antagonists in patients with lower urinary tract symptoms suggestive of benign prostatic obstruction. Eur Urol 1999;36(1):1–13.

29. Gormley GJ, Stoner E, Bruskewitz RC, et al. The effect of finasteride in men with benign prostatic hyperplasia. The Finasteride Study Group. N Engl J Med 1992; 327(17):1185–91.

30. McConnell JD, Bruskewitz R, Walsh P, et al. The effect of finasteride on the risk of acute urinary retention and the need for surgical treatment among men with benign prostatic hyperplasia. Finasteride Long-Term Efficacy and Safety Study Group. N Engl J Med 1998;338(9):557–63.

31. Roehrborn CG, Bruskewitz R, Nickel JC, et al. Sustained decrease in incidence of acute urinary retention and surgery with finasteride for 6 years in men with benign prostatic hyperplasia. J Urol 2004;171(3):1194–8.

32. Nickel JC, Gilling P, Tammela TL, et al. Comparison of dutasteride and finasteride for treating benign prostatic hyperplasia: the Enlarged Prostate International Comparator Study (EPICS). BJU Int 2011;108(3):388–94.

33. Foley SJ, Soloman LZ, Wedderburn AW, et al. A prospective study of the natural history of hematuria associated with benign prostatic hyperplasia and the effect of finasteride. J Urol 2000;163(2):496–8.

34. Thompson IM, Goodman PJ, Tangen CM, et al. The influence of finasteride on the development of prostate cancer. N Engl J Med 2003;349(3):215–24.

35. Andriole GL, Bostwick DG, Brawley OW, et al. Effect of dutasteride on the risk of prostate cancer. N Engl J Med 2010;362(13):1192–202.

36. Wessells H, Roy J, Bannow J, et al. Incidence and severity of sexual adverse ex-periences in finasteride and placebo-treated men with benign prostatic hyperpla-sia. Urology 2003;61(3):579–84.

37. Oelke M, Giuliano F, Mirone V, et al. Monotherapy with tadalafil or tamsulosin simi-larly improved lower urinary tract symptoms suggestive of benign prostatic

hyperplasia in an international, randomised, parallel, placebo-controlled clinical trial. Eur Urol 2012;61(5):917–25.

38. Porst H, Oelke M, Goldfischer ER, et al. Efficacy and safety of tadalafil 5 mg once daily for lower urinary tract symptoms suggestive of benign prostatic hyperplasia: subgroup analyses of pooled data from 4 multinational, randomized, placebo-controlled clinical studies. Urology 2013;82(3):667–73.

Evaluation and Treatment of Osteoporosis

Kim M. O'Connor, MD

KEYWORDS

- Osteoporosis • Postmenopausal women • Men • Screening • Diagnosis
- Treatment

KEY POINTS

- Screening for osteoporosis is recommend in all women more than 65 years of age or in women aged 50 to 64 years with certain risk factors.
- Treatment should be considered in postmenopausal women with osteoporosis on dual-energy x-ray absorptiometry scan, history of fragility fracture, or osteopenia plus a FRAX (Fracture Risk Assessment Tool) score of greater than or equal to 3% at the hip or greater than or equal to 20% at other sites.
- All of the osteoporosis agents decrease the risk of vertebral fractures but only some bisphosphonates, denosumab, and estrogen decrease hip fracture risk.
- Make sure the medication chosen to treat osteoporosis decreases fracture risk at the site of decreased bone mineral density or fracture. Also consider side effects, contraindications, secondary benefits, cost, and likelihood of adherence.
- Bisphosphonates should be first-line therapy in most cases.

INTRODUCTION

As the population ages, osteoporosis-related and osteoporosis-related fractures pose a significant public health concern. Although there has been a recent decline in hip fracture incidence in white women and men in the United States, rates are holding fairly steady in black, Asian, and Hispanic men and women.[1] Because of the aging of the population, fracture rates are expected to increase by 48% in the United States over the next 25 years to greater than 3 million fractures associated with a cost of $25.3 billion.[2] Seventy-one percent of all fractures and 75% of all fracture-related costs occur in women.[2] Approximately 20% of patients with a hip fracture do not survive for more than a year from diagnosis and more than 50% never completely regain

Conflict of Interest: The author has no conflicts of interest to report, and no financial disclosures.

Division of General Internal Medicine, Department of Internal Medicine, General Internal Medicine Clinic, University of Washington, Box 354760, 4245 Roosevelt Way Northeast, Seattle, WA 98105, USA

E-mail address: koconnor@u.washington.edu

Med Clin N Am 100 (2016) 807–826
http://dx.doi.org/10.1016/j.mcna.2016.03.016
0025-7125/16/$ – see front matter
medical.theclinics.com

their prefunction status.[3] Knowing these risks, the aim is for appropriate diagnosis and treatment of osteoporosis. The focus of this article is on the pharmacologic management of osteoporosis in postmenopausal women. It is important to recognize that nonpharmacologic interventions such as exercise, smoking cessation, fall prevention, and avoidance of heavy alcohol use are also recommended in the treatment of osteoporosis but these are not addressed in this article.

WHOM TO SCREEN

Most expert groups recommend screening with dual-energy x-ray absorptiometry (DXA) scan in postmenopausal women at age 65 years or older regardless of risk factors. For postmenopausal women between the ages of 50 and 64 years, differing screening recommendations exist. Organizations such as the National Osteoporosis Foundation (NOF), Endocrine Society, and Canadian Osteoporosis Society recommend screening in this age group when risk factors are present. Risk factors include advanced age, previous fracture, long-term glucocorticoid use, low body weight (less than 58 kg [127 lb]), family history of hip fracture, tobacco use, or excess alcohol use, with the most robust risk factors being age and previous low-trauma fracture[4] (**Box 1**). The United States Preventive Services Task Force (USPSTF) proposed the use of the FRAX calculator (https://www.shef.ac.uk/FRAX/) to determine need for screening in women aged 50 to 64 years.[5] If the FRAX 10-year major osteoporotic risk is greater than or equal to 9.3%, which is equivalent to a 65-year-old white woman without risk factors, then the USPSTF recommends screening with dual-energy x-ray absorptiometry (DXA) scan.[6] There are other, less complicated, screening tools, such as the Osteoporosis Risk Assessment Instrument (ORAI), Osteoporosis Self-assessment Tool (OST), Osteoporosis Index of Risk (OSIRIS), and Simple Calculated Risk Estimation Score (SCORE), which performed equally to FRAX in predicting fracture in comparison studies[7,8] (**Table 1**).

There are limited data to guide recommendations regarding rescreening if initial testing does not reveal osteoporosis. Most expert groups recommend rescreening in 1 to 2 years if women are at high risk for accelerated bone loss. In 2012, a prospective cohort study of almost 5000 women estimated the time interval for 10% of these women to develop osteoporosis before having a clinical hip or vertebral fracture. Based on this study the following rescreening recommendations can be considered. If baseline T score is −2.00 to −2.49 (advanced osteopenia) or if risk factors are present for accelerated bone loss regardless of T score, then repeat DXA every 2 years. If baseline T score is −1.50 to −1.99 (moderate osteopenia) with no risk factors for

---

Box 1
Risk factors for osteoporosis

Advanced age

Previous low-trauma fracture

Long-term glucocorticoid use

Low body weight (<58 kg [127 lb])

Family history of hip fracture

Tobacco use

Excess alcohol use

Table 1
Screening recommendations

Population	DXA Scan Screening Recommendations
Postmenopausal women aged ≥65 y	Screen regardless of risk factors
Postmenopausal women aged 50–64 y	• Screen if 1 or more risk factor present ○ National Osteoporosis Foundation (NOF) ○ Endocrine Society ○ Canadian Osteoporosis Society • Screen if FRAX 10-y major osteoporotic fracture risk ≥9.3% ○ USPSTF • Additional screening calculators ○ ORAI ○ OST ○ OSIRIS ○ SCORE
Men aged >70 y	• Insufficient evidence to screen ○ USPSTF • Screen regardless of risk factors ○ NOF ○ Endocrine Society ○ International Society for Clinical Densitometry
Men aged 50–70 y	• Insufficient evidence to screen ○ USPSTF • Screen if 1 or more risk factors present ○ NOF ○ Endocrine Society ○ International Society for Clinical Densitometry

Abbreviations: ORAI, Osteoporosis Risk Assessment Instrument; OSIRIS, Osteoporosis Index of Risk; OST, Osteoporosis Self-assessment Tool; SCORE, Simple Calculated Risk Estimation Score; USPSTF, US Preventive Services Task Force.

accelerated bone loss, then repeat DXA in 3 to 5 years. If baseline bone mineral density (BMD) is normal or T score is −1.01 to −1.49 (mild osteopenia) with no risk factors for accelerated bone loss, then consider repeating the DXA in 10 to 15 years[9] **(Table 2)**.

WHOM TO TREAT

Osteoporosis can be diagnosed based on BMD or the history of a fragility fracture. A fragility fracture is defined as a fracture occurring in the absence of major trauma such as a fall from standing height, coughing, or sneezing. The most common sites for fragility fracture involve the spine, ribs, hip, pelvis, wrist, or humerus. Based on DXA scan measurements, osteoporosis is defined as spinal or hip BMD 2.5 standard deviations or more less than the mean for healthy young women (T score −2.5 or less). Osteopenia is defined a spinal or hip BMD between 1 and 2.4 standard deviations less than the mean (T score −1.0 to −2.4) **(Table 3)**. Based on NOF recommendations, treatment should be considered in postmenopausal women with a history of hip or vertebral fracture or with osteoporosis on BMD measurements (T ≤ −2.5). In addition, it has been deemed cost-effective to consider treatment in postmenopausal women with osteopenia (T score between −1.0 and −2.4) if their 10-year probability of hip fracture reaches 3% or if major osteoporotic fracture (hip, shoulder, or wrist) risk is

Table 2
Rescreening recommendations

Baseline Screening DXA Results	Follow-up Plan
Normal	Consider recheck DXA in 10–15 y
Mild osteopenia, T −1.01 to −1.49	Consider recheck DXA in 10–15 y
Moderate osteopenia, T −1.5 to −1.99	Consider recheck DXA in 5 y
Advanced osteopenia, T −2.0 to −2.49 or if risk factors for accelerated bone loss regardless of baseline T score	Consider recheck DXA in 1–2 y
Osteoporosis	Discuss work-up ± treatment

greater than or equal to 20% based on the FRAX calculator.[10] Although it may be cost-effective, clinical trials have not assessed the benefit on absolute fracture risk using these FRAX-based treatment criteria (**Box 2**).

Cost-effectiveness analysis was based on the use of generic bisphosphonates for treatment of osteoporosis.[10] Additional studies are needed to determine at what level of risk it will remain cost-effective when the more expensive, newer agents are used. Clearly the emphasis on treatment in women with high absolute fracture risk rather than BMD criteria alone will increase the number of women treated. In a prospective cohort of community-dwelling white women greater than or equal to 65 years of age, recommendations for pharmacotherapy occurred for 72% of women more than 65 years old and 93% of women more than 75 years old when the revised NOF treatment guidelines were used.[11] When considering BMD criteria alone, only 50% of women in both age groups were recommended treatment. Shared decision making between provider and patient based on risks and benefits is needed to decide whether treatment is appropriate.

HOW TO CHOOSE A TREATMENT

Most medications available to treat osteoporosis are antiresorptives, which slow bone turnover by decreasing resorption. These antiresorptives include the bisphosphonates, selective estrogen receptor modulators (SERMs), denosumab, estrogen, and calcitonin. The only anabolic agent that stimulates bone formation is teriparatide. There are few head-to-head drug comparison trials to help determine efficacy.[12] Consequently, choice of drug should be based on site of diminished BMD and/or fracture, any secondary benefits, and contraindications. In the absence of contraindications, a generic oral bisphosphonate is recommended as first-line therapy because of low cost and availability of long-term safety data.

Table 3
Interpretation of DXA results

T Score	Interpretation
T +0.9 to −0.9	Normal
T −1.0 to −2.4	Osteopenia
T −2.5 or less	Osteoporosis
T −2.5 or less + fragility fracture	Severe osteoporosis

> **Box 2**
> **When to consider treatment of osteoporosis**
>
> - Osteoporosis based on DXA measurements of BMD
> - History of hip or vertebral fracture
> - Osteopenia on DXA scan + 10-year FRAX score of greater than or equal to 3% at hip or greater than or equal to 20% of major osteoporotic fracture

It is important to recognize that not all agents prevent fracture at all sites. Adequate data support vertebral fracture reduction with all the medications; however, at this time, data only support hip fracture reduction with most of the bisphosphonates, denosumab, and estrogen[13] (**Tables 4** and **5**).

CALCIUM AND VITAMIN D SUPPLEMENTATION

Controversy exists around the use of calcium and vitamin D supplementation for the prevention of osteoporosis because of the potential increased risks of cardiovascular outcomes and the small increased risk of kidney stones from supplemental calcium use. In 2015, with regard to primary prevention of osteoporosis, the USPSTF stated that there was insufficient evidence for higher-dose calcium (>1000 mg) and vitamin D supplementation in noninstitutionalized postmenopausal women, premenopausal women, and men. They recommended against low-dose (<1000 mg) supplementation in these same populations.[14] With regard to secondary prevention, there are some data that calcium plus vitamin D, but not vitamin D alone, decreases fractures in osteoporotic patients. Target calcium intake for patients with osteoporosis is 1200 mg/d, ideally through diet and 800 IU of vitamin D.[15,16] In order to increase calcium absorption, encourage patients to take their supplements with food and to take them in divided doses if using greater than 500 mg/d. Because calcium supplements can interfere with bisphosphonate absorption, make sure they are taken at least 1 hour after taking oral bisphosphonates. In general, calcium carbonate is recommended because of low cost. If patients are taking an H2 blocker or proton pump inhibitor, or plan to take the supplements on an empty stomach, they should use calcium citrate because an acidic environment is needed for absorption. It is important to make sure that vitamin D levels are replete before starting treatment because there is evidence that efficacy of bisphosphonate therapy is improved considerably in patients with serum 25-hydroxyvitamin D (25-OH) levels of greater than 33 ng/mL.

BISPHOSPHONATES

Bisphosphonates work by slowing bone turnover and they prevent fractures at all sites. The oral bisphosphonates alendronate and risedronate decrease the risk of vertebral and hip fractures by approximately 50% and nonvertebral fractures by 30%. Intravenous (IV) zoledronate reduces the risk of vertebral fractures by 70%, hip fractures by 40%, and nonvertebral fractures by 30%. Oral and IV ibandronate decrease vertebral fracture risk by 50% but there are insufficient data to support hip fracture and nonvertebral fracture reduction.[12,13] In general, the generic oral bisphosphonate alendronate is recommended as first-line therapy because of substantial data on fracture reduction and low cost. As mentioned previously, it is important that vitamin D levels are replete before starting treatment because there is evidence that bisphosphonates are more effective when 25-OH levels are greater

Table 4
Osteoporosis treatment options

Medication	Vertebral Fracture Risk Reduction (%)	Hip Fracture Risk Reduction (%)	Nonvertebral Fracture Risk Reduction (%)	Risks	Secondary Benefits
Bisphosphonates					
Alendronate, risedronate	50	50	30	GERD, esophagitis, jaw osteonecrosis, atypical femur fracture	—
Ibandronate	50	Not enough data	Not enough data		
Zoledronate	70	40	30		
SERMs					
Raloxifene	40	Not enough data	Not enough data	VTE, stroke	50% risk reduction of estrogen receptor–positive breast cancer in high-risk women with use of raloxifene
Bazedoxifene + CEE	—	—	—	Hot flashes (with raloxifene only)	Decrease in hot flashes and atrophic vaginitis with bazedoxifene + CEE
Teriparatide	70	Not enough data	50	Headaches, myalgias, hypercalcemia, hypercalciuria, hyperuricemia Use caution if history of kidney stones or gout	—
Denosumab	70	40	20	Hypocalcemia, hypercholesterolemia, musculoskeletal pain, cystitis, exacerbation of skin conditions, cellulitis	—
Estrogen	30	30	30	Estrogen + progestin: VTE, stroke, coronary heart disease, breast cancer Estrogen: VTE, stroke	—

Abbreviations: CEE, conjugated equine estrogen; GERD, gastroesophageal reflux disease; VTE, venous thromboembolism.

Table 5	
Special populations	
Population	**Medication Recommendations**
High risk for breast cancer	50% risk reduction of ER-positive breast cancer in high-risk patients with use of raloxifene
Hot flashes	Bazedoxefine + CEE

Chronic kidney disease	• If CrCl <35 mL/min
	  ○ Use denosumab (not renally cleared)
	  ○ Involve nephrologist/endocrinologist comfortable with CKD-MBD. May be able to use renally dosed bisphosphonates or SERM

Esophageal symptoms	• GERD/esophagitis
	  ○ Can use oral bisphosphonate if symptoms well controlled. Use H2 blocker rather than PPI for treatment of GERD symptoms
	  ○ IV zoledronate
	  ○ SERMs
	  ○ Teriparatide
	  ○ Denosumab
	• Barrett esophagus/esophageal stricture/achalasia
	  ○ Avoid oral bisphosphonates. Can use IV zoledronate
	  ○ SERMs
	  ○ Teriparatide
	  ○ Denosumab

Abbreviations: CKD-MBD, chronic kidney disease–induced metabolic bone disease; CrCl, creatinine clearance.

than 33 ng/mL.[17] It is recommended that all oral bisphosphonates be administered on an empty stomach 30 minutes before breakfast for the best absorption. Superior bioavailability and suppression of bone turnover was shown in a randomized controlled trial when taken before breakfast rather than at other times of fasting.[18] If patients have significant gastrointestinal side effects or if adherence is an issue then once-yearly IV zoledronate may be a better choice. Of note, only 50% of patients who were prescribed oral bisphosphonates were still taking them by 1 year, therefore it is important to inquire about adherence.[19]

There is concern about side effects of gastroesophageal reflux disease (GERD), esophagitis, and esophageal ulcers; however, if administered properly, these risks are low. In patients with well-controlled GERD it is appropriate to use a bisphosphonate if symptoms do not worsen. If treatment of GERD is needed it is probably better to use H2 blockers rather than proton pump inhibitors (PPIs) because of epidemiologic evidence that long-term, high-dose PPI use may increase fracture risk and that PPIs may blunt the effect of bisphosphonates.[20,21] An expensive, effervescent, dissolvable alendronate tablet is now available that may theoretically decrease gastrointestinal side effects compared with the traditional tablet formulation; however, no comparative studies are available.[19,22] Although data are inadequate to determine whether use of bisphosphonates increases risk of esophageal cancer, the US Food and Drug Administration (FDA) currently recommends against its use in patients with Barrett esophagus.[23]

IV formulations are associated with flulike symptoms and risks of hypocalcemia. Vitamin D stores should be replaced if 25-OH levels are less than 15 ng/mL and calcium replacement doses should be doubled 5 to 7 days before IV therapy. Bisphosphonates should be avoided in patients with a creatinine clearance of less than 35 mL/min.

The HORIZON (Health Outcomes and Reduced Incidence with Zoledronic acid Once Yearly) Pivotal Fracture trial raised concern about increased risk of atrial fibrillation in patients treated with IV zoledronate.[24] Several follow-up randomized-control and case-control studies both supported and refuted this concern.[25–27] The data for atrial fibrillation risk are conflicting but risk, if present, is likely small. The decision to treat with bisphosphonates should be weighed against the risk for atrial fibrillation versus osteoporotic fracture in the individual patient.

Rates of osteonecrosis are small, with 1 case per 10,000 to 100,000 person-years of treatment.[28] Risk is highest in patients receiving IV therapy in the setting of active cancer (especially metastatic breast cancer or myeloma) or cancer treatment, glucocorticoid use, poor dentition, and invasive dental procedures. In 2014, the American Association of Oral and Maxillofacial Surgeons updated their position paper on medication-related osteonecrosis of the jaw. Data are still limited but recommendations at this time include postponing initiation of bisphosphonates until after completion of invasive dental treatments. If already on a bisphosphonate, a drug holiday of 2 months before the procedure is recommended for patients who have been on bisphosphonates for longer than 4 years regardless of other risk factors. If patients are at high risk (concomitant corticosteroid or antiangiogenic cancer treatment medications) then consider a drug holiday even if bisphosphonate use is less than 4 years. In most cases the bisphosphonate should not be restarted until osseous healing has occurred.[29]

Bisphosphonate efficacy has been shown with up to 10 years of use. Determining length of therapy with bisphosphonates has become complicated because concerns arose about risk for atypical femur fractures (subtrochanteric or femoral shaft) with prolonged use. Although no direct causal evidence links long-term bisphosphonate use to atypical femur fractures (AFF), several case reports, case series, and cohort analyses show an association between the two. Bisphosphonate use for more than 5 years seems to be associated with an increased relative risk of AFF; however, the absolute risk is low (3.2–100 cases per 100,000 person-years), with the longer the duration, the higher the risk.[30,31]

At the same time, the benefit on typical hip fracture reduction generally outweighs the risk of AFF, especially in high-risk individuals. Although there is no consensus regarding length of therapy, clinicians might evaluate the need for a so-called drug holiday once the patient has been treated for 5 years.[32] At that time, if the patient is considered high risk (T score $\leq$ −2.5, history of previous hip or spine fracture, ongoing high-dose glucocorticoid use, or FRAX 10-year risk score at hip $\geq$3% or $\geq$20% at other sites) therapy should be continued for another 5 years. If moderate risk (T score now greater than −2.5, no prior hip or spine fracture, or FRAX score 10%–20%) consider a drug holiday. If low risk (does not meet criteria for treatment based on BMD, or FRAX score <10%) discontinue therapy[23] (**Table 6**).

If it is decided to take a drug holiday, there are no data to guide when to reinitiate therapy. A reasonable approach may be to reevaluate BMD via DXA scan every 2 to 3 years and consider restarting therapy if there is a rapid decline in BMD. An alternate approach would be to reevaluate fracture risk using the FRAX score and other risk factors every 2 years. Bone turnover markers may also be reasonable to use but there is no specific recommendation on target values or testing intervals[23] (**Box 3**).

If a patient who has been taking bisphosphonates for more than 3 years complains of a dull or aching pain in the groin or midthigh, plain radiographs are recommended to look for cortical thickening (**Fig. 1**) followed by MRI or bone scintigraphy looking for atypical fractures or stress reactions. A transverse-orientation fracture may also be noted on a plain film. If history or images are concerning, stop the bisphosphonate,

Table 6
Recommendation for drug holiday from bisphosphonates after 5 years of therapy: based on expert opinion

Patient Category	Recommendation
High risk: T score still ≤−2.5 at hip, previous fracture of hip or spine, ongoing high-dose glucocorticoids	Drug holiday not justified. Continue treatment for at least 5 more years
Moderate risk: T score now >−2.5, no prior hip or spine fracture	Consider drug holiday after 3–5 y of treatment with alendronate, risedronate or zoledronate[a]
Low risk: Did not meet current treatment criteria at time of treatment initiation	Discontinue therapy

[a] No information about ibandronate and drug holidays.

encourage adequate calcium and vitamin D supplementation, and refer to orthopedics urgently.

In a patient untreated for osteoporosis, the development of a fragility fracture should trigger a conversation about the importance of treatment because a history of hip fracture increase the risk of future fracture 3.2 times, especially during the first year after the fracture, and the risk remains increased for at least 5 years.[33] However, there is some concern that bisphosphonate therapy may disrupt bone remodeling and delay fracture repair. So how soon after a hip fracture surgery should a bisphosphonate be started? There is only 1 study of IV zoledronate that addresses this question. According to these results the ideal time to initiate a bisphosphonate after hip fracture in order to decrease rate of recurrent fracture and reduce all-cause mortality is between 2 weeks and 90 days.[34]

SELECTIVE ESTROGEN RECEPTOR MODULATORS

SERMs bind to estrogen receptors and have estrogen agonist and antagonist effects depending on the target organ. Raloxifene has more than 8 years of safety and fracture data and decreases the risk of vertebral fracture by approximately 40%.[13,35,36] There are inadequate data to support fracture reduction at hip and nonvertebral sites. Ideal recipients for raloxifene include women who cannot tolerate bisphosphonates but are not at high risk for venous thromboembolism (VTE) or stroke.[37] Raloxifene is dosed at 60 mg orally per day.

In addition, raloxifene reduces invasive, primarily estrogen receptor (ER)–positive, breast cancer risk by at least 50%.[37] This option may be good in women who are at high risk for breast cancer. In the studies on breast cancer reduction, the following constituted high risk: age greater than 60 years, age greater than 35 years with history of lobular carcinoma in situ, ductal carcinoma in situ or atypical ductal or lobular

Box 3
Monitoring drug holidays: empiric approaches to restarting treatment

- DXA and/or biochemical markers of bone turnover every 2 to 3 years
- Reevaluate risk every 2 to 3 years with FRAX calculator
- Any new fracture

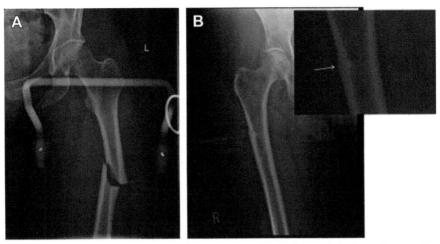

Fig. 1. (*A*) Completed atypical femur fracture. Note the beaking of the lateral cortex (*red arrow*) and short oblique nature of the fracture. There is also minimal comminution noted. (*B*) Incomplete atypical femur fracture. Note the lateral cortex beaking (*red arrow*). Also note the black line that represents the incomplete/nondisplaced fracture of the lateral cortex (*inset, white arrow*). (*From* Tyler W, Bukata S, O'Keefe R. Atypical femur fractures. Clin Geriatr Med 2014;30(2):350; with permission.)

hyperplasia, age 35 to 59 years with Gail model 5-year risk of breast cancer greater than 1.66%, or history of BRCA1 or BRCA2 mutation without prophylactic mastectomy.[38] As opposed to tamoxifen, raloxifene has not shown an increased risk of endometrial cancer so it presents less risk in women with an intact uterus.

Because of its risk of promoting VTE, SERMs should stopped at least 4 weeks before surgeries with moderate to high VTE risks. This recommendation is generally safe when SERMs are being used for the treatment of osteoporosis or breast cancer prevention. If a patient is on a SERM for treatment of breast cancer, then discuss the risks and benefits of stopping it with the patient's oncologist. Ideally, SERMs are restarted several weeks after surgery or when the VTE risk decreases.

One limiting side effect may be hot flashes. A new SERM formulation was recently introduced consisting of bazedoxifene plus conjugated equine estrogen (BZA/CE). Bazedoxifene alone has shown similar fracture reduction rates to raloxifene; however, this formulation is not available in the United States.[39,40] BZA/CE, which is available in the United States, has been shown to improve hot flashes and atrophic vaginitis but fracture and safety data have only been followed for 2 years. In addition, effects on breast cancer risk are unknown.

As opposed to the prolonged duration of action of bisphosphonates on BMD, when SERMs are discontinued BMD loss occurs fairly quickly and is similar to the loss in patients treated with placebo.[41] Consequently, unless side effects or contraindications develop, SERMs should probably be continued long term. Otherwise consider switching to an alternative osteoporosis treatment agent.

TERIPARATIDE

Teriparatide or recombinant human 1-34 parathyroid hormone is the only anabolic agent available for the treatment of osteoporosis. Dosing is a 20-μg subcutaneous injection given in the thigh or abdominal wall daily. It works by activating bone remodeling rather than slowing bone turnover. It decreases the risk of vertebral fractures by 70% and nonvertebral fractures by 50%; however, data are inadequate to determine hip fracture reduction.[42,43] BMD gains occur in the first few months of treatment; however, it takes at least 6 months before antifracture efficacy occurs.[42] Teriparatide should be stopped after 2 years of treatment because the benefits on BMD begin to level off after 18 months of therapy. In addition, animal studies and 1 human case report showed an increased risk of osteosarcoma with longer-term treatment, although causality between teriparatide and osteosarcoma was not established in the 1 case report.[44,45] Consequently, teriparatide should be avoided in patients at increased risk for osteosarcoma (history of Paget disease, bony radiation, skeletal metastases, and so forth).

Ideal candidates for teriparatide include postmenopausal women with severe vertebral osteoporosis (T < −3.5, or T < −2.5 plus fragility fracture). Because prior bisphosphonate use may blunt the effect of teriparatide, ideally it should be used first with a plan to transition to an antiresorptive such as a bisphosphonate or SERM after 2 years of treatment.[46] Teriparatide is extremely expensive and can cost up to $2000 per month without insurance. Teriparatide is covered by Medicare part D; however, patients need to show intolerance to or fail bisphosphonate therapy for coverage to be granted in most cases. Treatment with a bisphosphonate or SERM after discontinuation of teriparatide preserves or increases gains in BMD acquired with teriparatide alone. It is unclear how soon after an acute fracture teriparatide should be started because data are limited and conflicting about whether it accelerates or inhibits fracture repair.

Common side effects include headaches, myalgias, nausea, hypercalcemia, and hypercalciuria, so it should be avoided in patients with a history of kidney stones or persistent hypercalciuria. Uric acid levels can also increase and may precipitate a gout attack, therefore avoid the use of teriparatide until uric acid levels are controlled to less than 7.5 mg/dL in patients with a history of gout. Before initiating treatment check serum calcium, phosphate, creatinine, alkaline phosphatase, albumin, 25-OH, uric acid, and 24-hour urine calcium levels. If hypercalcemia or hypercalciuria present, evaluate for primary hyperparathyroidism. Replete vitamin D levels if low before initiating therapy.

DENOSUMAB

Denosumab is a monoclonal antibody that inhibits osteoclast formation and prevents resorption. Similar to bisphosphonates, it decreases fracture risk at all sites. Fracture risk decreases by 70% at the spine, 40% at the hip, and 20% at nonvertebral locations.[47,48] Ideal candidates for denosumab may include osteoporotic postmenopausal women who are intolerant or nonadherent to other medications or those with renal insufficiency (even if creatinine clearance is <35 mL/min). Dosing is 60 mg subcutaneously every 6 months and is only covered by Medicare part B, therefore it should be administered during a clinic visit in Medicare patients.

Most common side effects include musculoskeletal pain, hypercholesterolemia, and cystitis. There is a small increased risk of exacerbating eczema or causing cellulitis that requires hospitalization. Denosumab should be avoided in the setting of hypocalcemia until corrected and any vitamin D deficiency should be corrected before use. In the extension trial of denosumab after eight years of treatment with denosumab in 1546 postmenopausal women, one case of atypical femur fracture and five cases of osteonecrosis of the jaw (ONJ) occurred. There were three cases of ONJ and one atypical fracture in the 1457 cross-over group patients who received five years of denosumab therapy.[49] Longer-term safety data are needed to learn more about these risks.[49] Data are limited about the effect on acute fracture healing; however, at this time it seems that, even when administered within 6 weeks preceding or following a fracture, there is no delay in healing. There are few data on the idea duration of denosumab therapy or on sequential therapy with other osteoporosis agents. Denosumab has shown efficacy for 8 years.[50] BMD returns to baseline within 2 years after discontinuing therapy.

HORMONE REPLACEMENT THERAPY

Because of potential increased risks of breast cancer, stroke, VTE, and coronary heart disease (CHD), hormone replacement therapy (HRT) is no longer first line for the prevention or treatment of osteoporosis. Data from the Women's Health Initiative (WHI) showed an increase risk of CHD, stroke, VTE, and breast cancer in women on combination estrogen and progestin therapy. In women with hysterectomies who were treated with unopposed estrogen the risk of stroke and VTE was similar to combination therapy but there was no increased risk of CHD and a trend toward slightly lower rates of invasive breast cancer. However, some women who cannot tolerate other osteoporotic agents or who have hot flashes may consider using HRT. The best data for fracture reduction come from the WHI, which showed a 30% to 40% reduction in risk of hip, vertebral, and nonvertebral fractures.[51,52] BMD was not a criterion for randomization into the WHI, therefore baseline BMD may have differed between groups, thus making these results inconclusive. Maximum BMD improvement seems to occur when HRT is started shortly after menopause and continued long-term, but some studies suggest benefit even when started much later in life. Although HRT is not FDA approved for the treatment of osteoporosis, a few small studies have shown fracture reduction in osteoporotic women.[53] It seems that low-dose estrogen (0.3–0.45 mg/d) with or without progesterone is as effective as higher-dose estrogen (0.625 mg/d) in maintaining BMD.[54]

CALCITONIN

The Agency for Healthcare Research and Quality no longer recommends calcitonin for the treatment of osteoporosis because the quality of evidence for fracture reduction is only fair.[55,56] Probably the most beneficial use of calcitonin is for the treatment of acute compression fracture pain. Small studies show a reduction in pain within 4 days of starting the medication for up to 4 weeks of treatment.[57] It is not helpful for treatment of chronic compression fracture pain. Calcitonin, if used for treatment of acute compression fracture pain, is dosed 200 IU alternating nostrils every day or 100 units subcutaneously or intramuscularly every day or every other day. In general, the nasal formulation is recommended because side effects of nausea, vomiting, and flushing are less and analgesia is better compared with the injectable formulations.

STRONTIUM RANELATE

Strontium ranelate is available in Europe for the treatment of osteoporosis. In addition to its antiresorptive effects, strontium accumulates in the bone tissue, therefore the magnitude of BMD changes seen may not be representative of fracture risk reduction. Studies have shown a reduction in vertebral fracture risk by 40% and nonvertebral fracture risk by 15%. In high-risk groups, hip fracture risk may decrease by approximately 40%.[58–61] Strontium ranelate is not available in the Unites States and it is unclear whether the formulations available in the Unites States (citrate, gluconate, chloride) effectively treat osteoporosis. Side effects and complications, when they occur, can be severe and include diarrhea, VTE, myocardial infarction, drug reaction and eosinophilia and systemic symptoms, Stevens-Johnson, and toxic epidermal necrolysis. It is unclear how long patients should be treated but there are some safety data for up to 10 years.

MONITORING FOR RESPONSE TO THERAPY

There is no consensus on recommended follow-up after initiating treatment of osteoporosis. The controversy arises because it is unclear whether fracture risk reduction correlates with BMD changes while on therapy. Several studies have shown that the greater the improvement in BMD, the greater the fracture reduction.[62–65] However, other studies have suggested that fracture reduction occurs regardless of whether BMD increases or decreases with treatment.[66,67] Most subspecialist societies, including the NOF and the North American Menopause Society, recommend repeating a DXA scan 1 to 2 years after initiating therapy. How often to repeat after that depends on whether improvement or stability in BMD has been achieved or whether the patient is at high risk for more rapid decline of BMD caused by medication side effects or medical conditions. The alternative approach held by the Agency of Health Care Research and Quality is to not repeat a DXA scan after initiating therapy because treatment has been associated with a decreased fracture risk regardless of BMD changes on serial DXAs.[12,55] This option may be reasonable for patients who the clinicians thinks are adherent with medications and are at low risk for rapid decline of BMD caused by malabsorption or glucocorticoid use. If a follow-up DXA is obtained, what the clinician decides to do with the results depends on which philosophy the clinician holds. If BMD is decreasing, assessing for medication adherence and making sure patients are receiving adequate calcium and vitamin D supplementation is a good place to start.

Although in clinical trials bone turnover markers (BTMs) reflect the rate of bone turnover, it is not routinely recommended to check BTMs in patients on antiresorptives because of biological and laboratory variability confounding their use in clinical practice. In addition, there is insufficient evidence to support their use in deciding whether to change therapies based on the results. However, providers may choose to measure BTM in patients with conditions that might interfere with drug absorption or in patients reluctant to take these medications regularly. When using BTMs, measurements should be done at the same time of day in the same laboratory for a given patient in order to decrease risk of variability of results. BTMs cannot be used for patients on the anabolic agent, teriparatide. BTMs include fasting urinary N-telopeptide (NTX) or serum carboxy-terminal collagen cross-links (CTXs). These BTMs can be measured before initiating therapy and then 3 to 6 months later. A decrease in urinary NTX by at least 50% or serum CTX by at least 30% suggests adherence and efficacy. However, a decrease of less than this does not necessarily indicate treatment failure but may trigger the clinician to question the patient about medication adherence or malabsorption. Of note, insurance companies may not cover these tests.

GLUCOCORTICOID-INDUCED OSTEOPOROSIS

Glucocorticoids exposure, whether endogenous or exogenous, decreases bone density and increases the risk of fracture. Dosages as low at 2.5 to 7.5 mg of prednisone equivalents per day have been associated with increased vertebral and nonvertebral fractures, with higher daily doses likely more harmful.[68] Most BMD loss occurs within the first few months of therapy; however, continued use is associated with a slow and steady decline. Screening with DXA scan and vitamin D levels are recommended in all patients more than 30 years of age who are anticipated to be on glucocorticoids for greater than or equal to 3 months. These patients should also be encouraged to maintain calcium intake of 1200 mg/d and vitamin D intake of 800 IU/d through diet and/or supplements.

In 2010, the American College of Rheumatology (ACR) published recommendations on evaluation and management of glucocorticoid-induced osteoporosis (GIOP). In nonosteoporotic postmenopausal women and men greater than or equal to 50 years old, the FRAX calculator should be used to determine risk of fracture. In postmenopausal women and men greater than or equal to 50 years old with osteoporosis, history of fragility fracture, or a high-risk FRAX score (hip >3%, major osteoporotic >20%), treatment is recommended for patients on any dose of steroid for any period of time. If they are in the medium-risk category (FRAX score 10%–20% major osteoporotic), consider treatment if steroid use is anticipated for greater than or equal to 3 months. If low risk (FRAX score <10% major osteoporotic), consider treatment if steroids will extend past 3 months with at least 7.5 mg of prednisone equivalents per day. The 2010 ACR article provides a useful algorithm to determine need for treatment.[68] In premenopausal women and men less than 50 years old, treatment should be considered if there is a history of fragility fracture or evidence of accelerated bone loss. There are insufficient data to support treatment in this population if there is no history of fragility fracture (**Table 7**).

Bisphosphonates (alendronate, risedronate, zoledronate) or teriparatide are recommended for the treatment of GIOP in postmenopausal women, premenopausal women, and men of any age. In general, bisphosphonates are first-line agents because of their substantial data on fracture reduction and low cost. Because of higher cost and subcutaneous route of administration, teriparatide is generally not used as a first-line agent; however, there are some data suggesting that teriparatide

Table 7
Glucocorticoid-Induced Osteoporosis

Risk Categories	Consider Treatment	Which Treatment
Postmenopausal women and men ≥50 y old with osteoporosis, history of fragility fracture, or high-risk FRAX score (>3% hip, >20% major osteoporotic fracture risk)	Any patient on any dose of steroid for any period of time	Bisphosphonates (alendronate, risedronate, zoledronate) or teriparatide
Postmenopausal women and men ≥50 y old with medium-risk FRAX score (10%–20% major osteoporotic fracture risk)	If steroid treatment anticipated for ≥3 mo	Bisphosphonates (alendronate, risedronate, zoledronate) or teriparatide
Postmenopausal women and men ≥50 y old with low-risk FRAX score (<10% major osteoporotic fracture risk)	If steroids will extend past 3 mo with at least 7.5 mg prednisone equivalents per day	Bisphosphonates (alendronate, risedronate, zoledronate) or teriparatide
Premenopausal women and men <50 y old	If there is a history of fragility fracture or evidence of accelerated bone loss	Bisphosphonates (alendronate, risedronate, zoledronate) or teriparatide

leads to greater increases in BMD and lower rates of vertebral fractures compared with alendronate in high-risk patients treated with glucocorticoids.[69–71] Therefore, in patients with severe osteoporosis or those who cannot tolerate or fail other therapies, teriparatide may be the best option (**Box 4**).

TREATMENT OF OSTEOPOROSIS IN MEN

Bone density screening is uncommon in men. Most often DXA scans are obtained after the diagnosis of a low-trauma fracture or after osteopenia was incidentally noted on radiographs. Organizations such as the NOF, Endocrine Society, and International Society for Clinical Densitometry recommend screening all men more than 70 years of age and men between 50 and 70 years of age if certain risk factors are present. Risk factors may include history of fragility fracture, osteopenia on radiograph, loss of more than 37 mm (1.5 inches) of height, long-term glucocorticoid use, human immunodeficiency virus medications, androgen deprivation therapy for the treatment of prostate cancer, hypogonadism, primary hyperparathyroidism, and intestinal disorders. The same T-score classifications are used to diagnoses osteopenia and osteoporosis in men as in women. If osteoporosis is identified, then a work-up for secondary causes should be initiated because there is a high likelihood in men that a secondary cause will be identified. Men should be evaluated for hypogonadism, vitamin D deficiency, renal and liver disease, hyperparathyroidism, celiac disease and other causes of malabsorption, Cushing syndrome, and idiopathic hypercalciuria. Indications for treatment in men more than 50 years of age include osteoporosis on DXA scan, history of fragility fracture, or osteopenia plus high FRAX score (10-year probability of hip fracture $\geq$3% or if major osteoporotic fracture risk is $\geq$20%).[72]

Box 4
Common medications that may decrease BMD or increase fracture risk

- Glucocorticoids
- Antiepileptic drugs: phenobarbital, phenytoin, carbamazepine
- Antiretrovirals for human immunodeficiency virus
- Thiazolidinediones for diabetes
- Sodium-glucose cotransporter-2 inhibitors (canagliflozin) for diabetes
- High-dose medroxyprogesterone acetate for contraception (DepoProvera)
- Aromatase inhibitors
- Gonadotropin-releasing hormone agonists
- Methotrexate
- Cyclosporin and FK506 (tacrolimus)
- Proton Pump Inhibitors
- Lithium
- Antidepressants (selective serotonin reuptake inhibitors and tricyclic antidepressants)
- Loop diuretics
- Heparin (long-term use)
- Excessive thyroid HRT

In general, testosterone replacement therapy is recommended if hypogonadal and there are no contraindications; however, the effect of testosterone therapy on fracture risk has not been evaluated. Treatment options for men include bisphosphonates, teriparatide, and denosumab. All three agents have shown improvement in BMD in men. Only denosumab, when used for treatment of men with nonmetastatic prostate cancer on androgen deprivation therapy, and bisphosphonates have data supporting reduction in fracture risk.[73,74] When choosing between these therapies the same clinical indications, contraindications, and lengths of therapy apply as defined earlier. In general, oral bisphosphonates should be first-line therapy.

SUMMARY

As the population continues to age, the rates of osteoporotic fractures will increase. DXA scan screening is recommended in postmenopausal women more than 65 years of age or women aged 50 to 64 years with risk factors or at high risk of fracture based on FRAX score. DXA should also be considered for all men more than 70 years of age and men between 50 and 70 years of age if certain risk factors are present. Consider treatment if osteoporosis is present, there is a history of fragility fracture, or in the setting of osteopenia plus high risk for fracture based on a FRAX score of greater than or equal to 3% at the hip or greater than or equal to 20% at other sites. All the agents used to treat osteoporosis decrease fracture risk at the spine but only certain bisphosphonates, denosumab, and estrogen have data showing a reduction in hip fracture. The site of diminished BMD or fragility fracture, side effects, contraindications, secondary benefits, cost, and likelihood of adherence should influence the choice of treatment. In most cases, bisphosphonates should be first-line therapy.

REFERENCES

1. Wright NC, Saag KG, Curtis JR, et al. Recent trends in hip fracture rates by race/ethnicity among older US adults. J Bone Miner Res 2012;27(11):2325–32.
2. Cauley JA. Public health impact of osteoporosis. J Gerontol A Biol Sci Med Sci 2013;68(10):1243–51.
3. Boonen S, Laan RF, Barton IP, et al. Effect of osteoporosis treatments on risk of non-vertebral fractures: review and meta-analysis of intention-to-treat studies. Osteoporos Int 2005;16(10):1291–8.
4. Kanis JA, Borgstrom F, De Laet C, et al. Assessment of fracture risk. Osteoporos Int 2005;16(6):581–9.
5. Kanis J. FRAX. WHO fracture risk assessment tool. 2015. https://www.shef.ac.uk/FRAX/.
6. US Preventive Services Task Force. Screening for osteoporosis: U.S. preventive services task force recommendation statement. Ann Intern Med 2011;154(5):356–64.
7. Laya M. OsteoEd: Osteoporosis Education. 2015. http://depts.washington.edu/osteoed/.
8. Rubin KH, Abrahamsen B, Friis-Holmberg T, et al. Comparison of different screening tools (FRAX®, OST, ORAI, OSIRIS, SCORE and age alone) to identify women with increased risk of fracture. A population-based prospective study. Bone 2013;56(1):16–22.
9. Gourlay ML, Fine JP, Preisser JS, et al. Bone-density testing interval and transition to osteoporosis in older women. N Engl J Med 2012;366(3):225–33.
10. Cosman F, de Beur SJ, LeBoff MS, et al. Clinician's guide to prevention and treatment of osteoporosis. Osteoporos Int 2014;25(10):2359–81.

11. Donaldson MG, Cawthon PM, Lui LY, et al. Estimates of the proportion of older white women who would be recommended for pharmacologic treatment by the new U.S. National Osteoporosis Foundation guidelines. J Bone Miner Res 2009;24(4):675–80.

12. Crandall CJ, Newberry SJ, Diamant A, et al. Treatment To Prevent Fractures in Men and Women With Low Bone Density or Osteoporosis: Update of a 2007 Report [Internet]. Rockville (MD): Agency for Healthcare Research and Quality (US); 2012.

13. Crandall CJ, Newberry SJ, Diamant A, et al. Comparative effectiveness of pharmacologic treatments to prevent fractures: an updated systematic review. Ann Intern Med 2014;161(10):711–23.

14. Moyer VA, US Preventive Services Task Force. Vitamin D and calcium supplementation to prevent fractures in adults: U.S. Preventive Services Task Force recommendation statement. Ann Intern Med 2013;158(9):691–6.

15. Avenell A, Mak JC, O'Connell D. Vitamin D and vitamin D analogues for preventing fractures in post-menopausal women and older men. Cochrane Database Syst Rev 2014;(4):CD000227.

16. DIPART (Vitamin D Individual Patient Analysis of Randomized Trials) Group. Patient level pooled analysis of 68 500 patients from seven major vitamin D fracture trials in US and Europe. BMJ 2010;340:b5463.

17. Carmel AS, Shieh A, Bang H, et al. The 25(OH)D level needed to maintain a favorable bisphosphonate response is $\geq$33 ng/ml. Osteoporos Int 2012;23(10): 2479–87.

18. Agrawal S, Krueger DC, Engelke JA, et al. Between-meal risedronate does not alter bone turnover in nursing home residents. J Am Geriatr Soc 2006;54(5): 790–5.

19. Invernizzi M, Cisari C, Carda S. The potential impact of new effervescent alendronate formulation on compliance and persistence in osteoporosis treatment. Aging Clin Exp Res 2015;27(2):107–13.

20. FDA drug safety communication: possible increased risk of fractures of the hip, wrist, and spine with the use of proton pump. US Food and Drug Administration Web site. http://www.fda.gov/Drugs/DrugSafety/PostmarketDrugSafetyInformation forPatientsandProviders/ucm213206.htm. Accessed January 12, 2011.

21. Abrahamsen B, Eiken P, Eastell R. Proton pump inhibitor use and the antifracture efficacy of alendronate. Arch Intern Med 2011;171(11):998–1004.

22. In brief: effervescent alendronate. Med Lett Drugs Ther 2012;54(1401):84.

23. Brown JP, Morin S, Leslie W, et al. Bisphosphonates for treatment of osteoporosis: expected benefits, potential harms, and drug holidays. Can Fam Physician 2014; 60(4):324–33.

24. Black DM, Delmas PD, Eastell R, et al. Once-yearly zoledronic acid for treatment of postmenopausal osteoporosis. N Engl J Med 2007;356(18):1809–22.

25. Loke YK, Jeevanantham V, Singh S. Bisphosphonates and atrial fibrillation: systematic review and meta-analysis. Drug Saf 2009;32(3):219–28.

26. Sorensen HT, Christensen S, Mehnert F, et al. Use of bisphosphonates among women and risk of atrial fibrillation and flutter: population based case-control study. BMJ 2008;336(7648):813–6.

27. Heckbert SR, Li G, Cummings SR, et al. Use of alendronate and risk of incident atrial fibrillation in women. Arch Intern Med 2008;168(8):826–31.

28. Ruggiero SL, Dodson TB, Fantasia J, et al. American Association of Oral and Maxillofacial Surgeons position paper on medication-related osteonecrosis of the jaw–2014 update. J Oral Maxillofac Surg 2014;72(10):1938–56.

29. Shane E, Burr D, Ebeling PR, et al. Atypical subtrochanteric and diaphyseal femoral fractures: report of a task force of the American Society for Bone and Mineral Research. J Bone Miner Res 2010;25(11):2267–94.

30. Shane E, Burr D, Abrahamsen B, et al. Atypical subtrochanteric and diaphyseal femoral fractures: second report of a task force of the American Society for Bone and Mineral Research. J Bone Miner Res 2014;29(1):1–23.

31. Whitaker M, Guo J, Kehoe T, et al. Bisphosphonates for osteoporosis–where do we go from here? N Engl J Med 2012;366(22):2048–51.

32. Klop C, Gibson-Smith D, Elders PJ, et al. Anti-osteoporosis drug prescribing after hip fracture in the UK: 2000-2010. Osteoporos Int 2015;26(7):1919–28.

33. Seton M. How soon after hip fracture surgery should a patient start bisphosphonates? Cleve Clin J Med 2010;77(11):751–5.

34. Seeman E, Crans GG, Diez-Perez A, et al. Anti-vertebral fracture efficacy of raloxifene: a meta-analysis. Osteoporos Int 2006;17(2):313–6.

35. Ettinger B, Black DM, Mitlak BH, et al. Reduction of vertebral fracture risk in postmenopausal women with osteoporosis treated with raloxifene: results from a 3-year randomized clinical trial. Multiple Outcomes of Raloxifene Evaluation (MORE) Investigators. JAMA 1999;282(7):637–45.

36. Barrett-Connor E, Mosca L, Collins P, et al. Effects of raloxifene on cardiovascular events and breast cancer in postmenopausal women. N Engl J Med 2006;355(2): 125–37.

37. Visvanathan K, Chlebowski RT, Hurley P, et al. American Society of Clinical Oncology clinical practice guideline update on the use of pharmacologic interventions including tamoxifen, raloxifene, and aromatase inhibition for breast cancer risk reduction. J Clin Oncol 2009;27(19):3235–58.

38. Silverman SL, Christiansen C, Genant HK, et al. Efficacy of bazedoxifene in reducing new vertebral fracture risk in postmenopausal women with osteoporosis: results from a 3-year, randomized, placebo-, and active-controlled clinical trial. J Bone Miner Res 2008;23(12):1923–34.

39. Silverman SL, Chines AA, Kendler DL, et al. Sustained efficacy and safety of bazedoxifene in preventing fractures in postmenopausal women with osteoporosis: results of a 5-year, randomized, placebo-controlled study. Osteoporos Int 2012; 23(1):351–63.

40. Neele SJ, Evertz R, De Valk-De Roo G, et al. Effect of 1 year of discontinuation of raloxifene or estrogen therapy on bone mineral density after 5 years of treatment in healthy postmenopausal women. Bone 2002;30(4):599–603.

41. Neer RM, Arnaud CD, Zanchetta JR, et al. Effect of parathyroid hormone (1-34) on fractures and bone mineral density in postmenopausal women with osteoporosis. N Engl J Med 2001;344(19):1434–41.

42. Greenspan SL, Bone HG, Ettinger MP, et al. Effect of recombinant human parathyroid hormone (1-84) on vertebral fracture and bone mineral density in postmenopausal women with osteoporosis: a randomized trial. Ann Intern Med 2007;146(5):326–39.

43. Harper KD, Krege JH, Marcus R, et al. Osteosarcoma and teriparatide? J Bone Miner Res 2007;22(2):334.

44. Vahle JL, Sato M, Long GG, et al. Skeletal changes in rats given daily subcutaneous injections of recombinant human parathyroid hormone (1-34) for 2 years and relevance to human safety. Toxicol Pathol 2002;30(3):312–21.

45. Obermayer-Pietsch BM, Marin F, McCloskey EV, et al. Effects of two years of daily teriparatide treatment on BMD in postmenopausal women with severe

osteoporosis with and without prior antiresorptive treatment. J Bone Miner Res 2008;23(10):1591–600.

46. Cummings SR, San Martin J, McClung MR, et al. Denosumab for prevention of fractures in postmenopausal women with osteoporosis. N Engl J Med 2009; 361(8):756–65.

47. Boonen S, Adachi JD, Man Z, et al. Treatment with denosumab reduces the incidence of new vertebral and hip fractures in postmenopausal women at high risk. J Clin Endocrinol Metab 2011;96(6):1727–36.

48. Bone HG, Chapurlat R, Brandi ML, et al. The effect of three or six years of denosumab exposure in women with postmenopausal osteoporosis: results from the FREEDOM extension. J Clin Endocrinol Metab 2013;98(11):4483–92.

49. Papapoulos S, Lippuner K, Roux C, et al. The effect of 8 or 5 years of denosumab treatment in postmenopausal women with osteoporosis: results from the FREEDOM Extension study. Osteoporos Int 2015;26(12):2773–83.

50. Rossouw JE, Anderson GL, Prentice RL, et al. Risks and benefits of estrogen plus progestin in healthy postmenopausal women: principal results from the Women's Health Initiative randomized controlled trial. JAMA 2002;288(3):321–33.

51. Anderson GL, Limacher M, Assaf AR, et al. Effects of conjugated equine estrogen in postmenopausal women with hysterectomy: the Women's Health Initiative randomized controlled trial. JAMA 2004;291(14):1701–12.

52. Lufkin EG, Wahner HW, O'Fallon WM, et al. Treatment of postmenopausal osteoporosis with transdermal estrogen. Ann Intern Med 1992;117(1):1–9.

53. Lindsay R, Gallagher JC, Kleerekoper M, et al. Effect of lower doses of conjugated equine estrogens with and without medroxyprogesterone acetate on bone in early postmenopausal women. JAMA 2002;287(20):2668–76.

54. Levis S, Theodore G. Summary of AHRQ's comparative effectiveness review of treatment to prevent fractures in men and women with low bone density or osteoporosis: update of the 2007 report. J Manag Care Pharm 2012;18(4 Suppl B): S1–15 [discussion: S13].

55. Agency for Healthcare Research and Quality. Treatment to prevent fractures in men and women with low bone density or osteoporosis: update of a 2007 report. 2012. http://effectivehealthcare.ahrq.gov/index.cfm/search-for-guides-reviews-and-reports/?pageaction=displayproduct&productid=1007.

56. Knopp-Sihota JA, Newburn-Cook CV, Homik J, et al. Calcitonin for treating acute and chronic pain of recent and remote osteoporotic vertebral compression fractures: a systematic review and meta-analysis. Osteoporos Int 2012;23(1):17–38.

57. O'Donnell S, Cranney A, Wells GA, et al. Strontium ranelate for preventing and treating postmenopausal osteoporosis. Cochrane Database Syst Rev 2006;(3):CD005326.

58. Meunier PJ, Roux C, Seeman E, et al. The effects of strontium ranelate on the risk of vertebral fracture in women with postmenopausal osteoporosis. N Engl J Med 2004;350(5):459–68.

59. Reginster JY, Seeman E, De Vernejoul MC, et al. Strontium ranelate reduces the risk of nonvertebral fractures in postmenopausal women with osteoporosis: Treatment of Peripheral Osteoporosis (TROPOS) study. J Clin Endocrinol Metab 2005; 90(5):2816–22.

60. Reginster JY, Felsenberg D, Boonen S, et al. Effects of long-term strontium ranelate treatment on the risk of nonvertebral and vertebral fractures in postmenopausal osteoporosis: results of a five-year, randomized, placebo-controlled trial. Arthritis Rheum 2008;58(6):1687–95.

61. Hochberg MC, Ross PD, Black D, et al. Larger increases in bone mineral density during alendronate therapy are associated with a lower risk of new vertebral fractures in women with postmenopausal osteoporosis. Fracture Intervention Trial Research Group. Arthritis Rheum 1999;42(6):1246–54.

62. Hochberg MC, Greenspan S, Wasnich RD, et al. Changes in bone density and turnover explain the reductions in incidence of nonvertebral fractures that occur during treatment with antiresorptive agents. J Clin Endocrinol Metab 2002;87(4): 1586–92.

63. Eastell R, Vrijens B, Cahall DL, et al. Bone turnover markers and bone mineral density response with risedronate therapy: relationship with fracture risk and patient adherence. J Bone Miner Res 2011;26(7):1662–9.

64. Wasnich RD, Miller PD. Antifracture efficacy of antiresorptive agents are related to changes in bone density. J Clin Endocrinol Metab 2000;85(1):231–6.

65. Sarkar S, Mitlak BH, Wong M, et al. Relationships between bone mineral density and incident vertebral fracture risk with raloxifene therapy. J Bone Miner Res 2002;17(1):1–10.

66. Cummings SR, Karpf DB, Harris F, et al. Improvement in spine bone density and reduction in risk of vertebral fractures during treatment with antiresorptive drugs. Am J Med 2002;112(4):281–9.

67. Grossman JM, Gordon R, Ranganath VK, et al. American College of Rheumatology 2010 recommendations for the prevention and treatment of glucocorticoid-induced osteoporosis. Arthritis Care Res (Hoboken) 2010; 62(11):1515–26.

68. Langdahl BL, Marin F, Shane E, et al. Teriparatide versus alendronate for treating glucocorticoid-induced osteoporosis: an analysis by gender and menopausal status. Osteoporos Int 2009;20(12):2095–104.

69. Saag KG, Shane E, Boonen S, et al. Teriparatide or alendronate in glucocorticoid-induced osteoporosis. N Engl J Med 2007;357(20):2028–39.

70. Saag KG, Zanchetta JR, Devogelaer JP, et al. Effects of teriparatide versus alendronate for treating glucocorticoid-induced osteoporosis: thirty-six-month results of a randomized, double-blind, controlled trial. Arthritis Rheum 2009;60(11): 3346–55.

71. Watts NB, Adler RA, Bilezikian JP, et al. Osteoporosis in men: an Endocrine Society clinical practice guideline. J Clin Endocrinol Metab 2012;97(6):1802–22.

72. Joy M. Osteoporosis in men. N Engl J Med 2008;359(8):868 [author reply: 869].

73. Smith MR, Egerdie B, Hernandez Toriz N, et al. Denosumab in men receiving androgen-deprivation therapy for prostate cancer. N Engl J Med 2009;361(8): 745–55.

74. Smith MR, Saad F, Egerdie B, et al. Effects of denosumab on bone mineral density in men receiving androgen deprivation therapy for prostate cancer. J Urol 2009;182(6):2670–5.

Pharmacologic Therapies in Gastrointestinal Diseases

Rena K. Fox, MD[a],*, Thiruvengadam Muniraj, MD, PhD[b]

KEYWORDS

- Hepatitis C virus • Direct acting antivirals • Irritable bowel syndrome • GERD
- Peptic ulcer disease

KEY POINTS

- Treatment of hepatitis C virus has radically changed in recent years and most patients are now treatment candidates and have a high likelihood of permanent cure of the virus.
- First-line treatment of irritable bowel syndrome is lifestyle modification for patients with mild-moderate symptoms, and pharmacotherapy for patients with moderate to severe symptoms.
- Proton pump inhibitors (PPIs) are the mainstay of therapy in gastric and duodenal ulcers, and in gastroesophageal reflux disease, although long-term use of PPIs carries the risk of several side effects.

PHARMACOTHERAPY FOR HEPATITIS C VIRUS

In the United States, hepatitis C virus (HCV) is the leading case of liver-related deaths, hepatocellular carcinoma (HCC), and liver transplant.[1] Until recently, treatment of HCV consisted of pegylated interferon plus ribavirin, a regimen that was complicated, highly toxic, poorly efficacious, and had multiple contraindications.[1] Most patients were not treatment candidates, and in total only 5% to 6% of US patients with HCV were successfully treated in the interferon era.[2]

Clinical Benefit of Achieving Sustained Virologic Response

The goal of HCV antiviral treatment is to achieve a sustained virologic response (SVR), defined as HCV RNA levels at less than the limit of detection in the blood at 12 or more weeks after completing antiviral treatment. There is compelling evidence that an SVR has clinically meaningful improvements in outcomes. Among patients with cirrhosis

R.K. Fox has no disclosures.
[a] Division of General Internal Medicine, Department of Medicine, University of California, San Francisco School of Medicine, 1545 Divisadero St, Ste 307, San Francisco, CA, USA; [b] Section of Digestive Diseases, Department of Medicine, Yale University School of Medicine, 333 Cedar Street, 1080 LMP, New Haven, CT 06520-8019, USA
* Corresponding author.
E-mail address: rena.fox@ucsf.edu

Med Clin N Am 100 (2016) 827–850
http://dx.doi.org/10.1016/j.mcna.2016.03.009
medical.theclinics.com

who achieved an SVR, compared with patients who did not achieve an SVR, those with an SVR had a significantly reduced risk of HCC, liver failure, death related to liver disease, and all-cause mortality.[3,4]

Direct-acting Antivirals

HCV treatment has undergone radical changes since interferon. Novel treatments that target specific parts of the HCV lifecycle are called direct-acting antivirals (DAAs). Since late 2013, multiple DAAs have been introduced, such as sofosbuvir, simeprevir, ledipasvir, ombitasvir, dasabuvir, parataprevir, and daclatasvir. These drugs are used in combination with each other, or in combination with ribavirin. The new regimens are interferon free and all oral. The DAA regimens are generally short courses, usually 12 weeks in duration, but in some situations are 8 weeks or 24 weeks. In clinical trials, the cure rates with the DAAs are generally more than 90% and reach 100% in some subgroups.[5–16] In general, patients who are treatment naive achieve higher SVR rates, but, with DAA regimens, treatment-experienced patients are seen to still achieve SVR rates of more than 90%, although usually requiring at least a 12-week duration and sometimes longer, and/or often adding ribavirin, especially if there is also the presence of cirrhosis.[9,12,13,15] In large observational real-world studies, SVR rates are also greater than 90%, similar to trial outcomes.[17] The oral medicines have very mild and tolerable side effect profiles; when ribavirin is included in the regimen, there are higher side effect rates.[8–10,14] Discontinuation rates in real-world studies have also seemed to be low, especially when ribavirin is not needed.[17] Overall, these new interferon-free DAA regimens have dramatically changed HCV treatment, with most of the HCV population predicted to now be medically eligible, and to have a high likelihood of treatment success (**Table 1**).

Principles for Patient Selection for Hepatitis C Virus Treatment

All patients with chronic HCV who do not have medical contraindications are potential candidates for antiviral treatment. The natural history of untreated chronic HCV is variable; fibrosis progression is nonlinear, and it is estimated that 20% to 30% of patients with chronic HCV ultimately develop cirrhosis.[1] The urgency for treatment should be highest for patients with cirrhosis and advanced fibrosis, and also patients with HCC awaiting liver transplant, extrahepatic manifestations of HCV, after transplant, and women planning to conceive a child in the near term.[18,19]

Table 1
HCV-specific targets and antiviral medications: US Food and Drug Administration (FDA) approved or in phase II or III trials as of 2015

NS3/4A Protease Inhibitors	NS5B Polymerase Inhibitors Nucleoside/Nucleotide	NS5B Polymerase Inhibitors Non–Nucleoside/Nucleotide	NS5A Inhibitors
Simeprevir[a]	Sofosbuvir[a]	Dasabuvir[a]	Ledipasvir[a]
Paritaprevir[a]	Mericitabine	Beclabuvir	Ombitasvir[a]
Grazoprevir	ACH-3422	GS-9669	Daclatasvir[a]
ABT-493	MK/IDX-459	TMC-055	Elbasvir
Sovaprevir	MK-3682	MK-8876	Velpatasvir
GS-9857			ABT-530
Danoprevir			ACH-3102
Vedroprevir			Samatasvir
			GSK-2336805
			MK-8408

[a] Currently FDA approved.

Evaluating a patient's potential adherence to the prescribed regimen is crucial to the patient selection process. Providers should incorporate strategies for measuring and supporting adherence. Ongoing substance use, including drinking alcohol, using illicit drugs (including marijuana), or participating in opioid replacement programs should not be an exclusion for HCV treatment.[18,19]

Pretreatment Evaluation

Before initiating antiviral therapy in a patient with chronic HCV, the information listed in **Box 1** should be obtained.[18,19]

Principles of Regimen Selection

The most important pretreatment considerations for selection of DAA regimen are (1) genotype and subtype; (2) the presence or absence of cirrhosis and, if cirrhosis, then a determination of Child-Turcotte-Pugh (CTP) class A, B, or C; and (3) any prior history of treatment experience (**Table 2**).

Side Effects of Direct-acting Antiviral Regimens in Phase 3 Trials

Side effects of current DAAs are common but generally mild.[5–16] Periodic laboratory monitoring of levels of liver enzymes, bilirubin, and hemoglobin is recommended for patients receiving HCV antiviral therapy (**Table 3**).[18,19]

Box 1
HCV DAA pretreatment evaluation

- HCV genotype and subtype

- HCV RNA (quantitative viral load) ideally within 6 months before start of treatment

- Fibrosis assessment – may be done by 1 or more of the following:
  - Liver biopsy
  - Liver Fibrosis imaging such as transient elastography (FibroScan)
  - Serum markers of fibrosis such as FibroSure, FibroTest, FIBROSpect
  - Clinical calculators of fibrosis such APRI[20,21] or FIB-4[22]

- Determination of the absence/presence of cirrhosis – may be done by 1 or more of the following:
  - Physical exam findings (splenomegaly, spider angioma, other)
  - Routine laboratory findings (thrombocytopenia, hypoalbuminemia, other)
  - Abdominal imaging findings (nodular surface of liver, splenomegaly, other)
  - Liver biopsy documentation of cirrhosis
  - Non-invasive fibrosis assessment consistent with cirrhosis (e.g., APRI > 2.0, FIB-4 > 3.25, elastography > 1.25 kilopascals)

- If cirrhosis is detected, the CTP class should be determined

- If cirrhosis is detected, HCC should be excluded by imaging within the previous 6 months

- HCV treatment history and outcome

- Human immunodeficiency virus (HIV) status and, if HIV seropositive, current antiretroviral regimen and degree of viral suppression

Documented use of 2 forms of birth control in patient and sex partners in whom a ribavirin-containing regimen is chosen.
Abbreviations: APRI, AST to Platelet Ratio Index; FIB-4, Fibrosis-4 Calculator.

Table 2
CTP classification of the severity of cirrhosis

	Class A	Class B	Class C
Total points	5–6	7–9	10–15
Factor (points)	1	2	3
Total bilirubin (μmol/L)	<34	34–50	>50
Serum albumin (g/L)	>35	28–35	<28
Prothrombin time/ International Normalized Ratio	<1.7	1.71–2.30	>2.30
Ascites	None	Mild	Moderate–severe
Hepatic encephalopathy	None	Grade I–II (or suppressed with medication)	Grade III–IV (or refractory)

Assessing Hepatitis C Virus Treatment Response

Assessment of HCV RNA during and after therapy is critical to determining treatment response. The goal of treatment is to achieve an HCV RNA level less than the level of detection (ie, undetectable). Consider checking HCV RNA starting at week 2 or week 4, and every 2 weeks until the level becomes undetectable. End-of-treatment HCV RNA is recommended but optional. HCV RNA levels at 12 weeks after the completion of treatment need to be obtained to determine whether SVR was achieved (**Box 2**).

Interpretation of Hepatitis C Virus RNA Results

Several assays are available for quantifying HCV RNA levels, with different lower limits of quantification and ranges of detection. The US Food and Drug Administration (FDA) recommends use of a sensitive, real-time, reverse-transcription polymerase chain reaction (RT-PCR) assay for monitoring HCV RNA levels during treatment with DAA agents. To assess treatment response, commercial assays that have a lower limit of HCV RNA quantification of less than or equal to 25 IU/mL are strongly recommended. Some assays have a lower limit of HCV RNA quantification of 12 IU/mL. For results greater than the lower limit of quantification for the assay being used (eg, >25 IU/mL), the result is quantified, commonly referred to as the viral load. However, low levels of virus close to the limit of quantification may mean that HCV RNA is detected by the assay but not

Table 3
Side effects of DAAs in phase 3 trials

HCV DAA Regimen	Headache (%)	Fatigue (%)	Nausea (%)	Diarrhea (%)	Insomnia (%)	Skin Reactions (%)
Daclatasvir + sofosbuvir	20	19	12	9	6	NR
Ledipasvir/sofosbuvir	13–18	11–17	6–9	3–7	3–6	—
Ombitasvir/paritaprevir/ ritonavir + dasabuvir ± ribavirin	—	34	16–22	—	12–14	13–18
Sofosbuvir + simeprevir ± ribavirin	21	25	14	—	—	11

Abbreviation: NR, not reported.

Box 2
HCV treatment monitoring

Test the HCV RNA level assessed at week 4 of treatment.

If the HCV RNA is quantifiable at week 4 or at any time point thereafter, reassess HCV RNA in 2 weeks. If the repeated HCV RNA increases, discontinuation of all treatment should be strongly considered.

HCV RNA should be tested at end of treatment

HCV RNA must be tested at 12 weeks after completion of treatment or thereafter to determine whether SVR was achieved.

---

quantifiable, and often these are reported as detected. This result should be interpreted as extremely low level of virus but still detectable. In addition, when no HCV RNA can be detected by the assay, then the report may read either as "Target not detected," or as "Undetected," or simply as "Less than 25 IU/mL"; for example, when 25 IU/mL is the lower limit for that assay. It is important that treating providers understand how to interpret the reporting of HCV RNA results by their laboratories (**Box 3**).

Drug Resistance in Direct-acting Antivirals

DAAs target the HCV virus at the NS3, NS5A, and NS5B areas, but amino acid polymorphisms can exist within these areas causing reduced efficacy of DAAs.[23] These polymorphisms are termed resistance-associated variants (RAVs). NS5A inhibitors and NS3/4A protease inhibitors are particularly susceptible to resistance. Although a low percentage of patients treated with DAAs fail to achieve SVR, testing for RAVs may become part of planning for retreatment after a DAA failure. With further study, recommendations on who and when to test for RAVs are expected to be developed.

Genotype 1

Genotype 1 in the DAA era has had extremely high response rates, consistently 90% and higher. Some DAA studies have also uncovered that there are significant differences between genotype 1a and genotype 1b for some regimens, with genotype 1a having been shown to be more likely to contain baseline RAVs (eg, Q80K)

Box 3
Definitions of HCV treatment response

Rapid virologic response: undetectable HCV RNA at 4 weeks during treatment.

End-of-treatment response: HCV RNA less than lower limit of quantification (LLQ) at the end of treatment.

SVR: HCV RNA less than LLQ at least 12 weeks after treatment completion.

Relapse: HCV RNA less than LLQ during treatment and/or at the end of treatment, but subsequent quantifiable HCV RNA following treatment cessation.

Partial response: greater than or equal to 2 $\log_{10}$ reduction from baseline HCV RNA at week 12, but virus remains detectable through week 24 or treatment end with peginterferon and ribavirin.

Nonresponse: detectable HCV RNA throughout treatment.

Null response: less than 2 $\log_{10}$ reduction from baseline HCV RNA during peginterferon and ribavirin treatment.

---

and patients with genotype 1a requiring either a longer duration and/or the addition of ribavirin with some regimens, such as the regimen of paritaprevir/ritonavir/ombitasvir plus dasabuvir, compared with patients with genotype 1b.[11–14] Learning the subtype of a patients with genotype 1 can be relevant depending on which DAA is being used. By the end of 2015, there were 3 FDA-approved all-oral regimens for genotype 1: ledipasvir/sofosbuvir,[8–10] paritaprevir/ritonavir/ombitasvir plus dasabuvir plus/minus ribavirin,[11–14] and sofosbuvir plus simeprevir plus/minus ribavirin.[15] Other regimens are under FDA review and are anticipated to be introduced in 2016, and additional agents are also still in development at this time (**Table 4**).

Genotype 2

Current all-oral FDA-approved treatment of genotype 2 is sofosbuvir plus ribavirin for 12 weeks.[6,7] There are some data to show that extending to 16 weeks significantly improves outcomes for cirrhotics and treatment-experienced patients.[24] At this time, there have not been FDA-approved all-oral regimens that do not require ribavirin for genotype 2, but there are trials of ledipasvir/sofosbuvir and daclatasvir plus sofosbuvir for genotype 2,[25,26] both of which would not require ribavirin (**Table 5**).

Table 4 Genotype 1: 2015 recommended treatment options of FDA approved DAAs	
Treatment History and Cirrhosis Status	**Genotype 1 Recommended Regimens in 2015**

Treatment naive Without cirrhosis	Ledipasvir/sofosbuvir × 12 wk
	Ledipasvir/sofosbuvir × 8 wk: if baseline viral load <6 million IU/mL
	Ombitasvir/paritaprevir/ritonavir + dasabuvir × 12 wk
	  Genotype 1a: add ribavirin
	  Genotype 1b: ribavirin not required

Treatment naive Cirrhosis	Ledipasvir/sofosbuvir × 12 wk (CTP A, CTP B[a] and C[a])
	Ombitasvir/paritaprevir/ritonavir + dasabuvir (CTP A)[b]
	  Genotype 1a: add ribavirin; × 24 wk
	  Genotype 1b: ribavirin not required × 12 wk

Treatment experienced (prior peginterferon/ ribavirin experienced only) Without Cirrhosis	Ledipasvir/sofosbuvir × 12 wk
	Ombitasvir/paritaprevir/ritonavir + dasabuvir × 12 wk
	  Genotype 1a: add ribavirin
	  Genotype 1b: ribavirin not required

Treatment experienced (prior peginterferon/ ribavirin experienced only) Cirrhosis	Ombitasvir/paritaprevir/ritonavir + dasabuvir × 12 wk[b] (CTP A)
	  Genotype 1a: add ribavirin
	  Genotype 1b: ribavirin not required.
	Ledipasvir/sofosbuvir + ribavirin × 12 wk[a] (CTP A, B, C)

Treatment experienced (prior NS3/4A inhibitor or sofosbuvir + pegylated interferon + ribavirin) With or without cirrhosis	Ledipasvir/sofosbuvir + ribavirin × 12 wk[a]

[a] Not FDA approved.
[b] FDA warning against using in patients with advanced cirrhosis.

Table 5
Genotype 2: 2015 recommended treatment options of FDA approved DAAs

Treatment History and Cirrhosis Status	Genotype 2 Recommended Regimens in 2015
Treatment naive Without cirrhosis	Sofosbuvir + ribavirin × 12 wk
Treatment naive Cirrhosis	Sofosbuvir + ribavirin × 16 wk
Treatment experienced Without cirrhosis	Sofosbuvir + ribavirin × 12 wk[a]
Treatment experienced Cirrhosis	Sofosbuvir + ribavirin × 16 wk[a]

[a] FDA approved for 12 weeks. Not FDA approved for 16 weeks.

Genotype 3

Genotype 3 has had much more difficulty consistently achieving outstanding SVR rates.[27] Baseline and treatment emergent RAVs may be more relevant in patients with genotype 3, especially for NS5A RAVs,[23] and guidelines are now recommending baseline RAV testing for patients with genotype 3 to help guide selection of regimen.[18,19] At the end of 2015, the most effective interferon-free regimens for genotype 3 were daclatasvir plus sofosbuvir with ribavirin,[16] or ledipasvir/sofosbuvir with ribavirin, which is not FDA approved at this time.[28] These regimens have achieved 90% to 100% SVR among noncirrhotic patients, but in cirrhotic patients SVR rates have been much lower, and treatment must be extended to increase likelihood of SVR. Treatment with sofosbuvir plus pegylated interferon and ribavirin has the highest SVR rate for patients with genotype 3 with cirrhosis[24] and patients do not develop NS5A resistance, but the regimen requires interferon. At this time, patients with genotype 3 with cirrhosis and prior treatment experience are proving to be an especially challenging group, although more effective therapies are anticipated as early as 2016 (**Table 6**).[29]

Hepatitis C Virus–Human Immunodeficiency Virus Coinfection

Patients coinfected with HCV–human immunodeficiency virus (HIV) have SVR rates similar to those in patients not infected with HIV in the DAA era[30–34] and should receive the same HCV antiviral regimen as patients not infected with HIV, regardless of genotype.[18,19] Potential drug interactions are of greater concern for coinfected patients,

Table 6
Genotype 3: 2015 recommended treatment options of FDA approved DAAs

Treatment History and Cirrhosis Status	Genotype 3 Recommended Regimens in 2015
Treatment naive Without cirrhosis	Ledipasvir/sofosbuvir plus ribavirin × 12 wk[a] Daclatasvir + sofosbuvir × 12 wk
Treatment naive Cirrhosis	Daclatasvir + sofosbuvir + ribavirin × 12 wk (CTP A) Daclatasvir + sofosbuvir + ribavirin × 24 wk (CTP B and C)
Treatment experienced Without cirrhosis	Sofosbuvir + pegylated interferon + ribavirin × 12 wk[a] Ledipasvir/sofosbuvir + ribavirin × 12 wk[a]
Treatment experienced Cirrhosis	Sofosbuvir + pegylated interferon + ribavirin × 12 wk[a] Daclatasvir + sofosbuvir + ribavirin × 12 wk (CTP A) Daclatasvir + sofosbuvir + ribavirin × 24 wk (CTP B and C)

[a] Not FDA approved.

and the choice of HIV regimen and HCV DAA regimen need to be carefully considered to avoid toxicities and development of drug resistance (**Table 7**).

Summary

HCV treatment has undergone extensive change in the past 2 years. There are now multiple regimens of drugs that have extremely high success rates and that are all-oral, short courses with mild side effects. Physicians and providers who treat patients with HCV need to be familiar with the evaluation of patients with HCV for treatment and how to select treatment course and monitor appropriately, especially when the field is still rapidly evolving.

PHARMACOTHERAPY FOR IRRITABLE BOWEL SYNDROME

Irritable bowel syndrome (IBS) is one of the most common functional gastrointestinal (GI) disorders worldwide. Estimates of the US population prevalence of IBS have varied greatly across studies, ranging from 3.1% to 20.4%,[35] because of varying survey methodologies and the application of different diagnostic criteria. Chronic abdominal pain and altered bowel habits are the primary characteristic clinical features of IBS and these patients are broadly classified as those with constipation-predominant symptoms (IBS-C) and those with diarrhea-predominant symptoms (IBS-D).[36,37] IBS and other functional disorders account for substantial morbidity and cost.[38,39] Although lifestyle modifications and dietary manipulation remain as the initial management strategy for patients with mild to moderate symptoms that do not impair the quality of life, pharmacotherapy plays a significant role as an adjunctive treatment. This article focuses on the pharmacotherapy for IBS.

Approach to Pharmacotherapy for Irritable Bowel Syndrome

Pharmacologic therapy is initiated in patients with moderate to severe symptoms that impair quality of life. In the management of IBS, various treatments have been used, such as[35] fiber,[36] interventions that modify the microbiota (eg, probiotics, prebiotics, antibiotics),[37] antispasmodics,[38] antidiarrheals,[39] antidepressants,[40] psychological therapies,[41] prosecretory agents,[42] osmotic and stimulant laxatives,[43] narcotic and non-narcotic analgesics, and[44] antibiotics. The choice of agents depends on the dominant symptom and the subtype of IBS. Pharmacologic agents should be used to supplement lifestyle modifications as an adjunctive therapy (**Table 8**).

There are several trials comparing specific agents with placebo, resulting in mixed results. In a survey of 1966 patients with IBS by Drossman and colleagues,[40] patients with IBS took at least 2 drugs on average (range, 0–13), and the most commonly prescribed medications were non-narcotic analgesics (31%), antidepressants (30%), antidiarrheal agents (23%), antispasmodics (18%), and opiates (18%). The use of

Table 7			
Studies of DAA combination regimens in HIV-HCV coinfected patients			
Study	**N**	**Treatment**	**SVR Rates (%)**
ION-4	335	Ledipasvir/sofosbuvir × 12 wk	94–97
ALLY-2	127	Daclatasvir + sofosbuvir × 12 wk	91–98
TURQUOISE-1	63	Ombitasvir/paritaprevir/ritonavir + dasabuvir + ribavirin × 12–24 wk	83–95
C-EDGE	218	Grazoprevir/elbasvir × 12 wk	94–100

Table 8
Pharmacotherapy in IBS

Treatment	Benefits	Common Adverse Effects
Over-the-counter Agents		
Fiber: psyllium	Effective for IBS-C	Bloating, gas
Laxative	Beneficial for constipation in IBS-C, but not global symptoms	Bloating, gas, cramping, diarrhea
Antidiarrheal: loperamide	Beneficial for diarrhea in IBS-D, but not global symptoms	Constipation
Probiotics	Unclear benefit	Similar to placebo
Antispasmodic: peppermint oil	Beneficial for global symptoms and cramping	GERD, constipation
Prescription Drugs		
Antidepressants: TCAs, SSRIs, SNRIs	Improve global symptoms and pain	Dry eyes/mouth, sedation, constipation
Antispasmodics	Some benefit in global symptoms and pain	Dry eyes/mouth, sedation, constipation
Prosecretory agents Linaclotide Lubiprostone	Improve global abdominal and constipation symptoms in IBS-C	Nausea, diarrhea
Antibiotics: rifaxamin	Improve global abdominal and constipation symptoms in IBS-D	Similar to placebo
5-HT$_3$ antagonists Alosteron Ondansetron	Improve global abdominal and constipation symptoms in IBS-D	Constipation, rarely ischemic colitis
Eluxadoline	Improves abdominal pain and diarrhea with IBS-D	Constipation, nausea, rarely pancreatitis

Abbreviations: 5-HT$_3$, 5-hydroxytryptamine; GERD, gastroesophageal reflux disease; SNRIs, serotonin norepinephrine reuptake inhibitors; SSRIs, selective serotonin reuptake inhibitors.

pain medications (both narcotic and non-narcotic) and antidepressants reemphasizes that chronic pain is the predominant symptom reported by patients with IBS.[40] The adverse effects of these medications were greatest with narcotics, antidepressants, and anticonstipation drugs.

Pharmacotherapy in Constipation-predominant Irritable Bowel Syndrome

Bulking agents
Increased intake of dietary fiber is recommended to improve constipation-related symptoms in IBS-C. However, insoluble fiber (found in the seeds and skins of fruit) may exacerbate symptoms, causing more bloating, and provide little relief; soluble fiber (the type of fiber included in oatmeal, nuts, beans, apples, and blueberries) such as psyllium (ispaghula husk) in particular, provides relief in many patients. The authors suggest starting psyllium at a low dose of 1.2 gm daily and titrate up in dose and frequency based on the symptom response.[41] Psyllium should always be consumed mixed with water or other liquids, and not be swallowed dry because it may cause esophageal impaction.

If there is inadequate response to the initial management with dietary fiber, laxatives are the first choice for patients with IBS-C.

Osmotic laxatives

Polyethylene glycol Although there is no randomized controlled trial (RCT) showing a beneficial effect of polyethylene glycol (PEG) laxatives on IBS-related global symptom relief, the efficacy of PEG in increasing the frequency of bowel movements has been well shown and therefore PEG laxatives are useful in patients with IBS-C for specific symptom relief of constipation.[42,43] The usual dose is to start with 17 g of powder dissolved in 235 mL (8 oz) of water once daily and titrate up or down (to a maximum of 34 g daily) to effect. There are very few reported adverse effects with PEG and the cost is very low.

Other osmotic laxatives, such as lactulose and sorbitol, cause more bloating and flatulence and therefore should be avoided in patients with IBS.[44]

Stimulant laxatives

Stimulant laxatives include senna, bisacodyl, and sodium picosulfate. These laxatives cause fluid and electrolyte secretion by the colon mucosa and induce peristalsis, thereby producing a bowel movement. These drugs are used in chronic idiopathic constipation and are not indicated in IBS.[41]

Prosecretory agents

Linaclotide and lubiprostone are the two novel prosecretory agents that are FDA approved for use in IBS-C.[45,46] These drugs are similar in their pharmacokinetics and have negligible systemic absorption.[47]

Linaclotide Linaclotide is a peptide that activates guanylate cyclase-C receptors on the lumen of intestinal epithelium, which results in secretion of bicarbonate, chloride, and water into the lumen as well as stimulating colon transit. Linaclotide (Linzess) is administered at a dose of 290 μg daily and the most common adverse event is diarrhea.[46]

Lubiprostone Lubiprostone is a locally acting chloride channel activator that enhances chloride-rich intestinal fluid secretion. Lubiprostone (Amitiza) at dose of 8 μg twice daily is FDA approved to treat IBS-C in women 18 years and older.[45] The most common adverse effect is nausea.

The American Gastroenterological Association (AGA) recommends using linaclotide and lubiprostone (compared with using no drugs) in patients with IBS-C.[42]

Pharmacotherapy in Diarrhea-predominant Irritable Bowel Syndrome

Loperamide

Loperamide (Imodium) is a nonabsorbable opioid receptor agonist that acts on mu-opioid receptions in the myenteric plexus of the large intestine. The usual starting dose is 2 mg and can be titrated up to 12 mg safely.[48,49] Although the RCTs have not shown clear benefit in composite symptom end points in IBS, because of its low cost, wide availability, and minimal adverse effects, loperamide is widely used as an adjunct to other IBS-D therapies.[50]

Eluxadoline

Eluxadoline (Viberzi) is a novel mixed mu-opioid receptor agonist and delta-opioid receptor antagonist that acts locally in the GI tract with low systemic absorption.[51] Eluxadoline, at dosage of 100 mg twice daily, was shown to be effective in simultaneously relieving the symptoms of abdominal pain and diarrhea with IBS-D over 6 months in 2 large prospective phase 3 trials, and it was FDA approved in May 2015.[52,53] The most common side effects noted were constipation, nausea, and abdominal pain, and the most serious adverse effect noted was the risk of spasm in the sphincter of Oddi, which can result in pancreatitis.

Rifaximin

IBS is thought to be caused by alteration of gut microbial flora. Rifaximin, a minimally absorbed antibiotic, proved more effective than placebo for global symptoms and bloating, and was well tolerable, in patients with IBS.[54–56] Rifaxamin (Xifaxan) at a dosage of 550 mg 3 times daily has been recently approved by the FDA for IBS-D.[53] After a 2-week course, the efficacy persisted for up to 12 weeks.[55]

Tricyclic antidepressants and selective serotonin reuptake inhibitors

Antidepressants provide a statistically significant benefit compared with placebo for abdominal pain, global assessment, and IBS symptom score. Several RCTs showed a modest improvement in global symptom relief, with tricyclic antidepressants such as amitriptyline, desipramine, and imipramine. These are low-cost options that can be used as adjunctive therapy with caution, paying attention to the adverse effects such as sedation, prolongation of QT interval, urinary retention, and glaucoma.[42] Pooled results from 5 RCTs after durations of 6 to 12 weeks of selective serotonin re-uptake inhibitors (SSRIs) showed no improvement in symptoms in IBS. The AGA recommends against using SSRI for patients with IBS.[42]

Antispasmodics

Antispasmodics decrease the smooth muscle contractions and reduce motility and se-cretions, thereby giving relief for abdominal pain and diarrhea.[50] Spasmolytic agents compared with placebo provided a statistically significant benefit for abdominal pain, global assessment, and IBS symptom score. The commonly used antispasmodics agents are dicyclomine, hyoscine (ie, scopolamine), and L-hyoscyamine (ie, active L-iso-mer of atropine). These agents are preferably used to treat IBS-D because of the side effect of constipation, although they can also be used as add-on agents for IBD-C.

5-Hydroxytryptamine Receptor Antagonists

Alosetron

Alosetron, a 5-hydroxytryptamine (5-HT$_3$) receptor antagonist, has been shown to have good tolerability with clinical efficacy in women with refractory IBS-D symptoms that are severe and unresponsive to other agents.[57] Alosteron was initially approved by the FDA in 2000 at a dosage of 1 mg twice daily, and then, because of reports of complications such as constipation and ischemic colitis, it was withdrawn from the market, and has now been reintroduced for use only under a specific physician-based risk management program.[42,58]

Ondansetron

Patients with IBS-D have faster transit times than healthy controls.[59] Ondansetron, a 5-HT$_3$ receptor antagonist, a commonly used antiemetic, was shown to reduce colonic transit time in healthy individuals many years ago.[60] In a recent randomized trial of 120 patients, significant improvement in stool form and urgency was seen with ondansetron compared with placebo; however, there was no change in pain and bloating.[59] Considering the chronic nature of the disease, the results from this 5-week study should be approached with cautious optimism and could be considered when treating selected patients with IBS-D.[61]

Summary

Most recommendations on pharmacotherapy in IBS are based on low-quality to moderate-quality evidence. No single IBS therapy is uniformly effective for all patients, and the treatment should be personalized for each patient based on the symptom. Recognizing the risk of adverse effects, and the unclear benefit for global symptom relief, pharmacotherapy should be initiated only to patients with moderate to severe symptoms that impair the quality of life.

PHARMACOTHERAPY FOR GASTROESOPHAGEAL REFLUX DISEASE AND PEPTIC ULCER DISEASE

Gastroesophageal reflux disease (GERD) is one of the most prevalent diseases worldwide, and approximately 20% of the US population has GERD.[62–64] The prevalence of GERD is much less in Asia (5%) compared with the Western world.[63] Peptic ulcer disease (PUD) is another common GI disease with considerable morbidity and complications such as GI bleeding. Many environmental factors, such as nonsteroidal antiinflammatory drugs (NSAIDs), smoking, and *Helicobacter pylori*, have been strongly related to PUD. There is a downtrend in the incidence of PUD and related complications in recent decades because of better management of PUD.[65–69] Patients often have overlapping symptoms of GERD (ie, regurgitation and heartburn) and PUD (pain or discomfort localized to the upper abdomen) and it is important to distinguish between them, because this has important diagnostic and therapeutic implications. Lifestyle and dietary modification, and avoiding offending agents, are basic initial recommendations for both these diseases before initiating pharmacotherapy. This article focuses on pharmacotherapy for GERD and PUD.

Medical Management of Gastroesophageal Reflux Disease

Medical management of GERD should be initiated in patients who fail initial lifestyle interventions such as weight loss; head-of-bed elevation; avoidance of late evening meals; tobacco and alcohol cessation; and cessation of chocolate, caffeine, spicy foods, citrus, and carbonated beverages.[70–74]

Although antacids, histamine2-receptor antagonists (H$_2$RA), and proton pump inhibitors (PPIs) are the agents available to treat GERD, the cornerstone of GERD therapy is to decrease the esophageal acid exposure by decreasing gastric acid secretion.[75] Therefore PPIs remain the first-line therapy to achieve this goal[75] (**Table 9**).

Proton Pump Inhibitors

PPIs are the most potent inhibitors of gastric acid secretion by irreversibly inhibiting the final common step in acid secretion via hydrogen-potassium (H-K) ATPase pump. PPIs have been shown to be superior to H$_2$RA, antacids, and sucralfate in many clinical trials and meta-analyses.[75,76] PPIs have shown a significantly faster healing rate of peptic ulcers (12%/wk) versus H$_2$RAs (6%/wk) and provided faster, more complete heartburn relief (11.5%/wk) versus H$_2$RAs (6.4%/wk).[77] In patients who have erosive reflux disease, PPIs seem to give better relief than in patients with nonerosive reflux disease (NERD).[78] Even in patients with NERD, PPIs provided better heartburn relief than H$_2$RA.[78]

Which Proton Pump Inhibitor, When to Administer, What Dose, and How Long?

Among the 6 currently available PPIs (rabeprazole, pantoprazole, esomeprazole, dexlansoprazole, omeprazole, lansoprazole), omeprazole and lansoprazole can be obtained over the counter without a prescription. There is no significant difference in efficacy between different PPIs.[79] Although some studies show differences in esophageal reflux using pH monitoring, clinically superior outcomes have not yet been shown.[80,81]

Any form of PPI for an 8-week course is the initial first line of therapy for symptom relief in GERD. In general, PPIs are more effective when administered 30 to 60 minutes before

Table 9
Antisecretory agents in GERD and PUD

Drug Name	Dose (mg)	Interaction	Potential Adverse Effects
H₂RA	Dosage adjustment is required for patients with renal insufficiency	—	Cytopenias, rash, GI intolerance, and arrhythmias
Cimetidine	800 BID or 400 QID	Multiple drug interactions	—
Famotidine	20 BID or 40 QD	Multiple drug interactions	—
Nizatidine	150 BID or 300 QD	Multiple drug interactions	—
Ranitidine	150 BID or 300 QD	Multiple drug interactions	—
PPIs	No dosage adjustment needed for renal impairment May require lower dosage in hepatic impairment	—	GI symptoms (abdominal pain, diarrhea, nausea), headache, rash, liver toxicity, osteoporosis, community-acquired pneumonia
Omeprazole	20–40 QD	↓ Absorption of clopidogrel, ketoconazole ↑ Absorption of digoxin ↓ Clearance of diazepam, warfarin, phenytoin	—
Pantoprazole	40 QD or 40 BID	Not many drug interactions	—
Lansoprazole	15–30 QD or 30 BID	Not many drug interactions	—
Esomeprazole	20–40 QD	↓ Absorption of clopidogrel, ketoconazole ↓ Clearance of diazepam, warfarin, phenytoin	—
Dexlansoprazole	30–60 QD	Not many drug interactions	—

Abbreviations: BID, twice a day; QD, every day; QID, 4 times a day; TID, 3 times a day.

the first meal of the day for maximal pH control, because the amount of H-K–ATPase present in the parietal cell is greatest after a prolonged fast. However, the newer dexlansoprazole, which is in a dual delayed-release form, can be taken any time of the day regardless of food intake.[82] The PPI should be titrated down to the lowest possible effective dose based on the symptom control during long-term therapy.[83,84]

Can Proton Pump Inhibitors be Used as On-demand Therapy?

In general PPIs have a half-life of ~1 hour, although some newer PPIs, like lansoprazole, have slightly longer half-lives than the prototype omeprazole. Because only the actively acid-secreting proton pumps are inhibited, and only a few pumps may be active during the brief interval when PPIs are present (all PPIs have plasma half-lives of 1–2 hours), the antisecretory action increases on daily dosing and the full steady-state acid inhibition is achieved only after 4 to 5 days. Therefore, PPIs should be administered daily as a course rather than on demand, as in the case of antacids.[85]

Is Maintenance Therapy After the Initial 8 Weeks Necessary?

PPIs should be continued as daily maintenance therapy for patients who continue to have symptoms after PPIs are discontinued and in patients with complications, including erosive esophagitis and Barrett esophagus.[83,84,86] Almost two-thirds of patients with NERD and moderate to severe esophagitis have relapse of symptoms over a period of time when PPIs are discontinued.[87,88]

Histamine Receptor Antagonists

H_2RAs cause competitive (ranitidine) and noncompetitive (famotidine) inhibition of the histamine2 receptor on the gastric parietal cell and decrease the acid secretion. They soon develop tolerance, which limits their use in maintenance therapy for GERD.[89] The role of H2RAs in GERD is mainly as an adjunctive therapy, as additional bedtime H_2RA along with PPIs for patients with symptoms refractory to PPI. This bedtime H_2RA approach has been shown to be effective in decreasing nocturnal acid breakthrough in patients with GERD.[90] If clinical tolerance for H_2RA is encountered, intermittent or on-demand H_2RA could be helpful, although there are no data to support such a strategy.

Antacids

Antacids have a limited role in management of GERD. They tend to provide immediate short-term relief of heartburn by neutralizing the gastric acid, thereby limiting the acid reflux to the esophagus. However, this relief is temporary, lasting only for a few minutes to an hour and is therefore not recommended for definitive therapy.[91]

Pharmacotherapy for Nonresponders or Partial Responders to Proton Pump Inhibitors

For patients with refractory symptoms while on PPIs, the emphasis should be on lifestyle adjustments, and then referral for further evaluation with possible endoscopy. The initial step in management of refractory GERD is optimization of the dose and timing of administration of the PPI.[92] The dose could be doubled, nighttime H2RAs could be added along with the PPIs, and it could be reemphasized that patients should take the PPI 30 to 60 minutes before the first meal of the day. Sometimes a trial of switching to a PPI from a different group provides better relief to some patients.[93]

Baclofen for Refractory Gastroesophageal Reflux Disease

A small subset of patients with refractory GERD have nonacid reflux. Refractory GERD can be defined as failure of symptom resolution despite twice-daily PPIs and additional bedtime H_2RA therapy. In these patients, the gamma-aminobutyric acid B agonist baclofen has been shown to decrease reflux episodes and symptoms during PPI therapy.[94] Randomized trials comparing baclofen and surgical fundoplication are currently underway.[95]

Adverse Effects of Proton Pump Inhibitors

For minor common adverse effects, such as headache, dyspepsia, and diarrhea, clinicians should consider switching to a different class of PPI. During long-term PPI use, significant gastric acid reduction can lead to development of reactive hypergastrinemia and hypochlorhydria, which can result in development of atrophic gastritis, which is a precursor for gastric cancer.[96] There are convincing data establishing the association between PPI use with an increase in *Clostridium difficile* colitis, although the magnitude of risk is very low.[97] The FDA has issued a warning that long-term use of PPIs can decrease calcium absorption and increase the risk of osteoporotic fractures in the elderly.[96,98] The data on an increased risk for community-acquired pneumonia (CAP) in association with PPI therapy are still conflicting, and PPI therapy should not be withheld in patients requiring therapy because of a potential risk of CAP.[84,86,99] Although there are no worrisome issues, drug-to-drug interactions are to be considered when using PPIs. Recent studies have shown that PPI therapy does not need to be altered during concomitant clopidogrel use because no increased risk for adverse cardiovascular events has been found.[100–102] Because of the potential teratogenicity, PPIs should be avoided in pregnancy and instead sucralfate could be used.

Medical Management of Peptic Ulcer Disease

The initial management of PUD varies based on the clinical presentation and likely cause. The treatment options include empiric antisecretory therapy and empiric therapy for *H pylori* infection, along with avoiding the possible causative agents, such as NSAIDs.

Eradication of Helicobacter pylori

Apart from patients who are taking NSAIDs, most patients with duodenal ulcers and at least two-thirds of patients with gastric ulcers are infected with *H pylori*. Therefore, the current recommendation is to test for *H pylori* in all patients with active PUD and with confirmed history of peptic ulcer disease (not previously treated for *H pylori*).[103] First-line therapies for *H pylori* include a PPI, clarithromycin, and amoxicillin or metronidazole (triple therapy), and a bismuth/tetracycline-based quadruple therapy[103] (**Table 10**). In areas where clarithromycin resistance is high (>15%–20%), the effectiveness of this triple combination therapy is less than 70% to 80% and so metronidazole should be given instead of clarithromycin.

Table 10
First-line therapies for *H pylori*

Type of Regimen	Drugs	Frequency	Duration (d)
I	PPI	BID	10–14
	Clarithromycin 500 mg	BID	
	Amoxicillin 1 g or METRONIDAZOLE 500 mg	BID	
II	PPI	QD	10–14
	Tetracycline 500 mg	QID	
	Bismuth subsalicylate 525 mg	QID	
	Metronidazole 250 mg	QID	

Table 11
Sequential therapy for *H pylori*

Duration (d)	Drug	Frequency
First 5	PPI + amoxicillin 1 g	BID
Next 5	PPI + clarithromycin 500 mg + tinidazole 500 mg	BID

The treatment is usually recommended for 10 to 14 days, because shorter regimens are shown to have lesser eradication rates.[104] The eradication rates with PPI-based triple therapy and quadruple therapy are similar.[105,106] It is therefore reasonable to start empiric triple therapy (PPI, clarithromycin, and amoxicillin) in patients who have not previously received clarithromycin and who are not allergic to penicillin. If the patient is allergic to penicillin, metronidazole can be substituted for amoxicillin. If the patient is allergic to penicillin or has previously been treated with clarithromycin, bismuth quadruple therapy should be considered[105] (see **Table 10**).

In recent years, there has been a decline in eradication rates with clarithromycin-based triple therapy or bismuth-based quadruple therapy. Studies show eradication rates greater than 90% with sequential therapies based on PPIs, and amoxicillin for 5 days followed by a PPI, clarithromycin, and tinidazole for an additional 5 days[107] (**Table 11**).

Treatment of Persistent Helicobacter pylori Infection (Salvage Therapy)

After failed first-line therapy, a thorough review of the patient's previous treatment regimen is prudent to avoid the same antibiotics. Also, it is important to assess for medication nonadherence and to reinforce the importance of adhering to the regimen. because most patients are treated with clarithromycin-based triple therapy as first line, bismuth-based quadruple therapy is considered an accepted salvage therapy in patients not treated previously with metronidazole.[108] However, with persistent infection, levofloxacin-based therapy (levofloxacin, omeprazole, nitazoxanide, and doxycycline [LOAD]) for 10 days has been shown to be an alternate option, although no validation studies have so far been done in the United States[103,108,109] (**Table 12**).

Antisecretory Therapy

Antisecretory therapy is mandatory for all the patients with peptic ulcers, independent of cause, to aid ulcer healing. PPIs are a mainstay of antisecretory therapy because

Table 12
Salvage therapy for persistent *H pylori* infection

	Frequency	Duration (d)
Bismuth quadruple therapy		
PPI	QD	7–14
Tetracycline, bismuth, metronidazole	QID	—
LOAD	—	10
Levofloxacin 250 mg	QD	—
PPI	BID	—
Nitazoxinide 500 mg (Alinia)	BID	—
Doxycycline 100 mg	QD	—

> **Box 4**
> **Long-term maintenance PPI therapy in PUD**
>
> 1. Continued NSAID use
> 2. Failure to eradicate *H pylori*
> 3. Frequent recurrent peptic ulcers
> 4. Large ulcer (>2 cm) with multiple comorbid conditions

they are the most potent inhibitors of acid secretion and are superior to antacids, H_2RAs, prostaglandins, and sucralfate. There are 6 currently available PPIs (discussed earlier). As mentioned earlier, PPIs should be taken 30 to 60 minutes before the first meal of the day when the proton pumps and parietal cells are active. A longer duration of antisecretory therapy is recommended with gastric ulcers (8–12 weeks) compared with duodenal ulcers (4–6 weeks).

Long-term maintenance antisecretory therapy for an indefinite period is recommended in high-risk patients with complicated ulcers, and continued use of NSAIDs (**Box 4**).

Among the 4 H_2RAs available (cimetidine, ranitidine, famotidine, and nizatidine), only ranitdine (Zantac) and famotidine (Pepcid) are commonly used. Famotidine is a noncompetitive inhibitor of histamine and so is slightly more effective than the others, which are competitive inhibitors. Also, famotidine has the longest duration of action of them all. All the agents are renally excreted and therefore dose is to be adjusted in patients with renal failure. Tolerance to the antisecretory effects of H_2RAs develops quickly and frequently. Although PPIs are the first-line antisecretory medications, H_2RAs can be used when PPIs cannot be used for reasons such as adverse effects, allergies, and drug-drug interactions.[110] A single bedtime dose of an H_2RA can heal the peptic ulcers in 8 weeks.

Treatment of Nonsteroidal Antiinflammatory Drug Ulcers

NSAIDs should be discontinued wherever possible. If NSAID therapy cannot be discontinued, dose reduction of the NSAID should be considered, along with initiation of additional long-term-PPI therapy. PPIs have been shown to be more effective than $H_2$2RAs in reducing NSAID-induced ulcers.[110,111]

Misoprostol Use in Nonsteroidal Antiinflammatory Drug Ulcers

Misoprostol, a prostaglandin analogue, has been used as a gastroprotective agent during concomitant NSAID use. There is evidence that the ulcerogenic effect of NSAIDs correlates with prostaglandin synthesis. Misoprostol is the only prostaglandin analogue approved by the FDA for prevention of NSAID-induced ulcer disease. Misoprostol has been shown to be more effective than H_2RAs in preventing NSAID-induced mucosal injury.[112] Misoprostol at a dose of 800 µg daily is equally effective as PPI in ulcer prevention with NSAID use.[113] However, its usefulness is limited by its GI side effects; especially diarrhea.

Antacids

Antacids have no proven efficacy in healing ulcers. Some studies have shown ulcer healing with antacid alone, which is thought to be by binding bile, inhibiting pepsin, and promoting angiogenesis.[114] However, ulcer healing requires high doses of antacids, which often lead to adverse side effects and therefore are rarely used in practice to treat PUD.[115]

Summary

Although most patients respond well to pharmacologic agents, lifestyle modifications should be part of the initial management of GERD before initiating pharmacotherapy. Patients with refractory GERD who do not respond to any pharmacologic therapy may be considered for surgical antireflux procedures, such as Nissen fundoplication and laparoscopic sphincter augmentation. A subset of patients with PUD, such as *H pylori*–negative disease, NSAID-negative ulcer disease, refractory peptic ulcers, and recurrence of peptic ulcers, should be treated with indefinite maintenance antisecretory therapy and also be investigated for rare causes of ulcer disease, such as Zollinger-Ellison syndrome, Crohn disease, ischemia, sarcoid, lymphoma, eosinophilic gastroenteritis, and immunoglobulin G4–related sclerosing disease.

REFERENCES

1. Ghany MG, Strader DB, Thomas DL, et al. Diagnosis, management, and treatment of hepatitis C: an update. Hepatology 2009;49(4):1335–74.
2. Holmberg SD, Spradling PR, Moorman AC, et al. Hepatitis C in the United States. N Engl J Med 2013;368(20):1859–61.
3. Simmons B, Saleem J, Heath K, et al. Long-term treatment outcomes of patients infected with hepatitis C virus: a systematic review and meta-analysis of the survival benefit of achieving a sustained virological response. Clin Infect Dis 2015; 61(5):730–40.
4. Backus LI, Boothroyd DB, Phillips BR, et al. A sustained virologic response reduces risk of all-cause mortality in patients with hepatitis C. Clin Gastroenterol Hepatol 2011;9(6):509–16.e1.
5. Lawitz E, Mangia A, Wyles D, et al. Sofosbuvir for previously untreated chronic hepatitis C infection. N Engl J Med 2013;368(20):1878–87.
6. Jacobson IM, Gordon SC, Kowdley KV, et al. Sofosbuvir for hepatitis C genotype 2 or 3 in patients without treatment options. N Engl J Med 2013;368(20):1867–77.
7. Zeuzem S, Dusheiko GM, Salupere R, et al. Sofosbuvir and ribavirin in HCV genotypes 2 and 3. N Engl J Med 2014;370(21):1993–2001.
8. Afdhal N, Zeuzem S, Kwo P, et al. Ledipasvir and sofosbuvir for untreated HCV genotype 1 infection. N Engl J Med 2014;370(20):1889–98.
9. Afdhal N, Reddy KR, Nelson DR, et al. Ledipasvir and sofosbuvir for previously treated HCV genotype 1 infection. N Engl J Med 2014;370(16):1483–93.
10. Kowdley KV, Gordon SC, Reddy KR, et al. Ledipasvir and sofosbuvir for 8 or 12 weeks for chronic HCV without cirrhosis. N Engl J Med 2014;370(20):1879–88.
11. Feld JJ, Kowdley KV, Coakley E, et al. Treatment of HCV with ABT-450/r-ombitasvir and dasabuvir with ribavirin. N Engl J Med 2014;370(17):1594–603.
12. Zeuzem S, Jacobson IM, Baykal T, et al. Retreatment of HCV with ABT-450/r-ombitasvir and dasabuvir with ribavirin. N Engl J Med 2014;370(17):1604–14.
13. Poordad F, Hezode C, Trinh R, et al. ABT-450/r-ombitasvir and dasabuvir with ribavirin for hepatitis C with cirrhosis. N Engl J Med 2014;370(21):1973–82.
14. Ferenci P, Bernstein D, Lalezari J, et al. ABT-450/r-ombitasvir and dasabuvir with or without ribavirin for HCV. N Engl J Med 2014;370(21):1983–92.
15. Lawitz E, Matusow G, DeJesus E, et al. A phase 3, open-label, single-arm study to evaluate the efficacy and safety of 12 weeks of simeprevir (SMV) plus sofosbuvir (SOF) in treatment-naive or –experienced patients with chronic HCV genotype 1 infection and cirrhosis: OPTIMIST-2. Paper presented at: Program and

abstracts of the 50th Annual Meeting of the European Association for the Study of the Liver. Vienna, Austria, April 22–26, 2015, Abstract LP04.

16. Nelson DR, Cooper JN, Lalezari JP, et al. All-oral 12-week treatment with daclatasvir plus sofosbuvir in patients with hepatitis C virus genotype 3 infection: ALLY-3 phase III study. Hepatology 2015;61(4):1127–35.

17. Backus L, Belperio P, Shahoumian T, et al. Effectiveness of ledipasvir/sofosbuvir in treatment naïve genotype 1 patients treated in routine medical practice. Paper presented at: Program and abstracts of the 66th annual meeting of the American Association for the Study of Liver Diseases; San Francisco, California, November 15, 2015, Abstract 93.

18. American Association for the Study of Liver Diseases; Infectious Diseases Society of America. Recommendations for testing, managing, and treating hepatitis C. 2015. Available at: http://www.hcvguidelines.org. Accessed December 13, 2015.

19. Department of Veterans Affairs. Chronic hepatitis C virus (HCV) infection: treatment considerations. Department of Veterans Affairs National Hepatitis C Resource Center Program and Office of Public Health. 2014. Available at: http://www.hepatitis.va.gov/provider/guidelines/2014hcv/lab-monitoring.asp.Accessed December 13, 2015.

20. Lin ZH, Xin YN, Don QU, et al. Performance of the asparate aminotransferase-to-platelet ratio index for the staging of hepatitis C-related fibrosis: an updated meta-analysis. Hepatology 2011;53:726–36.

21. Chou R, Wasson N. Blood tests to diagnose fibrosis or cirrhosis in patients with chronic hepatitis C virus infection: a systematic review. Ann Intern Med 2013; 158:807–20.

22. Sterling RK, Lissen E, Clumeck N, et al. Development of a simple noninvasive index to predict significant fibrosis patients with HIV/HCV coinfection. Hepatology 2006;43:1317–25.

23. Sarrazini C. The importance of resistance to direct antiviral drugs in HCV infection in clinical practice. J Hepatol 2016;64(2):486–504.

24. Foster GR, Pianko S, Brown A, et al. Sofosbuvir plus Peg-IFN/RBV for 12 weeks vs sofosbuvir/RBV for 16 or 24 weeks in genotype 3 HCV-infected patients and treatment-experienced cirrhotic patients with genotype 2 HCV: the BOSON study. Paper presented at: The International Liver Congress™ 2015, 50th Annual Meeting of the European Association for the Study of the Liver (EASL). Vienna, Austria, April 22–26, 2015.

25. Gane EJ, Hyland RH, Yang Y, et al. Ledipasvir/sofosbuvir single tablet regimen is effective in patients with HCV genotype 2 infection. Paper presented at: ISVHLD 2015. Berlin, Germany, June 26-28, 2015.

26. Sulkowski MS, Gardiner DF, Rodriguez-Torres M, et al. Daclatasvir plus sofosbuvir for previously treated or untreated chronic HCV infection. N Engl J Med 2014; 370(3):211–21.

27. Zeuzem S, Dusheiko GM, Salupere R, et al. Sofosbuvir + ribavirin for 12 or 24 weeks for patients with HCV genotype 2 or 3: the VALENCE trial. Special Issue: The 64th Annual Meeting of the American Association for the Study of Liver Diseases: The Liver Meeting 2013. Hepatology 2013;58(4):733A–4A.

28. Gane EJ, Hyland RH, An D, et al. Efficacy of ledipasvir and sofosbuvir, with or without ribavirin, for 12 weeks in patients with HCV genotype 3 or 6 infection. Gastroenterology 2015;149(6):1454–61.e1.

29. Foster GR, Afdhal N, Roberts SK, et al. Sofosbuvir and velpatasvir for HCV genotype 2 and 3 infection. N Engl J Med 2015;373(27):2608–17.

30. Sulkowski MS, Naggie S, Lalezari J, et al. Sofosbuvir and ribavirin for hepatitis C in patients with HIV coinfection. JAMA 2014;312(4):353–61.

31. Wyles DL, Ruane PJ, Sulkowski MS, et al. Daclatasvir plus sofosbuvir for HCV in patients coinfected with HIV-1. N Engl J Med 2015;373(8):714–25.

32. Naggie S, Cooper C, Saag M, et al. Ledipasvir and sofosbuvir for HCV in patients coinfected with HIV-1. N Engl J Med 2015;373(8):705–13.

33. Sulkowski MS, Eron JJ, Wyles D, et al. Ombitasvir, paritaprevir co-dosed with ritonavir, dasabuvir, and ribavirin for hepatitis C in patients co-infected with HIV-1: a randomized trial. JAMA 2015;313(12):1223–31.

34. Rockstroh JK, Nelson M, Katlama C, et al. Efficacy and safety of grazoprevir (MK-5172) and elbasvir (MK-8742) in patients with hepatitis C virus and HIV co-infection (C-EDGE CO-INFECTION): a non-randomised, open-label trial. Lancet HIV 2015;2(8):e319–27.

35. Canavan C, West J, Card T. The epidemiology of irritable bowel syndrome. Clin Epidemiol 2014;6:71–80.

36. Longstreth GF, Thompson WG, Chey WD, et al. Functional bowel disorders. Gastroenterology 2006;130:1480–91.

37. Moayyedi P, Ford AC, Quigley EM, et al. The American College of Gastroenterology irritable bowel syndrome monograph: translating systematic review data to clinical practice. Gastroenterology 2010;138:789–91 [author reply: 791–2].

38. Sandler RS, Everhart JE, Donowitz M, et al. The burden of selected digestive diseases in the United States. Gastroenterology 2002;122:1500–11.

39. Peery AF, Crockett SD, Barritt AS, et al. Burden of gastrointestinal, liver, and pancreatic diseases in the United States. Gastroenterology 2015;149(7):1731–41.e3.

40. Drossman DA, Morris CB, Schneck S, et al. International survey of patients with IBS: symptom features and their severity, health status, treatments, and risk taking to achieve clinical benefit. J Clin Gastroenterol 2009;43:541–50.

41. Ford AC, Moayyedi P, Lacy BE, et al. American College of Gastroenterology monograph on the management of irritable bowel syndrome and chronic idiopathic constipation. Am J Gastroenterol 2014;109(Suppl 1):S2–26 [quiz: S7].

42. Weinberg DS, Smalley W, Heidelbaugh JJ, et al. American Gastroenterological Association Institute guideline on the pharmacological management of irritable bowel syndrome. Gastroenterology 2014;147:1146–8.

43. Bharucha AE, Pemberton JH, Locke GR 3rd. American Gastroenterological Association technical review on constipation. Gastroenterology 2013;144(1):218–38.

44. Lee-Robichaud H, Thomas K, Morgan J, et al. Lactulose versus polyethylene glycol for chronic constipation. Cochrane Database Syst Rev 2010;(7):CD007570.

45. Available at: http://www.fda.gov/NewsEvents/Newsroom/PressAnnouncements/2008/ucm116889.htm. Accessed December 7, 2015.

46. Available at: http://www.fda.gov/NewsEvents/Newsroom/PressAnnouncements/ucm317505.htm. Accessed December 7, 2015.

47. Thomas RH, Luthin DR. Current and emerging treatments for irritable bowel syndrome with constipation and chronic idiopathic constipation: focus on prosecretory agents. Pharmacotherapy 2015;35(6):613–30.

48. Brandt LJ, Chey WD, Foxx-Orenstein AE, et al. An evidence-based position statement on the management of irritable bowel syndrome. Am J Gastroenterol 2009;104(Suppl 1):S1–35.

49. Efskind PS, Bernklev T, Vatn MH. A double-blind placebo-controlled trial with loperamide in irritable bowel syndrome. Scand J Gastroenterol 1996;31(5): 463–8.

50. Lacy BE, Chey WD, Lembo AJ. New and emerging treatment options for irritable bowel syndrome. Gastroenterol Hepatol 2015;11:1–19.

51. Wade PR, Palmer JM, McKenney S, et al. Modulation of gastrointestinal function by MuDelta, a mixed micro opioid receptor agonist/micro opioid receptor antagonist. Br J Pharmacol 2012;167:1111–25.

52. Garnock-Jones KP. Eluxadoline: first global approval. Drugs 2015;75:1305–10.

53. Available at: http://www.fda.gov/NewsEvents/Newsroom/PressAnnouncements/ucm448328.htm. Accessed December 7, 2015.

54. Menees SB, Maneerattannaporn M, Kim HM, et al. The efficacy and safety of rifaximin for the irritable bowel syndrome: a systematic review and meta-analysis. Am J Gastroenterol 2012;107(1):28–35 [quiz: 36].

55. Pimentel M, Lembo A, Chey WD, et al. Rifaximin therapy for patients with irritable bowel syndrome without constipation. N Engl J Med 2011;364(1):22–32.

56. Schoenfeld P, Pimentel M, Chang L, et al. Safety and tolerability of rifaximin for the treatment of irritable bowel syndrome without constipation: a pooled analysis of randomised, double-blind, placebo-controlled trials. Aliment Pharmacol Ther 2014;39(10):1161–8.

57. Camilleri M, Northcutt AR, Kong S, et al. Efficacy and safety of alosetron in women with irritable bowel syndrome: a randomised, placebo-controlled trial. Lancet 2000;355(9209):1035–40.

58. Chang L, Tong K, Ameen V. Ischemic colitis and complications of constipation associated with the use of alosetron under a risk management plan: clinical characteristics, outcomes, and incidences. Am J Gastroenterol 2010;105(4): 866–75.

59. Garsed K, Chernova J, Hastings M, et al. A randomised trial of ondansetron for the treatment of irritable bowel syndrome with diarrhoea. Gut 2014;63(10): 1617–25.

60. Talley NJ, Phillips SF, Haddad A, et al. GR 38032F (ondansetron), a selective 5HT3 receptor antagonist, slows colonic transit in healthy man. Dig Dis Sci 1990;35(4):477–80.

61. Luthra P, Ford AC. The fall and rise of 5-hydroxytryptamine receptor antagonists in irritable bowel syndrome with diarrhea. Gastroenterology 2014; 147(2):527–8.

62. DeVault KR, Castell DO. Updated guidelines for the diagnosis and treatment of gastroesophageal reflux disease. Am J Gastroenterol 2005;100(1):190–200.

63. Dent J, El-Serag HB, Wallander MA, et al. Epidemiology of gastro-oesophageal reflux disease: a systematic review. Gut 2005;54(5):710–7.

64. Camilleri M, Dubois D, Coulie B, et al. Prevalence and socioeconomic impact of upper gastrointestinal disorders in the United States: results of the US upper gastrointestinal study. Clin Gastroenterol Hepatol 2005;3(6):543–52.

65. Anand BS, Raed AK, Malaty HM, et al. Low point prevalence of peptic ulcer in normal individuals with *Helicobacter pylori* infection. Am J Gastroenterol 1996; 91(6):1112–5.

66. el-Serag HB, Sonnenberg A. Opposing time trends of peptic ulcer and reflux disease. Gut 1998;43(3):327–33.

67. Sonnenberg A. Time trends of ulcer mortality in Europe. Gastroenterology 2007; 132(7):2320–7.

68. Sung JJ, Kuipers EJ, El-Serag HB. Systematic review: the global incidence and prevalence of peptic ulcer disease. Aliment Pharmacol Ther 2009; 29(9):938–46.
69. Laine L, Yang H, Chang SC, et al. Trends for incidence of hospitalization and death due to GI complications in the United States from 2001 to 2009. Am J Gastroenterol 2012;107(8):1190–5 [quiz: 1196].
70. Jacobson BC, Somers SC, Fuchs CS, et al. Body-mass index and symptoms of gastroesophageal reflux in women. N Engl J Med 2006;354(22):2340–8.
71. Fraser-Moodie CA, Norton B, Gornall C, et al. Weight loss has an independent beneficial effect on symptoms of gastro-oesophageal reflux in patients who are overweight. Scand J Gastroenterol 1999;34(4):337–40.
72. Hamilton JW, Boisen RJ, Yamamoto DT, et al. Sleeping on a wedge diminishes exposure of the esophagus to refluxed acid. Dig Dis Sci 1988;33(5): 518–22.
73. Orr WC, Harnish MJ. Sleep-related gastro-oesophageal reflux: provocation with a late evening meal and treatment with acid suppression. Aliment Pharmacol Ther 1998;12(10):1033–8.
74. Kadakia SC, Kikendall JW, Maydonovitch C, et al. Effect of cigarette smoking on gastroesophageal reflux measured by 24-h ambulatory esophageal pH monitoring. Am J Gastroenterol 1995;90(10):1785–90.
75. Chiba N, De Gara CJ, Wilkinson JM, et al. Speed of healing and symptom relief in grade II to IV gastroesophageal reflux disease: a meta-analysis. Gastroenterology 1997;112(6):1798–810.
76. Robinson M, Sahba B, Avner D, et al. A comparison of lansoprazole and ranitidine in the treatment of erosive oesophagitis. Multicentre Investigational Group. Aliment Pharmacol Ther 1995;9(1):25–31.
77. Sifrim D, Castell D, Dent J, et al. Gastro-oesophageal reflux monitoring: review and consensus report on detection and definitions of acid, non-acid, and gas reflux. Gut 2004;53(7):1024–31.
78. van Pinxteren B, Sigterman KE, Bonis P, et al. Short-term treatment with proton pump inhibitors, H2-receptor antagonists and prokinetics for gastro-oesophageal reflux disease-like symptoms and endoscopy negative reflux disease. Cochrane Database Syst Rev 2010;(11):CD002095.
79. Gralnek IM, Dulai GS, Fennerty MB, et al. Esomeprazole versus other proton pump inhibitors in erosive esophagitis: a meta-analysis of randomized clinical trials. Clin Gastroenterol Hepatol 2006;4(12):1452–8.
80. Gerson LB, Mitra S, Bleker WF, et al. Control of intra-oesophageal pH in patients with Barrett's oesophagus on omeprazole-sodium bicarbonate therapy. Aliment Pharmacol Ther 2012;35(7):803–9.
81. Sharma P, Shaheen NJ, Perez MC, et al. Clinical trials: healing of erosive oesophagitis with dexlansoprazole MR, a proton pump inhibitor with a novel dual delayed-release formulation–results from two randomized controlled studies. Aliment Pharmacol Ther 2009;29(7):731–41.
82. Metz DC, Vakily M, Dixit T, et al. Review article: dual delayed release formulation of dexlansoprazole MR, a novel approach to overcome the limitations of conventional single release proton pump inhibitor therapy. Aliment Pharmacol Ther 2009;29(9):928–37.
83. Kahrilas PJ, Shaheen NJ, Vaezi MF. American Gastroenterological Association Institute technical review on the management of gastroesophageal reflux disease. Gastroenterology 2008;135(4):1392–413, 1413.e1-5.

84. Kahrilas PJ, Shaheen NJ, Vaezi MF, et al. American Gastroenterological Association Medical Position Statement on the management of gastroesophageal reflux disease. Gastroenterology 2008;135(4):1383–91, 1391.e1-5.

85. Stedman CA, Barclay ML. Review article: comparison of the pharmacokinetics, acid suppression and efficacy of proton pump inhibitors. Aliment Pharmacol Ther 2000;14(8):963–78.

86. Katz PO, Gerson LB, Vela MF. Guidelines for the diagnosis and management of gastroesophageal reflux disease. Am J Gastroenterol 2013;108(3):308–28 [quiz: 329].

87. Schindlbeck NE, Klauser AG, Berghammer G, et al. Three year follow up of patients with gastrooesophageal reflux disease. Gut 1992;33(8):1016–9.

88. Vigneri S, Termini R, Leandro G, et al. A comparison of five maintenance therapies for reflux esophagitis. N Engl J Med 1995;333(17):1106–10.

89. Komazawa Y, Adachi K, Mihara T, et al. Tolerance to famotidine and ranitidine treatment after 14 days of administration in healthy subjects without *Helicobacter pylori* infection. J Gastroenterol Hepatol 2003;18(6):678–82.

90. Fackler WK, Ours TM, Vaezi MF, et al. Long-term effect of H2RA therapy on nocturnal gastric acid breakthrough. Gastroenterology 2002;122(3):625–32.

91. Sontag SJ. The medical management of reflux esophagitis. Role of antacids and acid inhibition. Gastroenterol Clin North Am 1990;19(3):683–712.

92. Hatlebakk JG, Berstad A. Pharmacokinetic optimisation in the treatment of gastro-oesophageal reflux disease. Clin Pharmacokinet 1996;31(5):386–406.

93. Fass R, Sontag SJ, Traxler B, et al. Treatment of patients with persistent heartburn symptoms: a double-blind, randomized trial. Clin Gastroenterol Hepatol 2006;4(1):50–6.

94. Koek GH, Sifrim D, Lerut T, et al. Effect of the GABA(B) agonist baclofen in patients with symptoms and duodeno-gastro-oesophageal reflux refractory to proton pump inhibitors. Gut 2003;52(10):1397–402.

95. VA Office of Research and Development. ClinicalTrials.gov [Internet]. Bethesda (MD): National Library of Medicine (US). 2000- [cited 2015 Dec 7]. Available from: https://clinicaltrials.gov/ct2/show/NCT01265550. NLM Identifier: NCT01265550.

96. Lodato F, Azzaroli F, Turco L, et al. Adverse effects of proton pump inhibitors. Best Pract Res Clin Gastroenterol 2010;24(2):193–201.

97. Bavishi C, Dupont HL. Systematic review: the use of proton pump inhibitors and increased susceptibility to enteric infection. Aliment Pharmacol Ther 2011; 34(11–12):1269–81.

98. Available at: http://www.fda.gov/Drugs/DrugSafety/PostmarketDrugSafety InformationforPatientsandProviders/ucm213206.htm. Accessed December 7, 2015.

99. Johnstone J, Nerenberg K, Loeb M. Meta-analysis: proton pump inhibitor use and the risk of community-acquired pneumonia. Aliment Pharmacol Ther 2010;31(11):1165–77.

100. Sibbing D, Morath T, Stegherr J, et al. Impact of proton pump inhibitors on the antiplatelet effects of clopidogrel. Thromb Haemost 2009;101(4):714–9.

101. Ho PM, Maddox TM, Wang L, et al. Risk of adverse outcomes associated with concomitant use of clopidogrel and proton pump inhibitors following acute coronary syndrome. JAMA 2009;301(9):937–44.

102. Bhatt DL, Cryer BL, Contant CF, et al. Clopidogrel with or without omeprazole in coronary artery disease. N Engl J Med 2010;363(20):1909–17.

103. Chey WD, Wong BC. American College of Gastroenterology guideline on the management of *Helicobacter pylori* infection. Am J Gastroenterol 2007;102(8): 1808–25.
104. Paoluzi P, Iacopini F, Crispino P, et al. 2-week triple therapy for *Helicobacter pylori* infection is better than 1-week in clinical practice: a large prospective single-center randomized study. Helicobacter 2006;11(6):562–8.
105. Laine L. Is it time for quadruple therapy to be first line? Can J Gastroenterol 2003;17(Suppl B):33b–5b.
106. Luther J, Higgins PD, Schoenfeld PS, et al. Empiric quadruple vs. triple therapy for primary treatment of *Helicobacter pylori* infection: systematic review and meta-analysis of efficacy and tolerability. Am J Gastroenterol 2010;105(1):65–73.
107. Moayyedi P, Malfertheiner P. Editorial: sequential therapy for eradication of *Helicobacter pylori*: a new guiding light or a false dawn? Am J Gastroenterol 2009;104(12):3081–3.
108. Malfertheiner P, Megraud F, O'Morain C, et al. Current concepts in the management of *Helicobacter pylori* infection–the Maastricht 2-2000 consensus report. Aliment Pharmacol Ther 2002;16(2):167–80.
109. Basu PP, Rayapudi K, Pacana T, et al. A randomized study comparing levofloxacin, omeprazole, nitazoxanide, and doxycycline versus triple therapy for the eradication of *Helicobacter pylori*. Am J Gastroenterol 2011;106(11):1970–5.
110. Yeomans ND, Tulassay Z, Juhasz L, et al. A comparison of omeprazole with ranitidine for ulcers associated with nonsteroidal antiinflammatory drugs. Acid suppression trial: ranitidine versus omeprazole for NSAID-associated ulcer treatment (ASTRONAUT) Study Group. N Engl J Med 1998;338(11):719–26.
111. Agrawal NM, Campbell DR, Safdi MA, et al. Superiority of lansoprazole vs ranitidine in healing nonsteroidal anti-inflammatory drug-associated gastric ulcers: results of a double-blind, randomized, multicenter study. NSAID-Associated Gastric Ulcer Study Group. Arch Intern Med 2000;160(10):1455–61.
112. Koch M, Dezi A, Ferrario F, et al. Prevention of nonsteroidal anti-inflammatory drug-induced gastrointestinal mucosal injury. A meta-analysis of randomized controlled clinical trials. Arch Intern Med 1996;156(20):2321–32.
113. Graham DY, Agrawal NM, Campbell DR, et al. Ulcer prevention in long-term users of nonsteroidal anti-inflammatory drugs: results of a double-blind, randomized, multicenter, active- and placebo-controlled study of misoprostol vs lansoprazole. Arch Intern Med 2002;162(2):169–75.
114. Weberg R, Berstad A, Lange O, et al. Duodenal ulcer healing with four antacid tablets daily. Scand J Gastroenterol 1985;20(9):1041–5.
115. Lauritsen K, Bytzer P, Hansen J, et al. Comparison of ranitidine and high-dose antacid in the treatment of prepyloric or duodenal ulcer. A double-blind controlled trial. Scand J Gastroenterol 1985;20(1):123–8.

Pharmacologic Therapies in Pulmonology and Allergy

Andrew G. Ayars, MD[a,b,*], Matthew C. Altman, MD[a,b]

KEYWORDS

- Asthma • Chronic rhinitis • Allergic rhinitis • Angioedema • Acute urticaria
- Chronic urticaria

KEY POINTS

- Although conditions such as chronic rhinitis, urticaria, angioedema, and asthma have markedly different clinical presentations, a core group of medications such as antihistamines, corticosteroids (systemic and topical), leukotriene blockers, and anticholinergic medications are often used to treat these conditions, and knowing the indications and side-effect profiles of each can allow for maximum efficacy.
- Chronic rhinitis symptoms often respond to first-line agents such as second-generation H1 antihistamines, topical antihistamines, and nasal steroids, but other therapies such as leukotriene blockers, nasal anticholinergics agents, and nasal decongestants can be used depending on patient symptoms and cause of rhinitis being treated.
- Urticaria is generally divided into acute (<6-week duration) and chronic (>6-week duration) because they often have different causes based on this distinction. Although medications used to treat urticaria can be similar to atopic conditions, the dosing regimens can differ significantly.
- Angioedema can often be differentiated into mast cell and complement-mediated forms, and this distinction is important given the medications used to treat each form are significantly different.
- Although medications such as inhaled corticosteroids, β-agonists, and leukotriene blockers used according to National Heart Lung and Blood Institute are effective for most patients, there are biologic therapies available to treat uncontrolled asthma according to the asthma phenotypes.

Drs A.G. Ayars and M.C. Altman do not have any financial conflicts of interest to disclose.
[a] Division of Allergy and Infectious Diseases, University of Washington School of Medicine, Seattle, WA 98195, USA; [b] Center for Allergy and Inflammation, UW Medicine at South Lake Union, 750 Republican Street, Box 358061, Seattle, WA 98109-4725, USA
* Corresponding author. Center for Allergy and Inflammation, UW Medicine at South Lake Union, 750 Republican Street, Box 358061, Seattle, WA 98109-4725.
E-mail address: dayars@u.washington.edu

Med Clin N Am 100 (2016) 851–868
http://dx.doi.org/10.1016/j.mcna.2016.03.010
0025-7125/16/$ – see front matter © 2016 Elsevier Inc. All rights reserved.

medical.theclinics.com

RHINITIS

Rhinitis is characterized by 1 or more of the following nasal symptoms: congestion, rhinorrhea, sneezing, and itching. Rhinitis symptoms are one of the most common causes of primary care physician visits and can result in a decrease in quality of life, decreased productivity, missed work/school days, and significant treatment costs.[1] There are different causes of rhinitis symptoms, and it is important to try and elucidate a specific diagnosis because the treatment varies.

Seasonal and perennial allergic rhinitis are reactions to aeroallergens due to an immunoglobulin E (IgE) antibody-mediated sensitivity. Allergic rhinitis is one of the most common chronic illnesses in developed countries with significant morbidity to patients and substantial treatment-related costs with loss of workplace productivity.[1,2] Allergic rhinitis most commonly develops before 20 years of age, whereas nonallergic forms of rhinitis can have similar symptoms but often affects an older population and may involve sensitivity to triggers, such as strong odors and other non-IgE-mediated irritants.[3–5] Different forms include nonallergic rhinitis (NAR), nonallergic rhinitis with eosinophilia (NARES), infectious rhinitis, and medication-induced rhinitis. **Table 1** reviews some of the common forms of rhinitis and lists treatments that are often effective.

H1 Antihistamines

H1 antihistamines act as inverse agonists that combine with and stabilize the inactive conformation of the H1 receptor (**Table 2**).[5] H1 antihistamines represent a first-line treatment for many conditions such as allergic rhinitis and urticaria. This class of medications offers an inexpensive, safe, and effective therapy in many different conditions.

First-generation H1 antihistamines were introduced for clinical use in the 1940s and are one of the more commonly used medication classes available. This group of antihistamines readily crosses the blood-brain barrier, which accounts for sedation that is often seen with this group of medications. First-generation H1 antihistamines should be prescribed cautiously in the elderly or patients with occupations for which alertness is essential. More than 40 H1 antihistamines are available, and adverse effects can include dry eyes, dry mouth, constipation, and urinary hesitancy and retention, increased appetite and weight gain, and dizziness.[5]

In the 1980s, relatively nonsedating second-generation H1 antihistamines were introduced.

Table 1 Different types of rhinitis and common treatment	
Common Types of Rhinitis	**Common Treatments**
Allergic rhinitis	Oral antihistamines, nasal steroids, nasal antihistamines, antileukotriene agents
NAR	Nasal antihistamines, nasal steroids
NARES	Nasal steroids
Gustatory rhinitis	Nasal anticholinergics[63]
Medication induced[a]	Treat symptoms or discontinue medication
Infectious rhinitis	Supportive therapy or antibiotics
Atrophic rhinitis	Difficult to treat, often use lubrication and removal of crusts

[a] Oral contraceptives, antihypertensives, aspirin/NSAIDs, ACE inhibitors, phosphodiesterase-5-selective inhibitors, α-receptor antagonists.

Table 2
Common rhinitis medications

Drug Type	Examples/Common Trade Names	Discussion
Antihistamines		
First-generation H1 antihistamines	Diphenhydramine (Benadryl) Doxepin (Deptran, Sinequan) Hydroxyzine (Vistaril) Chlorpheniramine (Chlor-Trimeton)	The use of first-generation H1 antihistamines should be used with caution in most patients given associated sedation
Second-generation H1 antihistamines	Loratadine (Claritin) Fexofenadine (Allegra) Cetirizine (Zyrtec) Levocetirizine (Xyzal) Desloratadine (Clarinex)	Second-generation H1 antihistamines are effective, inexpensive first-line options for allergic rhinoconjunctivitis
Intranasal antihistamines	Azelastine (Astelin, Astepro) Olopatadine (Patanase)	Intranasal antihistamines work well in many allergic rhinitis patients and are often effective in other conditions such as NAR
Intranasal corticosteroids	Beclomethasone (Beconase) Budesonide (Rhinocort) Ciclesonide (Omnaris) Flunisolide (Nasarel) Fluticasone furoate (Veramyst) Fluticasone propionate (Flonase) Mometasone (Nasonex) Triamcinolone (Nasacort)	Another first-line agent for chronic rhinitis patients Safe long-term treatment for both allergic and NAR No one medication has been shown to be superior to other members of this class; treatment depends on cost and individual patient preference Although side effects are minimal, nasal dryness, irritation, and epistaxis can occur
Combination nasal sprays		
Intranasal corticosteroid + intranasal antihistamine	Azelastine/Fluticasone (Dymista)	There is thought to be a synergistic effect with ICS and nasal antihistamines
Intranasal anticholinergics		
Ipratropium	Ipratropium (Atrovent)	Not a first-line agent in most cases but works well for rhinorrhea; not as effective for congestion and postnasal drip
Leukotriene blockers		
LTRAs 5-LO inhibitors	Montelukast (Singulair) Zafirlukast (Accolate) Zileuton (Zyflo)	These medications are not a first-line treatment for rhinitis but can have a role as an add-on therapy or in patients with associated asthma

(continued on next page)

Drug Type	Examples/Common Trade Names	Discussion
		LTRAs are generally preferred over 5-LO inhibitors due to the need to monitor liver function with zileuton
Nasal/oral decongestants		
α-Adrenergic agonists	Oxymetazoline (Afrin, Neo-Synephrine) Phenylephrine (Neo-Synephrine) Pseudoephedrine (Sudafed)	These agents work well for short-term relief of congestion but should not be used long term given side-effect profile Prolonged use of high-dose nasal decongestants can lead to rebound worsening of symptoms, which is called rhinitis medicamentosa Some think that once-daily dosing can be an effective add-on therapy without the rebound symptoms

Table 2 (continued)

These medications do not cross the blood-brain barrier as readily as first-generation H1 antihistamines and are generally preferred for the treatment of allergic rhinitis given the side-effect profile.[1] There are slight differences among the second-generation H1 antihistamines in regard to their sedative properties. Fexofenadine is the least likely to cross the blood-brain barrier; cetirizine and loratadine may cause sedation at increased doses, although most patients do not experience this side effect.[1] Although increasing the dose of antihistamine for allergic rhinitis has not in general been shown to improve efficacy, some patients do respond better to increased doses of these medications, and a 2- to 3-fold increase in the second-generation H1 antihistamines is generally well tolerated.

Antihistamines can be delivered as intranasal sprays and are an effective treatment for both allergic rhinitis and NAR with a rapid onset of action and equal or superior efficacy compared with oral antihistamines.[1] Although these medications are generally thought to be less effective than intranasal corticosteroids for treatment of allergic rhinitis, they can work well as an add-on therapy. Intranasal antihistamines rarely cause sedation and are generally well tolerated. Many patients use them on an as-needed basis given the onset of action is more rapid than intranasal corticosteroids.

Corticosteroids

Corticosteroids are produced in the adrenal cortex and are involved in the regulation of inflammation, electrolyte levels, physiologic stress response, and behavior, among other actions. Glucocorticoids control carbohydrate, fat, and protein metabolism and are anti-inflammatory. Mineralocorticoids are involved in electrolyte balance and intravascular volume. Derivatives such as dexamethasone, prednisone, and fludrocortisone have differing amounts of glucocorticoid and mineralocorticoid action. Side effects of these medications are broad and are usually separated into those occurring with short- or long-term treatments. Short-term effects include neuropsychiatric changes, fluid retention, hyperglycemia, and insulin resistance. Long-term effects include fat redistribution (moon facies and buffalo hump), muscle wasting, osteoporosis, cataracts, and increased risk of infections. Although oral corticosteroids are very effective in relieving symptoms of most allergic conditions when used for short periods, every effort should be made to avoid frequent or prolonged administration given the side-effect profile.

It is well known that systemic and topical corticosteroids differ significantly in their side-effect profile. Intranasal corticosteroids are considered the most effective medication class for controlling symptoms of allergic rhinitis, such as congestion, rhinorrhea, and postnasal drip, and do not have the systemic side effects of oral corticosteroids.[1] The regular use of intranasal corticosteroids is generally preferred over as-needed use. These medications are generally well tolerated; common side effects include nasal irritation, dryness, epistaxis, and in rare cases, ulceration or septal perforation.[6] Anecdotal evidence suggests that a more lateral application has the potential to reduce the frequency of epistaxis, and patients should be instructed to aim toward the outside of the nose bilaterally.[7,8] Although a definitive risk of cataracts or glaucoma has not been clearly demonstrated, patients should be asked if they have a history of either of these conditions before prescribing nasal corticosteroids, and if so, monitoring by an ophthalmologist is recommended.[9,10] Although there are multiple options available, there are no head-to-head studies showing superiority of one nasal steroid agent versus another.

Anticholinergic Agents

The use of anticholinergic medications dates back many years when plants containing atropine, hyoscyamine, and scopolamine were consumed.[11] Competitive antagonists of acetylcholine act in the central and the peripheral nervous system to inhibit the parasympathetic nerve impulses through a variety of receptors.[12] In the human respiratory tract, muscarinic receptors are expressed by smooth muscle cells, and antimuscarinic agents are bronchodilators and are also thought to have an anti-inflammatory function.

Topical anticholinergics are used in nasal preparations and may reduce rhinorrhea but have minimal effect on other nasal symptoms.[1] Although the side-effect profile is minimal, these agents should not be considered first line for conditions such as allergic rhinitis but can be used as an add-on therapy or as monotherapy in patients that do not respond to nasal steroids and oral antihistamines when the most bothersome symptom is rhinorrhea.

Decongestants

α-Adrenergic agonists relieve congestion by constricting the blood vessels in the nasal cavity and can be administered by oral and nasal preparations. Oral decongestants not only constrict the blood vessels in the nasal cavity but also can cause other unwanted symptoms such as hypertension, insomnia, and anxiety.[13,14] Continuous use of these medications is generally discouraged, but they are often effective for short-term relief of nasal congestion.[1] Examples of these mediations include oxymetazoline, pseudoephedrine, and phenylephrine. Phenylephrine is available as an oral medicine or as a nasal spray and is a common ingredient in over-the-counter decongestants. Similar to oral preparations, consistent use of nasal decongestants is discouraged due to the development of rhinitis medicamentosa, which is a syndrome of rebound nasal congestion due to overuse of nasal decongestants.[15] Although it is known that multiple daily doses of oxymetazoline can result in rebound symptoms, many think that once-daily dosing is safe and can be an effective therapy when used with nasal steroids.[16]

Antileukotriene Agents

Leukotrienes are products of the 5-lipoxygenase (5-LO) pathway of arachidonic acid metabolism and are often involved in airway inflammation. Cysteinyl leukotrienes promote allergic inflammation by enhancing immune responses and can increase adhesion, migration, and survival of inflammatory cells.[17] Leukotrienes promote nasal mucous secretion, congestion, and inflammation and increase the generation of an array of other proinflammatory mediators. There are 2 classes of leukotriene blockers: leukotriene receptor antagonists (LTRAs) and 5-LO inhibitors. Both block the effects of leukotrienes and were approved for use in the late 1990s.

The LTRAs available in the United States are montelukast and zafirlukast. These drugs can lessen rhinorrhea, sneezing, and pruritus in patients with allergic rhinitis and are often used if patients have concurrent asthma that is exercise induced or in patients that do not like using nasal sprays. Although these medications are effective in some cases of allergic rhinitis, they are generally not recommended as first-line agents.[18] These medications are generally well tolerated with minimal side effects. There have been reports of a possible link between the use of leukotriene blockers and an increased suicide risk, although this has not been firmly established. It is currently recommended that LTRAs be indicated unless the patient expresses severe depression or suicidal thoughts.[19,20] The use of the 5-LO inhibitor zileuton can be complicated by hepatitis, and liver function tests should be monitored. Given the risk of hepatitis in addition to the frequency of administration, zileuton is not generally used in allergic rhinitis.

Environmental Controls

When a sensitivity to aeroallegens has been established by history and skin testing/serum IgE testing, then efforts should be made to decrease exposure to the specific aeroallergens. Environmental controls have been shown to be effective in decreasing exposure and symptoms due to perennial allergens, such as dust mites, pets, and cockroaches.[21–25]

Allergen Immunotherapy

Allergen immunotherapy (allergy shots) should be considered for patients with allergic rhinitis and documented allergic sensitivities (IgE mediated) to aeroallergens with an appropriate history. Allergen immunotherapy is the only treatment that has been shown to alter the immune response to aeroallergens.[26] Subcutaneous immunotherapy (SCIT) and sublingual immunotherapy (SLIT) are both available and have each been shown to be effective. Head-to-head studies are limited, and although it is generally thought that SCIT provides greater clinical and immunologic responses than SLIT, treatment depends on patient preference and clinical history.[27] Immunotherapy should only be administered by health care professionals experienced in treating anaphylaxis given this reaction can occur even when used at appropriate doses.

One of the manifestations of chronic rhinitis can be chronic cough, which is a very challenging symptom to treat. Because therapies for chronic rhinitis are generally quite safe, they should be considered in patients with unexplained chronic cough.

URTICARIA

Urticaria is a common condition that is often categorized by duration into acute (<6 weeks) and chronic (>6 weeks) forms.[28] The reason for classification is that causes and treatments are generally different.

Acute Urticaria

Acute urticaria is defined as hives that have been present for less than a 6-week duration. Common causes of acute urticaria include infections, foods, and medications such as nonsteroidal anti-inflammatory drugs (NSAIDs). In these cases, a detailed history should be taken to evaluate for possible triggers. In some cases, evaluation with skin-prick testing or serum-specific IgE testing for possible triggers can help identify a cause.

Chronic Urticaria

Chronic urticaria is defined as hives that have been present most days of the week for more than 6 weeks. Common causes of chronic urticaria include autoimmune forms, physical urticarias, and idiopathic urticaria, which is a diagnosis of exclusion. Specific allergens interacting with IgE rarely cause chronic urticaria. Forms of physical urticaria include cholinergic, aquagenic, pressure, cold, solar, heat, dermatographism, and exercise induced. These forms of urticaria are best diagnosed by a detailed clinical history and testing for specific causes such as the ice cube test for cold urticaria.

For patients with chronic urticaria, testing for allergic triggers to inhalants/foods and extensive laboratory testing are not recommended because most often it does not lead to changes in treatment or outcome.[28,29] Although the treatment of acute and chronic urticaria involves the use of medications that are often used in other atopic disorders, the indications and doses used can differ significantly.

Antihistamines

First- and second-generation H1 antihistamines can be used in both acute and chronic urticaria and are effective in most patients.[28] Although first-generation H1 antihistamines are frequently used for acute urticaria, second-generation H1 antihistamines are often just as efficacious, and the dose can typically be advanced further given the lower side-effect profile of these medications. It has been shown that a 2- to 4-fold increase in the US Food and Drug Administration (FDA)–approved dose of second-generation antihistamines can be effective for achieving control in some patients.[28] An example regimen is cetirizine 10-mg tablets, 1 to 2 pills twice a day. Although this seems like a significant increase from the recommended doses, this dose is usually well tolerated and available as an inexpensive generic without prescription. Even at these doses, most patients do not experience significant sedation. If patients experience sedation with cetirizine, switching to fexofenadine is the next agent often used given that sedation is not associated with this medication. Up to 30-fold overdoses of second-generation H1 antihistamines have not been associated with serious adverse events or fatality.[5] For many conditions, such as chronic urticaria, where difficulty sleeping may be an issue due to pruritus, the sedation associated with first-generation agents may be useful when used with scheduled second-generation agents.

Corticosteroids

Although there is a lack of studies documenting the efficacy of oral corticosteroids in urticaria, it is well known that these medications are effective, although not ideal for long-term use given their side-effect profile. Alternatively, there is no role for topical corticosteroids in acute or chronic urticaria given the transient and migratory nature of this rash. If topical corticosteroids are effective in treating a rash, then an alternative diagnosis such as atopic dermatitis needs to be considered.

Other Agents

When the standard agents are not effective for patients with chronic urticaria, there are other medications available that can be more effective but often have more potential side effects or cost. Omalizumab is a monoclonal anti-IgE treatment that has been shown to be effective in refractory urticaria patients that do not respond to treatments such as high-dose antihistamines.[20,30] Omalizumab is administered as a subcutaneous injection every 4 weeks. This treatment needs to be given in a monitored setting because anaphylaxis has very rarely been reported.[31] Other agents used to treat refractory urticaria are reviewed in **Table 3**.

ANGIOEDEMA

Angioedema is defined as localized subcutaneous swelling that results from extravasation of fluid into interstitial tissues that often will affect the face, lips, mouth, throat, larynx, extremities, and genitalia.[32] Clinically significant angioedema is often divided into mast cell–mediated versus complement-mediated causes.

Bradykinin is the primary mediator in the complement-mediated form or angioedema and is typically slower in onset and often more severe than mast cell forms and is generally not associated with urticaria.[32] In this disease, there is an absence or nonfunction of an important enzyme called C1 esterase inhibitor, and this abnormality leads to overproduction of the vasodilator bradykinin. This distinction is important because this process can lead to airway compromise and possibly death.

The classic complement-mediated form of severe angioedema is hereditary angioedema (HAE), which usually presents during childhood, and a family history is often present.[33] Other forms of complement-mediated angioedema include acquired angioedema (AAE) and angiotensin-converting enzyme (ACE) inhibitor-induced angioedema, which often present later in life. AAE is often due to autoantibodies against the C1 inhibitor. ACE inhibitor-induced angioedema is a well-known cause of this condition and occurs due to decreased production of angiotensin II in susceptible individuals. The medication list of any patient presenting with angioedema should be screened for ACE inhibitors. Other patients can have a history consistent with HAE and a family history, but normal laboratory results. These patients are often classified as type III HAE patients or C1-inhibitor normal HAE if there is a family history, or idiopathic angioedema if there is no family history. There are some reports that type III HAE and idiopathic angioedema patients might respond to many of the same medications used in type I and type II HAE.[34] Differentiation of the type of angioedema is based on clinical history and laboratory evaluation (**Table 4**). Treatment of

Table 3 Treatments for refractory chronic urticaria		
Other Agents Often Used in Refractory Cases	Omalizumab Cyclosporine Methotrexate Dapsone Mycophenolate mofetil Sulfasalazine Hydroxycholoroquine	These agents should only be discussed if symptoms are not controlled with standard agents such as high-dose antihistamines Given there are often more risks and/or costs associated with these agents, a long discussion regarding risks and benefits needs to take place Should only be administered by health care professionals with experience is using these medications

Table 4
Laboratory classification of the different forms of angioedema

Type of Angioedema	C4	C1 Inhibitor Level	C1 Inhibitor Function	C1q
Type I HAE	Low	Low	Low	Normal
Type II HAE	Low	Normal	Low	Normal
Type III HAE	Normal	Normal	Normal	Normal
AAE	Low	Low	Low	Low
Idiopathic angioedema	Normal	Normal	Normal	Normal
ACE inhibitor induced angioedema	Normal	Normal	Normal	Normal

complement-mediated angioedema can be difficult because patients do not often respond to typical therapies such as antihistamines, epinephrine, and oral corticosteroids. The treatment of HAE can be classified into 2 approaches: treatment of acute attacks and prophylactic treatment (short term and long term). Treatment options available are often unique to this condition and are discussed in **Table 5**.

Mast cell–mediated angioedema often comes on rapidly and can be associated with urticaria and pruritus. If urticaria is present with angioedema, then a mast cell–mediated cause should be suspected. In addition to urticaria, there can be other systemic symptoms of mast cell–mediated angioedema, such as bronchospasm, abdominal pain/diarrhea, and hypotension, and if this is the case, then investigation into anaphylaxis should take place. The mast cell–mediated form often responds to medications used to treat urticaria, as discussed in the previous section. If a mast cell–mediated cause is suspected, then second-generation H1 antihistamines can be used either in the setting of an event or as prophylactic therapy. As discussed previously, these medications offer a low-cost option with minimal risk.

ASTHMA

Asthma is a heterogeneous chronic inflammatory disease resulting in variable obstruction of the lower airways. The diagnosis of asthma is similar to other conditions, such as arthritis or anemia, in the fact that there are many different forms that can lead to a similar clinical phenotype.[35–38] Examples of the asthma phenotype include eosinophil- or neutrophil-driven asthma, allergic bronchopulmonary aspergillosis (ABPA), autoimmune conditions such as Churg-Strauss, and aspirin exacerbated respiratory disease (AERD). Asthma management is consistent with other chronic disease management: periodic assessment with continual clinical reassessment and individualization of therapy is necessary for optimal management. Patient reports do not always accurately reflect airway obstruction so peak flow measurement or spirometry should be performed.[39] For many asthmatic patients, the management strategy outlined in the National Heart Lung and Blood Institute (NHLBI) Guidelines is effective (**Table 6**). Common medications used to treat asthma are discussed in **Table 7**.

Rescue Medications

Short-acting β2-agonists
β2-Agonists interact with the β2 adrenoreceptor to work as bronchodilators, causing a direct relaxation effect on airway smooth muscle cells.[40] Isoproterenol and isoetharine were used until the 1970s, but had substantial cardiovascular effects, including tachycardia, increased blood pressure, and central nervous system stimulation. Short-acting β2-agonists (SABAs) are the standard rescue medications used to treat asthma

Table 5
Treatments for bradykinin-mediated angioedema

Type of Therapy	Agents	Mechanism of Action	Discussion
Acute treatment			
Fresh frozen plasma	NA	Contains high circulating levels of C1 Inhibitor (C1INH) protein; also contains plasma prekallikrein, coagulation factor XII, and high-molecular-weight kininogen	Fresh frozen plasma is often effective in abrogating HAE attacks given it contains the C1INH protein; however, fresh frozen plasma might acutely exacerbate some attacks given the other factors that it contains and caution is required[32]
C1 inhibitor concentrate	Berinert	Derived from C1-esterase inhibitor concentrate, can be used to abort angioedema attacks	Treatment within <6 h after start of an attack results in shorter time to resolution of symptoms[32] Made from human plasma and theoretically may contain infectious agents such as viruses and prion disease Self-administered, does not need to be given under observation
Bradykinin receptor antagonist	Icatibant (Firazyr)	A competitive antagonist selective for the bradykinin B2 receptor, which reduces smooth muscle contraction and vascular permeability	Shown to decrease the median time to clinically significant relief of symptoms[64,65] Does not have to be given under medical observation
Kallikrein inhibitor	Ecallantide (Kalbitor)	Inhibits kallikrein by blocking the plasma-binding site, thereby stopping production of bradykinin	Has been shown to decrease symptom scores in patients with angioedema[66] Due to the risk of anaphylaxis, medication must be given under observation

Chronic treatment

Antifibrinolytics	Tranexamic acid Epsilonaminocaproic acid	Antifibrinolytics interfere with the formation of the fibrinolytic enzyme plasmin	Relatively safe and can be effective in some patients[67] Thought to be generally less effective than androgens[33] but are often used in patients who cannot tolerate androgens Do not administer if patients are at risk for thrombotic events
Androgenic steroids	Danazol	The mechanism of androgenic steroids controlling angioedema is unknown	Shown to be effective, but appropriate patients need to be selected due to side effects of this medication[32] Side effects can include weight gain, acne, virilization, menstrual irregularities, and changes in lipid profile, and hepatotoxicity
C1 inhibitor concentrate	Cinryze	Derived from C1-esterase inhibitor concentrate	Can be administered every 3–4 d for routine prophylaxis or for preprocedure prophylaxis Appropriate for home administration

Table 6
National Heart Lung and Blood Institute guidelines for asthma management

Asthma Classification	Treatment	
Mild intermittent asthma • Symptoms ≤2 d/wk • Nighttime awakenings ≤2 times/mo • SABA use ≤2 d/wk • No interference with daily activities • FEV1 ≥80%	Step 1 SABA as needed	⬆

Mild persistent asthma
• Symptoms >2 d/wk
• Nighttime awakenings 3–4 times/mo
• SABA use >2 d/wk
• Minor interference with daily activities
• FEV1 ≥80%
• Systemic oral corticosteroids 0–1 time per year
	Step 2
	  Low-dose ICS
	
	Step 3
	  Low dose-ICS + either LABA or LTRA
		Step down if asthma remains controlled for >3 mo

Moderate persistent asthma • Symptoms daily • Nighttime awakenings >1 time/wk • SABA use daily • "Some limitation" with daily activities • FEV1 >60% but <80% • Systemic oral corticosteroids ≥2 times per year	Step 4 • Medium-dose ICS + LABA • Alternative: medium dose ICS + LTRA Step 5 High-dose ICS + LABA	Step up if asthma control guidelines are not being met
Severe persistent asthma • Symptoms throughout the day • Nighttime awakenings nightly • SABA use several times per day • "Extreme limitation" with daily activities • FEV1 <60% • Systemic oral corticosteroids ≥2 times per y	Step 6 • High-dose ICS + LABA • Oral corticosteroids or biologic agent (Omalizumab)	⬇

Abbreviation: FEV1, forced expiratory volume in 1 second.
Each visit includes patient education, environmental controls, and management of comorbidities. Step down if asthma is well controlled for at least 3 mo.
From National Heart, Lung and Blood Institute. Expert Panel Report 3 (EPR3): guidelines for the diagnosis and management of asthma. Bethesda (MD): NHLBI; 2007.

exacerbations and should be supplied for all asthmatics. These medications should only be used as a rescue medication for asthma exacerbations/symptoms or before exercise, not as a scheduled medication.[41] β2-Agonists exist as isomers and levalbuterol is the R isomer of racemic albuterol. Levalbuterol has been shown to cause less tremor and heart-rate changes but has not been shown to be more efficacious or safer than albuterol.[42]

Maintenance Therapy

Inhaled corticosteroids

Inhaled corticosteroids (ICS) form the cornerstone of asthma management. They have been shown to result in fewer symptoms, reduced albuterol use, reduced

Table 7
Common asthma medications

Drug	Examples/Trade Names	Discussion
Rescue medications		
SABA	Albuterol (Ventolin, Proventil, ProAir)	Used as monotherapy for mild intermittent asthma
	Pirbuterol (Maxair)	Should only be used as a rescue medication in all forms of asthma
	Levalbuterol (Xopenex)	
Controller medications		
ICS	Beclomethasone (Qvar)	Gold-standard therapy in patients with mild-severe persistent asthma
	Budesonide (Pulmicort)	If asthma symptoms are not controlled, increasing the ICS dose is
	Ciclesonide (Alvesco)	often effective
	Flunisolide (Aerobid)	
	Fluticasone (Flovent)	
	Mometasone (Asmanex)	
	Triamcinolone (Azmacort)	
LABA	Salmeterol (Serevent)	Should not be a monotherapy in asthma patients
	Formoterol (Foradil)	Work well as an add-on therapy to ICS
Combination ICS/LABA	Budesonide/Formoterol (Symbicort)	Combination ICS/LABA therapy is an effective therapy in asthmatic patients
	Fluticasone/Salmeterol (Advair)	Although ICS therapy is effective in many asthmatics, the combination
	Mometasone/Formoterol (Dulera)	ICS/LABA has been shown to be an effective step-up therapy
Leukotriene blockers	Montelukast (Singulair)	Add on therapy to ICS
	Zafirlukast (Accolate)	First-line agent for exercise-induced asthma
	Zileuton (Zyflo)	
Extended therapy for uncontrolled moderate/severe asthma		
Anticholinergic	Tiotropium (Spiriva)	Can be effective as an add-on therapy in patients with low FEV1 to decrease exacerbations
Biologic agents (monoclonal antibodies)	Omalizumab (Xolair)	Omalizumab (anti-IgE) can improve symptoms and decrease exacerbations in patients with uncontrolled asthma despite maximal medical therapy; indicated in patients with sensitivity to perennial aeroallergens and an IgE level >20
	Mepolizumab (Nucala)	Mepolizumab (anti-IL-5) can decrease exacerbations and improve symptoms in severe persistent asthma patients with an eosinophilic phenotype

hospitalizations, fewer urgent care visits, and decreased courses of oral corticoste-roids.[43–45] ICS are the first step in pharmacotherapy to reduce asthma impairment and risk in patients with persistent symptoms that are uncontrolled with SABA therapy. Side effects include hoarseness and sore throat, especially when used at higher doses.[46] There is also a risk for oropharyngeal candidiasis, and patients should be encouraged to rinse their mouth out after administration. Although an increased risk of osteoporosis and fracture has not been consistently shown, every effort should be made to maintain the patient on the lowest dose of ICS necessary to control symptoms.[47]

Controller Medications

Long-acting β-Agonists

Long-acting β2-agonists (LABA) have a slower dissociation from the β2-receptor lead-ing to prolonged action.[48] A landmark trial involving LABAs was the SMART (Salme-terol Multicenter Asthma study Research Trial), which evaluated outcomes in subjects receiving usual asthma pharmacotherapy alone versus usual asthma therapy plus salmeterol.[49] There were slight but statistically significant increases in respiratory-related and asthma-related deaths or life-threatening experiences in the salmeterol group in African American patients. Because of this study, it is not recom-mended that patients with asthma be on an LABA without an ICS unless the risks are clearly laid out and documented.

Combination inhaled corticosteroids/long-acting β-agonists

Although LABA monotherapy is not indicated in asthmatic patients, the role of LABA in addition to ICS is well established and recommended per guidelines. Adding an LABA to ICS has been shown to decrease exacerbations, improve asthma symptoms, and improve lung function.[50,51] Both the addition of LABA to ICS therapy and increasing ICS dose have been shown to be effective options when trying to optimize asthma control.[52]

Leukotriene Antagonists

LTRAs are often used in asthmatic patients as an add-on treatment to ICS in mild to moderate asthma.[53] The other role for LTRAs is in exercise-induced asthma patients, where it has been shown to help prevent exercise-induced bronchoconstriction.[54,55] Another patient population where this medication works well is in patients with allergic rhinitis and asthma. A different option is the 5-LO inhibitor zileuton. As discussed pre-viously, this medication is used less frequently for asthma patients, given the need to monitor liver function and dosing frequency. It is unclear whether this drug offers a sig-nificant benefit beyond LTRAs, but it is an option in patients that are not controlled with standard therapies.

Anticholinergics

Tiotropium has mainly been used in chronic obstructive pulmonary disease patients and is not a standard medication for asthmatics; however, it may have a role in some moderate to severe asthmatics. It has been shown to improve lung function and reduce the frequency of exacerbations when used in addition to standard thera-pies in this patient population.[56,57]

Omalizumab

In patients with uncontrolled allergic asthma despite high-dose ICS/LABA treatment, the monoclonal anti-IgE treatment omalizumab has been shown to decrease exacerbations and decrease asthma symptoms.[58–60] Patients should be sensitized to a perennial aeroallergen and have a total IgE level greater than 30. Dosing is based on weight and total IgE level.

Mepolizumab

Mepolizumab is a monoclonal antibody directed against interleukin-5 (IL-5), which acts to decrease eosinophil production and was FDA approved in 2015 for treatment of severe asthma with an eosinophilic phenotype. Although there is not a definitive cut-off for a level of peripheral eosinophilia, a peripheral eosinophil count of greater than 150/µL is often cited. This medication has been shown to decrease exacerbations and improve symptoms in patients with severe persistent asthma and either peripheral or sputum eosinophilia.[61,62]

SUMMARY

Although the clinical presentations of chronic rhinitis, urticaria, angioedema, and asthma are distinct, a limited core group of medications is used in these conditions. Each of these conditions is a heterogeneous group of disorders and distinguishing the different forms can help guide appropriate therapies. Common medications used in these conditions include antihistamines, antileukotrienes, corticosteroids (both systemic and topical), and anticholinergics. Knowing the indications for use, forms of administration, and side-effect profiles of these medications can help improve patient outcome.

REFERENCES

1. Wallace DV, Dykewicz MS, Bernstein DI, et al. The diagnosis and management of rhinitis: an updated practice parameter. J Allergy Clin Immunol 2008;122(2 Suppl):S1–84.
2. Schoenwetter WF, Dupclay L Jr, Appajosyula S, et al. Economic impact and quality-of-life burden of allergic rhinitis. Curr Med Res Opin 2004;20(3):305–17.
3. Settipane RA. Rhinitis: a dose of epidemiological reality. Allergy Asthma Proc 2003;24:147–54.
4. Singh K, Axelrod S, Bielory L. The epidemiology of ocular and nasal allergy in the United States, 1988-1994. J Allergy Clin Immunol 2010;126(4):778.
5. Simons FE, Simons KJ. Histamine and H1-antihistamines: celebrating a century of progress. J Allergy Clin Immunol 2011;128(6):1139–50.
6. Rosenblut A, Bardin PG, Muller B, et al. Long-term safety of fluticasone furoate nasal spray in adults and adolescents with perennial allergic rhinitis. Allergy 2007;62(9):1071–7.
7. Benninger MS. Epistaxis and its relationship to handedness with use of intranasal steroid spray. Ear Nose Throat J 2008;87(8):463–5.
8. Benninger MS, Hadley JA, Osguthorpe JD, et al. Techniques of intranasal steroid use. Otolaryngol Head Neck Surg 2004;130(1):5–24.
9. Derby L, Maier WC. Risk of cataract among users of intranasal corticosteroids. J Allergy Clin Immunol 2000;105(5):912–6.
10. Bui CM, Chen H, Shyr Y, et al. Discontinuing nasal steroids might lower intraocular pressure in glaucoma. J Allergy Clin Immunol 2005;116(5):1042–7.
11. López-Muñoz F, Alamo C, García-García P. Psychotropic drugs in the Cervantine texts. J R Soc Med 2008;101(5):226–34.
12. Brann MR, Jørgensen HB, Burstein ES, et al. Studies of the pharmacology, localization, and structure of muscarinic acetylcholine receptors. Ann N Y Acad Sci 1993;20(707):225–36.

13. Salerno SM, Jackson JL, Berbano EP. The impact of oral phenylpropanolamine on blood pressure: a meta-analysis and review of the literature. J Hum Hypertens 2005;19(8):643–52.

14. Laccourreye O, Werner A, Giroud JP, et al. Benefits, limits and danger of ephedrine and pseudoephedrine as nasal decongestants. Eur Ann Otorhinolaryngol Head Neck Dis 2015;132(1):31–4.

15. Graf P. Adverse effects of benzalkonium chloride on the nasal mucosa: allergic rhinitis and rhinitis medicamentosa. Clin Ther 1999;21(10):1749–55.

16. Baroody FM, Brown D, Gavanescu L, et al. Oxymetazoline adds to the effectiveness of fluticasone furoate in the treatment of perennial allergic rhinitis. J Allergy Clin Immunol 2011;127(4):927–34.

17. Peters-Golden M, Henderson WR Jr. Leukotrienes. N Engl J Med 2007;357(18): 1841–54.

18. Seidman MD, Gurgel RK, Lin SY, et al, Guideline Otolaryngology Development Group. AAO-HNSF. Clinical practice guideline: allergic rhinitis. Otolaryngol Head Neck Surg 2015;152(1 Suppl):S1–43.

19. Bisgaard H, Skoner D, Boza ML, et al. Safety and tolerability of montelukast in placebo-controlled pediatric studies and their open-label extensions. Pediatr Pulmonol 2009;44(6):568–79.

20. Manalai P, Woo JM, Postolache TT. Suicidality and montelukast. Expert Opin Drug Saf 2009;8(3):273–82.

21. de Blay F, Chapman MD, Platts-Mills TA. Airborne cat allergen (Fel d I): environmental control with the cat in situ. Am Rev Respir Dis 1991;143:1334–9.

22. Arbes SJ Jr, Sever M, Archer J, et al. Abatement of cockroach allergen (Bla g 1) in low-income, urban housing: a randomized controlled trial. J Allergy Clin Immunol 2003;112:339–45.

23. Woodcock A, Forster L, Matthews E, et al. Medical Research Council general practice research framework control of exposure to mite allergen and allergen-impermeable bed covers for adults with asthma. N Engl J Med 2003;349(3):225.

24. Sheikh A, Hurwitz B. House dust mite avoidance measures for perennial allergic rhinitis. Cochrane Database Syst Rev 2010;(7):CD001563.

25. Tovey ER, Taylor DJ, Mitakakis TZ, et al. Effectiveness of laundry washing agents and conditions in the removal of cat and dust mite allergen from bedding dust. J Allergy Clin Immunol 2001;108:369–74.

26. Calderon MA, Alves B, Jacobson M, et al. Allergen injection immunotherapy for seasonal allergic rhinitis. Cochrane Database Syst Rev 2007;(1):CD001936.

27. Nelson HS. Subcutaneous immunotherapy versus sublingual immunotherapy: which is more effective? J Allergy Clin Immunol Pract 2014;2(2):144–9.

28. Bernstein JA, Lang DM, Khan DA, et al. The diagnosis and management of acute and chronic urticaria: 2014 update. J Allergy Clin Immunol 2014;133(5):1270–7.

29. Tarbox JA, Gutta RC, Radojicic C, et al. Utility of routine laboratory testing in management of chronic urticaria/angioedema. Ann Allergy Asthma Immunol 2011; 107(3):239–43.

30. Maurer M, Rosén K, Hsieh HJ, et al. Omalizumab for the treatment of chronic idiopathic or spontaneous urticaria. N Engl J Med 2013;368(10):924–35.

31. Harrison RG, MacRae M, Karsh J, et al. Anaphylaxis and serum sickness in patients receiving omalizumab: reviewing the data in light of clinical experience. Ann Allergy Asthma Immunol 2015;115(1):77–8.

32. Zuraw BL, Bernstein JA, Lang DM, et al, American Academy of Allergy, Asthma and Immunology, American College of Allergy, Asthma and Immunology. A focused parameter update: hereditary angioedema, acquired C1 inhibitor

deficiency, and angiotensin-converting enzyme inhibitor-associated angioe-dema. J Allergy Clin Immunol 2013;131(6):1491–3.

33. Zuraw BL. Clinical practice. Hereditary angioedema. N Engl J Med 2008;359(10): 1027–36.

34. Shroba J, Hanson J, Portnoy J. Current treatment options for idiopathic angioe-dema. Ann Allergy Asthma Immunol 2015;115(5):429–33.

35. Nair P, Dasgupta A, Brightling CE, et al. How to diagnose and phenotype asthma. Clin Chest Med 2012;33(3):445–57.

36. Rajan JP, Wineinger NE, Stevenson DD, et al. Prevalence of aspirin-exacerbated respiratory disease among asthmatic patients: a meta-analysis of the literature. J Allergy Clin Immunol 2015;135(3):676–81.

37. Groh M, Pagnoux C, Baldini C, et al. Eosinophilic granulomatosis with polyangiitis (Churg-Strauss) (EGPA) consensus task force recommendations for evaluation and management. Eur J Intern Med 2015;26(7):545–53.

38. Silkoff PE, Strambu I, Laviolette M, et al. Asthma characteristics and biomarkers from the airways disease endotyping for personalized therapeutics (ADEPT) lon-gitudinal profiling study. Respir Res 2015;16(1):142.

39. Joint Task Force on Practice Parameters, American Academy of Allergy, Asthma and Immunology, American College of Allergy, Asthma and Immunology and Joint Council of Allergy, Asthma and Immunology. Attaining optimal asthma con-trol: a practice parameter. J Allergy Clin Immunol 2005;116(5):S3–11.

40. Cazzola M, Page CP, Calzetta L, et al. Pharmacology and therapeutics of bron-chodilators. Pharmacol Rev 2012;64(3):450–504.

41. Walters EH, Walters J. Inhaled short acting beta2-agonist use in asthma: regular vs as needed treatment. Cochrane Database Syst Rev 2000;(4):CD001285.

42. Jat KR, Khairwa A. Levalbuterol versus albuterol for acute asthma: a systematic review and meta-analysis. Pulm Pharmacol Ther 2013;26(2):239–48.

43. Chipps BE. Inhaled corticosteroid therapy for patients with persistent asthma: learnings from studies of inhaled budesonide. Allergy Asthma Proc 2009;30(3): 217–28.

44. Donahue JG, Weiss ST, Livingston JM, et al. Inhaled steroids and the risk of hos-pitalization for asthma. JAMA 1997;277(11):887.

45. Long-term effects of budesonide or nedocromil in children with asthma. The Child-hood Asthma Management Program Research Group. N Engl J Med 2000;343: 1054–63.

46. Yang IA, Fong KM, Sim EH, et al. Inhaled corticosteroids for stable chronic obstruc-tive pulmonary disease. Cochrane Database Syst Rev 2007;(2):CD002991.

47. Johnell O, Pauwels R, Löfdahl CG, et al. Bone mineral density in patients with chronic obstructive pulmonary disease treated with budesonide Turbuhaler. Eur Respir J 2002;19(6):1058–63.

48. Cazzola M, Page CP, Rogliani P, et al. β2-agonist therapy in lung disease. Am J Respir Crit Care Med 2013;187(7):690–6.

49. Nelson HS, Weiss ST, Bleecker ER, et al, SMART Study Group. The salmeterol multicenter asthma research trial: a comparison of usual pharmacotherapy for asthma or usual pharmacotherapy plus salmeterol. Chest 2006;129(1):15–26.

50. Pauwels RA, Löfdahl CG, Postma DS, et al. Effect of inhaled formoterol and bu-desonide on exacerbations of asthma. Formoterol and Corticosteroids Establish-ing Therapy (FACET) International Study Group. N Engl J Med 1997;337(20): 1405–11.

51. Ducharme FM, Ni Chroinin M, Greenstone I, et al. Addition of long-acting beta2-ag-onists to inhaled steroids versus higher dose inhaled steroids in adults and children with persistent asthma. Cochrane Database Syst Rev 2010;(4):CD005533.

52. Greenstone IR, Ni Chroinin MN, Masse V, et al. Combination of inhaled long-acting beta2-agonists and inhaled steroids versus higher dose of inhaled steroids in children and adults with persistent asthma. Cochrane Database Syst Rev 2005;(4):CD005533.

53. Joos S, Miksch A, Szecsenyi J, et al. Montelukast as add-on therapy to inhaled corticosteroids in the treatment of mild to moderate asthma: a systematic review. Thorax 2008;63(5):453–62.

54. Leff JA, Busse WW, Pearlman D, et al. Montelukast, a leukotriene-receptor antag-onist, for the treatment of mild asthma and exercise-induced bronchoconstriction. N Engl J Med 1998;339(3):147–52.

55. Reiss TF, Hill JB, Harman E, et al. Increased urinary excretion of LTE4 after exer-cise and attenuation of exercise-induced bronchospasm by montelukast, a cys-teinyl leukotriene receptor antagonist. Thorax 1997;52(12):1030–5.

56. Peters SP, Kunselman SJ, Icitovic N, et al, National Heart, Lung, and Blood Insti-tute Asthma Clinical Research Network. Tiotropium bromide step-up therapy for adults with uncontrolled asthma. N Engl J Med 2010;363(18):1715–26.

57. Rodrigo GJ, Castro-Rodríguez JA. Tiotropium for the treatment of adolescents with moderate to severe symptomatic asthma: a systematic review with meta-analysis. Ann Allergy Asthma Immunol 2015;115(3):211–6.

58. Busse W, Corren J, Lanier BQ, et al. Omalizumab anti-IgE recombinant human-ized monoclonal antibody, for the treatment of severe allergic asthma. J Allergy Clin Immunol 2001;108(2):184–90.

59. Busse WW, Morgan WJ, Gergen PJ, et al. Randomized trial of omalizumab (anti-IgE) for asthma in inner-city children. N Engl J Med 2011;364(11):1005–15.

60. Hanania NA, Alpan O, Hamilos DL, et al. Omalizumab in severe allergic asthma inadequately controlled with standard therapy: a randomized trial. Ann Intern Med 2011;154:573–82.

61. Nair P, Pizzichini MM, Kjarsgaard M, et al. Mepolizumab for prednisone-dependent asthma with sputum eosinophilia. N Engl J Med 2009;360(10): 985–93.

62. Ortega HG, Liu MC, Pavord ID, et al. Mepolizumab treatment in patients with se-vere eosinophilic asthma. N Engl J Med 2014;371(13):1198–207.

63. Jovancevic L, Georgalas C, Savovic S, et al. Gustatory rhinitis. Rhinology 2010; 48(1):7–10.

64. Cicardi M, Banerji A, Bracho F, et al. Icatibant, a new bradykinin-receptor antag-onist, in hereditary angioedema. N Engl J Med 2010;363(6):532–41.

65. Lumry WR, Li HH, Levy RJ, et al. Randomized placebo-controlled trial of the bra-dykinin B2 receptor antagonist icatibant for the treatment of acute attacks of he-reditary angioedema: the FAST-3 trial. Ann Allergy Asthma Immunol 2011;107: 529–37.

66. Sheffer AL, Campion M, Levy RJ, et al. Ecallantide (DX-88) for acute hereditary angioedema attacks: integrated analysis of 2 double-blind, phase 3 studies. J Allergy Clin Immunol 2011;128(1):153–9.

67. Wintenberger C, Boccon-Gibod I, Launay D, et al. Tranexamic acid as mainte-nance treatment for non-histaminergic angioedema: analysis of efficacy and safety in 37 patients. Clin Exp Immunol 2014;178(1):112–7.

Pharmacologic Therapies in Musculoskeletal Conditions

Melinda S. Loveless, MD*, Adrielle L. Fry, MD

KEYWORDS

- Musculoskeletal pain • Medications • Acute pain • Back pain • Osteoarthritis
- Neuropathy • Tendinopathy

KEY POINTS

- There are a wide variety of pharmacologic options for musculoskeletal conditions from the traditional anti-inflammatories and analgesics to topical preparations and nutraceuticals.
- The research regarding effectiveness of medications for musculoskeletal conditions is mixed and limited. Many of the studies are of poor quality.
- Evaluation of an individual's medical comorbidities as well as chronicity and distribution of pain can assist in choosing the most appropriate pharmacologic therapies.
- Different medications are used for acute and chronic pain and for neuropathic versus musculoskeletal pain.

INTRODUCTION

Musculoskeletal (MSK) conditions are common complaints of individuals seeking medical care. Osteoarthritis and back problems are in the top 3 reasons for visits to health care providers.[1,2] The World Health Organization estimates that 25% of adults age 65 or older suffer from MSK conditions.[2] In addition, osteoarthritis affects approximately 9% of American adults by the age of 60.[3] In the population 20 to 89 years of age, back pain and sciatica are present in up to 27% of individuals.[2] Treatments for these conditions are often multimodal, including modification of activity, modalities such as ice or heat, physical therapy, and medications. This article reviews the pharmacologic therapy options for treatment of MSK conditions.

Disclosure Statement: The authors have nothing to disclose.
Department of Rehabilitation Medicine, University of Washington, 325 Ninth Avenue, Box 359721, Seattle, WA 98104, USA
* Corresponding author.
E-mail address: mlovel@uw.edu

Med Clin N Am 100 (2016) 869–890
http://dx.doi.org/10.1016/j.mcna.2016.03.015
0025-7125/16/$ – see front matter © 2016 Elsevier Inc. All rights reserved.

ACUTE MUSCULOSKELETAL PAIN

Acute MSK pain is common, and there are many causes, including muscle strains, ligament sprains, tendonitis, bony injuries, and joint or cartilage injuries. By definition, acute pain does not require long-term treatment with analgesic medications,[4] but analgesic medications can be effective for relieving pain and improving function. The most commonly used analgesic medications are oral and topical nonsteroidal anti-inflammatory drugs (NSAIDs), acetaminophen, tramadol, and opioids. Oral NSAIDs and acetaminophen are available over the counter and are generally effective for most mild-to-moderate pain. Acetaminophen and NSAIDs have been found to be fairly equivalent for most MSK pain, but may be more effective in combination.[5] Tramadol can be useful in individuals in whom NSAIDs and acetaminophen are either not indicated or not effective and in whom opioids are not indicated. Opioid medications are more potent analgesics and appropriate in the setting of more severe pain. Combining opioids with acetaminophen or NSAIDs can also provide added benefit.[4]

Oral Nonsteroidal Anti-Inflammatory Drugs

NSAIDs are very effective medications with known anti-inflammatory, analgesic, anti-pyretic, and antiplatelet effects.[6,7] NSAIDs reversibly inhibit the cyclooxygenase (COX) -1 and -2 enzymes, which block prostaglandin synthesis.[7] Different NSAIDs have varying degrees of effect on COX-1 and COX-2. Traditional NSAIDs are nonselective, each with varying degrees of COX-1 and COX-2 activity, while newer NSAIDs have been formulated to be COX-2 selective. Although the different NSAIDs have proven equivalent in clinical studies, it is important to remember that individual treatment responses may vary, and different NSAIDs may need to be tried if the response to one NSAID is inadequate.[6,8] NSAIDs are effective in soft tissue impingement, tenosynovitis, sprains, and other soft tissue injuries.[7,9] **Table 1** lists appropriate doses for the most commonly used NSAIDs and considerations in prescribing. The lowest effective dose should be prescribed for the shortest duration necessary.[8]

NSAIDs are known to have many undesirable adverse effects from mild to severe and the adverse effects are generally dose-dependent. All NSAIDs have a black box warning regarding the possible gastrointestinal (GI) and cardiovascular (CV) risks.[10] GI adverse effects, caused by COX-1 inhibition, are most common and include dyspepsia, abdominal discomfort, and ulcer with risk of bleeding and perforation.[6,11] Coadministration of a proton pump inhibitor (PPI), H_2-receptor blocker, or misoprostol with nonselective NSAIDs can reduce the risk of duodenal ulcers, but does not necessarily prevent lower GI tract events.[4,6] There are also risks of renal impairment and increased blood pressure. Last, CV risks of myocardial infarction (MI) and cerebrovascular accident (CVA) increase with NSAIDs, and the risk is thought to be greatest with diclofenac. Naproxen has generally been considered the safest NSAID for those with CV risk, but it also has the potential to reduce the cardioprotective anti-platelet effects of aspirin.[6,12] For those with high CV risk taking aspirin and in whom NSAIDs are deemed necessary, low-dose celecoxib ($\leq$200 mg/d) may be the safest.[6] NSAIDs should be avoided in individuals with a history of MI, coronary artery bypass grafting, congestive heart failure, and CVA.[13] **Table 2** reviews a suggested prescribing algorithm based on CV and GI risk. As older individuals have a higher risk of adverse effects of NSAIDs, the American Geriatrics Society recommends lower doses or avoidance of NSAIDs in individuals over the age of 75.[14] In certain individuals, topical NSAIDs represent a safer and possibly equally efficacious option.

Table 1
Most commonly used nonsteroidal anti-inflammatory drugs, usual dose range, maximum daily dose, and considerations in use

NSAID	Usual Dosing for Pain	Maximum Daily Dose	Considerations
Nonselective			
Aspirin	325–650 mg QID	4000 mg	Mainly used for antiplatelet effects
Diclofenac	50–75 mg BID	200 mg	Highest risk of elevated liver enzymes; better GI risk, higher CV risk
Etodolac	200–400 mg TID–QID	1200 mg	—
Ibuprofen	200–800 mg TID–QID	3200 mg	Less GI risk than naproxen; reduces cardioprotective antiplatelet effect of aspirin when taken before aspirin
Indomethacin	25–50 mg TID	200 mg	Headache in 15%–25% of patients
Ketorolac	10 mg QID	40 mg oral	Higher analgesic effect, often given IM or IV
Meloxicam	7.5–15 mg daily	15 mg	—
Nabumetone	1000 mg daily	2000 mg	Less GI effects
Naproxen	250–500 mg BID	1500 mg	Better for individuals with high CV risk, but reduces cardioprotective antiplatelet effect of aspirin
Piroxicam	20 mg daily	40 mg	Higher GI risk, especially at higher dose
Sulindac	150–200 mg BID	400 mg	Can elevate liver enzymes
COX-2 Selective			
Celecoxib	100–200 mg BID	400 mg	Lower GI risk Can interact with warfarin; can cause rash (sulfonamide)

Abbreviations: BID, twice daily; IM, intramuscular; IV, intravenous; QID, four times daily; TID, three times daily.
    Data from Scarpignato C, Lanas A, Blandizzi C, et al. Safe prescribing of non-steroidal anti-inflammatory drugs in patients with osteoarthritis—an expert consensus addressing benefits as well as gastrointestinal and cardiovascular risks. BMC Med 2015;13:55; and Malanga GA, Dennis RL. Treatment of acute low back pain: use of medications. J Musculoskelet Med 2005;22:79–89.

Topical Nonsteroidal Anti-Inflammatory Drugs

Many NSAIDs are available in topical preparations, but diclofenac is the only option available in the United States. The mechanism of action is similar to oral NSAIDs, but with significantly lower plasma drug concentrations compared with oral NSAIDs.[10] These medications are good options in individuals who have increased risk of adverse effects from oral NSAIDs who present with a focal area of pain. Topical agents penetrate the skin and distribute to the underlying tissue; therefore, they are only effective for treating more superficial structures.[10] A 2015 Cochrane Review on the use of topical NSAIDs for acute MSK pain concluded that topical NSAIDs are effective and provide pain relief similar to oral NSAIDs. Diclofenac gel was found to be one of the most effective formulations.[16] In addition to improved pain, there has been demonstrated improvement in function, mobility, and soft tissue swelling.[10]

Table 2
Nonsteroidal anti-inflammatory drug algorithm based on cardiovascular and gastrointestinal risk factors

		Cardiovascular Risk		
		Low risk	High risk (eg, age >65, known CV disease, hypertension, heart failure, diabetes)	High risk and taking aspirin
Gastrointestinal Risk	Low risk	Nonselective NSAID	Avoid NSAIDs if possible Naproxen or Celecoxib 200 mg/d	Avoid NSAIDs if possible Celecoxib 200 mg/d
	High risk (eg, Age >60, history of ulcer, GI bleeding, dual anti-platelet therapy, *Helicobacter pylori*)	Nonselective NSAID + PPI or Celecoxib ± PPI	Avoid NSAIDs if possible Naproxen + PPI or Celecoxib 200 mg/d + PPI	Avoid NSAIDs if possible Celecoxib 200 mg/d + PPI

Data from Refs.[6,12,13,15]

The dosing for topical NSAIDs is outlined in **Table 3**. Topical preparations have been found to be effective within 2 to 3 days and achieve steady state within 2 to 5 days.[10,17] The primary adverse effect is local skin irritation. Systemic adverse effects are rare compared with oral NSAIDs, but the topical formulations still have the black box warning regarding GI and CV risks.[4,10] Similar to the oral formulation, it is recommended to check liver function studies within 4 to 8 weeks of initiating diclofenac due to risk of hepatotoxicity.[10] Topical NSAIDs should only be applied to intact skin.[10,16]

Table 3
Topical nonsteroidal anti-inflammatory drugs, US Food and Drug Administration–approved indications, and dosing

Topical NSAID	FDA-Approved Indication	Dose
Diclofenac sodium 1% gel	Osteoarthritis pain	Lower extremities: 4 g topically QID Upper extremities: 2 g topically QID MAX: 32 g/d overall affected joints
Diclofenac epolamine topical patch 1.3%	Acute pain due to minor strains, sprains, and contusions	Apply one patch (180 mg) twice daily
Diclofenac sodium topical solution 1.5%, 2%	Osteoarthritis of the knee	1.5%: 40 drops (~19 mg) topically to each knee QID 2%: 2 pumps (40 mg) BID

Data from Refs.[10,18,19]

Acetaminophen

Acetaminophen is an effective analgesic and antipyretic. The mechanism of action is central and peripheral. It inhibits prostaglandin synthesis through inhibition of COX-1 and COX-2 enzymes and also affects neurotransmitters in the central nervous system (CNS). It has a weak anti-inflammatory effect compared with NSAIDs.[5] Recommended dosing of acetaminophen is 325 to 650 mg every 4 to 6 hours, or 1000 mg 3 times daily. The daily maximum is 4000 mg or 2000 mg in patients at higher risk for hepatotoxicity. However, some recommend a lower maximum of 3000 or 3250 mg.[5,20] Patients should be counseled to avoid alcohol and other medications containing acetaminophen while taking acetaminophen for pain. The US Food and Drug Administration (FDA) recently enacted labeling changes to make it clear which over-the-counter medications contain acetaminophen to reduce the risk of overdose.[5,20]

Acetaminophen has been used as first-line treatment because of its perceived safety compared with NSAIDs, but some studies demonstrated that acetaminophen may be less efficacious than NSAIDs for pain. In addition, recent studies have found that acetaminophen is less safe than originally thought, including its use during pregnancy.[5] It is well known that acetaminophen is hepatotoxic, and its use is the leading cause of acute liver failure in adults in the United States, with most of these cases due to unintentional overdose.[5,20] In addition to hepatic risk, there are possible GI and CV risks similar to NSAIDs.[6] It has also been found to increase the effect of warfarin, increase blood pressure in patients with coronary artery disease, increase the risk of asthma in children, and increase the risk of hematologic malignances with chronic use.[5,6] A patient's individual risk factors should be considered when recommending acetaminophen for pain.

Tramadol

Tramadol is an analgesic medication that has weak affinity for μ-opioid receptors and also blocks norepinephrine and serotonin reuptake.[4,21] It is an effective alternative for patients with intolerance to or insufficient relief with NSAIDs or acetaminophen. In the setting of insufficient pain relief, it can be combined with NSAIDs or acetaminophen to supplement analgesia.[21,22] The recommended dosing is 50 to 100 mg orally up to 4 times daily with lower doses in older individuals and those with renal impairment or cirrhosis.[14,21,23] At these levels, it has been shown to suppress nociceptive pain and is effective when compared with placebo.[21,24] In contrast to other μ-opioid receptor agonists, tramadol has only minor GI transit delay and respiratory depression potential.[21] The most frequent adverse effects are nausea, dizziness, drowsiness, fatigue, sweating, vomiting, and dry mouth.[21,22] It is also safer than opioids because of low abuse and dependence potential.[4,21] It should not be administered along with other medications that increase serotonin, such as monoamine oxidase inhibitors, tricyclic antidepressants (TCAs), selective serotonin reuptake inhibitors, and serotonin and norepinephrine reuptake inhibitors (SNRIs) due to risk of serotonin syndrome.[4,23]

Opioids

Opioids are a class of analgesics that primarily bind the μ-opioid receptors centrally and peripherally. They are usually reserved for severe pain not relieved by acetaminophen, NSAIDs, and tramadol.[11,24] They are best for acute pain, and there is evidence that prolonged high-dose therapy is likely neither safe nor effective.[25] Prescribing opioid medications should be very patient specific and undertaken with caution. **Table 4** lists suggested starting doses. Similar to other medications, lower doses

Table 4
Dosing for opioid medications

Opioid Medication	Typical Starting Dose
Codeine	30 mg every 3–4 h
Hydrocodone	10 mg every 3–4 h
Morphine	15 mg every 3–4 h
Morphine SR	15 mg every 8–12 h
Oxycodone	5 mg every 3–4 h
Oxycodone CR	10 mg every 8–12 h
Hydromorphone	2–4 mg every 3–4 h
Fentanyl	25 µg patch every 72 h

Data from Ballantyne JC, Mao J. Opioid therapy for chronic pain. N Engl J Med 2003;349:1943–53.

are recommended in older individuals.[14] For acute pain, short-acting opioids are recommended.[8]

A significant reason for the recommended caution in prescribing opioid medications is due to the wide array of potentially serious adverse effects. Common side effects of opioid medications are somnolence, nausea, vomiting, constipation, and itching. Hypotension, bradycardia, and respiratory depression can also occur.[11,23,26,27] Caution should be used before prescribing these medications beyond the acute period due to the potential for addiction or abuse and developing opioid-induced hyperalgesia, a nociceptive sensitization caused by opioid use that causes the individual to become more sensitive to pain. The pain can be felt as worsening of the underlying pain or a distinct and different pain.[25,28]

Mixed Opioid and Nonopioid Medications

Combination medications, such as acetaminophen with hydrocodone, oxycodone, or tramadol, have similar mechanisms to their individual components. There is a synergistic effect due to the different mechanisms of action for each component, which allows for lower doses of the medications to be used. Studies regarding these medications are limited, but the opioid combinations have proven to provide effective analgesia in both acute and chronic MSK pain conditions.[4,29] One study has also demonstrated efficacy of tramadol with acetaminophen over placebo for improving pain and function in chronic low back pain when administered for 3 months.[30] Although these medications are effective for analgesia, they carry potential adverse effects of both acetaminophen and opioids. Because of the risk of hepatic injury with acetaminophen, the FDA now prohibits combination medications with more than 325 mg of acetaminophen per dosage unit (tablet or capsule).[5]

NECK AND BACK PAIN

Back and neck pain account for the top 2 MSK reasons for visits to primary care[31] and are in the top 10 overall reasons for primary care visits.[24] It is estimated that 60% to 80% of individuals will experience back pain during their lifetime.[24] Neck and back pain can present as either acute or chronic pain complaints.[24]

Despite the prevalence of neck pain, studies evaluating noninjectable pharmacologic treatment options for neck pain are limited. In studies of acute whiplash, the only medication studied is intravenous methylprednisolone, which demonstrates no difference at 2 weeks compared with placebo. In studies of interventions for nonspecific neck pain, there were positive short-term benefits in those who received NSAIDs or a combination of acetaminophen and muscle relaxer. However, those who received medication plus advice and mobilization or other treatments demonstrated greater benefits than medication alone.[32]

Similarly, the evidence for use of medications in acute low back pain is limited, and most treatments only demonstrate small benefit.[8,33] Overall, in addition to education and exercise, acute spine pain is managed with acetaminophen or NSAIDs as first-line medications with addition of opioids or skeletal muscle relaxants as a second- or third-line option.[8,33–35] The addition of a skeletal muscle relaxant to acetaminophen or an NSAID may be superior to the analgesic medication alone.[4,8,36] For low back pain, topical NSAIDs do not have proven efficacy, but they can be used for the cervical spine given its more superficial anatomy.[16,24] Analgesic medications have been reviewed previously in this article. Skeletal muscle relaxants are classified into 2 categories, antispasmodics and true antispasticity medications; however, benzodiazepines are also used off-label for similar effect.[37] Use of these medications can be limited by adverse effects such as sedation.[8] Last, in the case of acute radiculopathy or radiculitis in the upper or lower extremities, oral steroids are often prescribed.[8,34,38]

In the setting of chronic pain, the recommendations are for education and advice to stay active with analgesic medications used episodically to treat acute flares of pain.[8,33,39] Opioids do have proven efficacy in chronic pain,[8] but there are associated risks and likely small functional benefit.[23] If using opioids for chronic pain, a pain contract and regular monitoring can be useful.[23] Recent studies support the use of antidepressant medications, such as TCAs or SNRIs, but the benefit may be small with high risk of adverse effects.[33,39]

Skeletal Muscle Relaxants

Antispasmodics

The antispasmodics are cyclobenzaprine, metaxalone, methocarbamol, and carisoprodol. They are thought to reduce muscle spasms that can accompany acute MSK pain. The mechanism of action is not completely known but generally thought to be related to central sedation.[23,40] Studies have found these medications to be superior to placebo and as efficacious as NSAIDs in management of acute painful MSK conditions such as low back pain, but have little effect on chronic pain.[8,36] This group is the preferred group of muscle relaxants for MSK conditions.[40]

Cyclobenzaprine, which is similar to TCAs, has the most consistent evidence supporting its effectiveness for MSK conditions.[24,40] Methocarbamol has been shown to have an effect on skeletal muscle, but there are limited data to support this.[40] The limited evidence to support the use of metaxalone is from the 1960s and 1970s, and there are no high-quality trials.[35,36] The last medication to be classified into this category, carisoprodol, has not been shown to be more efficacious than the other medications. It has a risk of withdrawal and high risk for abuse and addiction. Unlike the other medications in this group, it is now a schedule IV medication. It is not recommended for use in MSK pain.[4,8,35] **Table 5** reviews dosing for the recommended medications. The most common side effects are central sedation, drowsiness, and headache.[35]

Antispasticity medications

The antispasticity medications baclofen, tizanidine, and dantrolene are primarily used in the setting of spasticity due to CNS injury. Of these medications, tizanidine has

Table 5
Dosing for recommended antispasmotic medications

Medication	Typical Dosing Regimen	Individual Considerations
Cyclobenzaprine	5 mg TID equivalent to 10 mg TID with less adverse effects	Can have anticholinergic adverse effects Caution in those with CV risk
Methocarbamol	1000–1500 mg TID or QID	—
Metaxalone	400–800 mg TID or QID	Less sedation Can cause jaundice, hemolytic anemia, leukopenia, and rash Liver function monitoring recommended with long-term use

Data from Refs.[4,11,23,35,41]

shown possible efficacy in short-term treatment of acute low back pain.[8,37] However, these medications are used less commonly than the antispasmodic medications for MSK issues.

Baclofen is a γ-aminobutyric acid (GABA$_B$) agonist and reduces the release of excitatory neurotransmitters from the CNS. It has been shown to be effective in acute management of low back pain to reduce pain and interference with daily activities.[40,42] Usual starting dose is 5 mg 3 times daily with titration up to a maximal dose of 80 mg per day.[41] However, in acute pain, studies have used higher doses of 20 mg 4 times daily.[42] Common adverse effects are drowsiness, dizziness, weakness, confusion, nausea, and hypotension. Abrupt discontinuation should be avoided because of risk of hallucinations, psychiatric disturbances, and seizures.[41]

Tizanidine is an α-2 adrenergic receptor agonist that reduces release of excitatory neurotransmitters in the CNS.[36,40] It has demonstrated efficacy for pain relief and reduction of muscle spasm in acute low back pain.[37] The usual starting dose is 2 mg nightly or up to 3 times per day and can be titrated up to 16 mg per day divided in 3 to 4 doses as needed.[40] The most common adverse effects are dry mouth, somnolence, dizziness, and headache.[40] Hepatic injury and liver failure are possible.[36]

Dantrolene is the only medication in the antispasmodic and antispasticity medication classes that acts peripherally on muscle; it reduces calcium release from sarcoplasmic reticulum of skeletal muscle.[40,41] Dantrolene has been shown in one small study to improve pain and spasm in low back pain.[37] However, it is not more effective than either baclofen or tizanidine, and due to risk of fatal hepatotoxicity, it is not recommended for MSK pain and related muscle spasm.[8,41]

Benzodiazepines

Benzodiazepines act as GABA$_A$ receptor agonists[8,36] and provide sedative and anxiolytic effects.[8] They are often used off-label as skeletal muscle relaxants. Diazepam is the most studied medication from this class because of its longer half-life. Numerous studies have compared diazepam with placebo and other skeletal muscle relaxants with mixed results.[8,36,41] It is generally superior to placebo, but equivalent to other muscle relaxers.[24,37] Dosing of diazepam is 2 to 10 mg 3 to 4 times daily, starting with low doses and titrating up only if needed.[41] The most common adverse effects are sedation, confusion, dizziness, GI upset, behavioral changes, rebound anxiety, dependence, memory impairment, and withdrawal reactions.[41,43] Given the potential for abuse or addiction, benzodiazepines should be used for a short period or avoided.[8,34]

Oral Corticosteroids

Corticosteroids inhibit phospholipase A2, preventing the inflammatory cascade.[11] Oral corticosteroids are often used as a potent anti-inflammatory in the setting of acute upper or lower extremity radicular pain. In addition to their anti-inflammatory effects, there may be added antinociceptive benefits.[27] However, studies demonstrate little improvement in function and pain.[8,11,23,38,44,45] Despite this lack of evidence, oral steroids are often used clinically for radiculopathy.[11,27] Prednisone and methylprednisolone are most commonly prescribed. Prednisone dosing varies by practitioner but is generally given as a short burst or taper with doses starting at 40 mg or 60 mg daily. Methylprednisolone is often administered as a 6-day taper starting at 24 mg and decreasing by 4 mg each day.[11] The most common adverse effects include insomnia, nervousness, increased appetite, fluid retention, increased blood sugar, psychological changes, facial flushing, and suppression of cortisol production.[38,46,47]

Antidepressants

For chronic MSK pain, TCAs and SNRIs can be used. There have been more studies on the use of TCAs for chronic MSK pain, but evidence for efficacy in reducing pain and improving function is mixed.[8] TCAs are often recommended as second-line treatment after analgesic medications for chronic MSK pain.[23] Studies evaluating SNRIs have mostly focused on neuropathic pain, but newer studies have evaluated SNRIs for back pain, and there was significant improvement in pain, depression, and function compared with placebo.[48,49] Many individuals with chronic pain are also depressed and that should be assessed and treated appropriately; antidepressant medications can provide the benefit of improving both mood and pain. However, the doses used for pain are generally lower than the doses for depression.[8,23] Dosing and adverse effects are reviewed in **Table 6**.

TCAs inhibit the reuptake of serotonin and norepinephrine.[27] The secondary amine TCAs nortriptyline and desipramine are favored over tertiary amine TCAs amitriptyline and imipramine due to fewer adverse effects, which include dry mouth, urinary retention, constipation (anticholinergic side effects), and orthostatic hypotension. TCAs should be continued for at least 6 weeks to determine efficacy. Caution should be used in those with CV risk, especially at doses greater than 100 mg per day due to risk of arrhythmia or sudden death.[8,50] The Neuropathic Pain Special Interest Group recommends a screening electrocardiogram in individuals aged 40 and older before initiating treatment with TCAs.[51]

The SNRIs duloxetine and venlafaxine inhibit reuptake of both serotonin and norepinephrine.[27] In patients with depression and pain, there has been improvement in both symptoms.[23] Nausea is the most common side effect of SNRIs. SNRIs should be continued for at least 4 weeks to determine efficacy. Withdrawal can occur with abrupt cessation.[51]

VERTEBRAL COMPRESSION FRACTURES

Osteoporosis-related fractures are unfortunately very common, with expectation that 50% of women and 25% of men over the age of 50 will have an osteoporosis-related fracture in their lifetime,[52] about half of which will be vertebral compression fractures.[53] These fractures often occur with minimal trauma and can cause severe pain.[53,54] For pain relief, analgesic medications such as acetaminophen, NSAIDs, tramadol, and opioids can be used,[52–54] but the evidence for efficacy in the setting of vertebral compression fractures is inconclusive[55] and there is concern for reduced

Table 6
Dosing recommendations for tricyclic antidepressants and serotonin and norepinephrine reuptake inhibitors

Medication	Starting Dose	Titration	Usual Therapeutic Dose	Maximum Daily Dose	Adverse Effects	Other Considerations
Nortriptyline Desiprimine	25 mg QHS	25 mg every 3–7 d	50–150 mg QHS	150 mg or 100 mg/mL blood level	Sedation, anticholinergic, orthostatic hypotension	Caution with significant CV disease, glaucoma
Duloxetine	30 mg daily	30 mg weekly	60 mg daily or 60 mg BID	120 mg	Nausea, somnolence, anticholinergic, dizziness	Caution with hepatic dysfunction or renal insufficiency
Venlafaxine	37.5 mg daily or BID	75 mg weekly	150–225 mg once daily or divided BID	225 mg		Caution in those with CV risk

Abbreviation: QHS, at bedtime.

Data from Dworkin RH, O'Connor AB, Audette J, et al. Recommendations for the pharmacological management of neuropathic pain: an overview and literature update. Mayo Clin Proc 2010;85(3):S3–14; and Attal N, Cruccu G, Baron R, et al. EFNS guidelines on the pharmacological treatment of neuropathic pain: 2010 revision. Eur J Neurol 2010;17(9):1113–e88.

bone healing with NSAIDs.[53] Another medication, calcitonin, is used primarily for treating the pain of vertebral compression fractures. It is better tolerated and safer than traditional analgesic medications, especially in this older population.[52,54]

Calcitonin is produced in the body by the thyroid gland and plays a role in bone and calcium metabolism. Calcitonin binds receptors on osteoclasts, decreasing their activity. In addition, it is thought to have a role in reducing pain through central and peripheral mechanisms by increasing central β-endorphin production and inhibiting prostaglandin and cytokine production peripherally.[52,54] With use of calcitonin for vertebral compression fractures, many studies have demonstrated improvement in pain and mobility.[52,54] It is most effective in the acute phase,[54] and the American Academy of Orthopaedic Surgeons clinical practice guidelines recommend treatment for 4 weeks in individuals presenting within 5 days of painful fractures.[55] Dosing is 1 spray (200 IU) daily, alternating nostrils each day.[56] Adverse effects include nasal irritation, flushing, nausea, diarrhea, and dizziness.[54–56] The intranasal formulation is salmon derived and is more potent and longer lasting than human calcitonin.[52] It is contraindicated in individuals with salmon or seafood allergies.[56]

NEUROPATHIC PAIN

Neuropathic pain, which is caused by a lesion or disease in the somatosensory system,[57] arises from many causes, including CNS injury (ie, stroke, spinal cord injury), nerve root injury (ie, radiculitis, radiculopathy), postherpetic neuralgia, peripheral neuropathy, and peripheral nerve injury.[23,50] In addition to treating the underlying cause of neuropathy, there are pharmacologic options for managing pain. Acetaminophen and NSAIDs generally do not provide adequate relief of neuropathic pain. Certain antidepressants, anticonvulsants, and topical medications are considered first-line options.[45,57] These medications can be used alone or in combination.[50,51] These medications have greatest proven efficacy in the setting of diabetic peripheral neuropathy and postherpetic neuralgia with limited proven efficacy in chronic radicular pain. However, they are generally thought to be effective for all types of neuropathic pain with the exception of trigeminal neuralgia.[58] For patients with severe acute neuropathic pain or exacerbations of pain, analgesic medications such as tramadol or opiates may be necessary due to their shorter onset of action.[45] These medications can be used as needed while titrating first-line medications to a therapeutic dose and then discontinued. Refer to the earlier section, Acute Musculoskeletal Pain, for dosing and adverse effects of analgesic medications.

Antidepressants

The secondary amine class of TCAs is considered to be a first-line option, whereas the SNRIs are first- or second-line depending on the guidelines referenced.[51,58,59] Both TCAs and SNRIs inhibit serotonin and norepinephrine reuptake, and TCAs additionally have direct serotonin antagonism. These medications can be valuable in patients with comorbid depression, but as stated previously, doses for pain relief are lower than doses used to treat depression.[8,23] TCAs have demonstrated efficacy in placebo-controlled trials and systematic reviews. Generally, 40% to 60% of patients obtain partial relief of pain with these medications, but evidence is better in diabetic peripheral neuropathy and postherpetic neuralgia than chronic radicular pain.[51] Duloxetine and venlafaxine are also effective for neuropathic pain based on placebo-controlled trials for diabetic neuropathy with less evidence for use in other types of neuropathic pain.[23,51] Caution should be used when combined with tramadol due to risk of serotonin syndrome.[51] Refer to **Table 6** for dosing and adverse effects.

Anticonvulsants

Gabapentin and pregabalin are GABA analogues that bind the α2-δ subunit of voltage-gated calcium channels in the CNS, decreasing the release of glutamate, norepinephrine, and substance P.[23,51] In addition to benefits on pain, they can also improve disturbed sleep. These medications are generally safe options in those with medical comorbidities because there are no interactions with other medications, but they do require dose reduction in renal insufficiency.[51] Unlike TCAs, gabapentin demonstrates efficacy in most causes of neuropathic pain, including radiculopathy. Pregabalin has not been studied as extensively but demonstrates efficacy in diabetic peripheral neuropathy and postherpetic neuralgia as well as pain related to spinal cord injury and radiculopathy.[23,27,45,51]

Common side effects include dizziness, somnolence, nausea, GI upset, peripheral edema, and weight gain. Dizziness and somnolence often subside within 10 days and may be lessened by starting with low doses and titrating slowly. An adequate trial can take up to 2 months with gabapentin because of slow titration and delayed onset of action, but pregabalin can be effective within 4 weeks.[51] **Table 7** lists dosing and adverse effects.

Topical Medications

Lidocaine

Lidocaine is a local anesthetic that prevents action potential propagation by blocking voltage-gated sodium channels. It is thought to act on abnormally firing afferents.[60] It is effective in those with a focal area of pain such as a peripheral nerve injury. Topical lidocaine in the form of a 5% patch or 5% gel is the only topical medication considered a first- or second-line treatment option for neuropathic pain.[51,58,59] Adverse effects include mild skin reactions such as erythema or rash and dizziness. Although there is likely minimal systemic absorption, topical lidocaine should not be used in individuals receiving class I antiarrhythmic medications and in those with severe hepatic dysfunction due to theoretic toxicity. The patches have been studied the most, and a maximum of 3 patches can be used for 12 to 18 hours per day.[51]

Capsaicin

Capsaicin is derived from chili peppers and binds skin nociceptors, causing a period of enhanced sensitivity followed by a refractory period with reduced pain sensation due to possible depletion of substance P. With prolonged use, there is persistent desensitization.[17,61,62] Although generally thought to be more effective in neuropathic

Table 7 Dosing recommendations for anticonvulsants				
Medication	Starting Dose	Titration	Usual Therapeutic Dose	Maximum Daily Dose
Gabapentin	100–300 mg QHS or TID	100–300 mg TID every 1–7 d	600–1200 mg TID	3600 mg
Pregabalin	75 mg daily or BID	75 mg BID every 3–7 d	150 or 300 mg BID	600 mg

Data from Dworkin RH, O'Connor AB, Audette J, et al. Recommendations for the pharmacological management of neuropathic pain: an overview and literature update. Mayo Clin Proc 2010;85(3):S3–14; and Attal N, Cruccu G, Baron R, et al. EFNS guidelines on the pharmacological treatment of neuropathic pain: 2010 revision. Eur J Neurol 2010;17(9):1113–e88.

pain,[51] a 2004 meta-analysis found that capsaicin was significantly better than placebo for treating both neuropathic and MSK pain.[62]

Because of inconsistent results in randomized controlled trials, topical capsaicin is considered a third-line agent for neuropathic pain.[51] However, it has more proven efficacy for postherpetic neuralgia and can be considered earlier in treatment for those individuals.[58] There are multiple over-the-counter formulations available as creams, gels, lotions, or patches with potency ranging from 0.025% to 0.1%.[61] It can take up to 6 weeks of regular application 3 or 4 times per day to achieve optimal pain relief.[23] Primary adverse effects are burning pain and local skin irritation.[17,62]

OSTEOARTHRITIS

Osteoarthritis affects most individuals over the age of 65 and most commonly involves the hands, knees, hips, and spine.[23] There are multiple published guidelines[63–72] regarding the pharmacologic and nonpharmacologic management of osteoarthritis. First-line treatment of osteoarthritis includes nonpharmacologic measures, such as activity modification, physical therapy, exercise, weight loss, bracing, and use of assistive devices as indicated. If those measures fail to provide adequate pain relief, medications can be used. It is important to acknowledge that osteoarthritis is a chronic condition, and many of the medications recommended for osteoarthritis are not recommended for long-term use.

Most guidelines list acetaminophen as the first-line medication, but some recent guidelines[66,67] suggest it may not be as efficacious as previously thought and raise concerns regarding risk of GI and hepatic adverse effects. Topical NSAIDs are often recommended as a safer first-line medication or as second-line treatment after acetaminophen. Evidence suggests they are as effective as oral NSAIDs and generally safer, but only effective for more superficial joints such as hands and knees.[19] The American College of Rheumatology recommends topical NSAIDs over oral NSAIDs in individuals age 75 or older for hand and knee osteoarthritis.[69] In the setting of multiple or deep arthritic joints, oral NSAIDs are easier to use and more efficacious. NSAIDs can improve rest and walking pain in osteoarthritis.[7,9] As reviewed previously, one must consider a patient's comorbidities when selecting the appropriate NSAID (see **Tables 1** and **2**). Acetaminophen and NSAIDs can also be used in combination if each provides insufficient relief alone. Tramadol and opioid medications can be added if there is insufficient pain relief with acetaminophen and NSAIDs or if those medications are contraindicated due to comorbidities. Refer to the earlier section, the Acute Musculoskeletal Pain, for review of these analgesic medications.

Although there is limited evidence for their use, other medications that can be considered in the setting of osteoarthritis are topical lidocaine or capsaicin for pain relief and the nutraceuticals glucosamine and chondroitin for pain relief and disease modification. Last, injectable medications are used in the management of osteoarthritis. These medications are generally considered for use when there are flares of osteoarthritis pain not controlled by analgesic medications.[64,67,70–72]

Nutraceuticals: Glucosamine and Chondroitin

Glucosamine and chondroitin are important components of the extracellular matrix of articular cartilage involved in maintaining the viscosity of synovial fluid and providing the support in cartilage to withstand loading.[73] Both are used to treat osteoarthritis pain and slow the progression of joint space narrowing. Results of clinical trials and meta-analyses are variable, but overall there is possibly a small benefit on both pain and disease progression with glucosamine or the combination of glucosamine and chondroitin.[73–76]

Glucosamine is available in hydrochloride and sulfate formulations. Most studies have used glucosamine sulfate, and some reviews suggest that the sulfate component is important, either from glucosamine sulfate[77,78] or with a combination of glucosamine hydrochloride and chondroitin sulfate.[76] Recommended dosing is 1500 mg/d of glucosamine and 800 mg per day of chondroitin.[75,78] Doses up to 2000 mg per day of glucosamine and 1200 mg per day of chondroitin have been safe in trials.[74] These supplements should be continued for at least 1 to 2 months before determining effectiveness in reducing pain.[73,76,78] Adverse effects are similar to placebo with occasional GI disturbance.[73,76] There is concern for interaction with diabetes medications and warfarin so these individuals should be monitored appropriately.[73] In addition, glucosamine is derived from shellfish and caution is advised in patients with shellfish allergies, but there have been no reports of allergic reaction.[73,78]

Injectable Medications

Corticosteroids

Injected steroids reduce inflammation, swelling, and pain through several mechanisms, including decreasing the inflammatory cascade and altering several aspects of synovial fluid within joints.[79,80] In the setting of osteoarthritis, corticosteroids may provide some short-term benefits in pain and function. There are several steroids available with varying potencies and durations. **Table 8** lists details and recommended dosing. Most recommend no more than 4 injections in a joint per year.[81–83] Steroids are often mixed with a local anesthetic or normal saline to dilute the steroid and allow local spread of the medication.[80] A 24- to 48-hour period of relative rest after injection is often recommended.[82] Contraindications to injection include local infection, open skin, and acute fracture.[46,80] Adverse effects are similar to

Table 8 Dosing for injectable corticosteroids			
Corticosteroid	Available Strengths	Usual Dose Range[a]	Notes
Betamethasone	6 mg/mL	Large: 6–12 mg Intermediate: 1.5–6 mg Small: 1.5–3 mg	Most soluble Possibly more toxic to chondrocytes
Dexamethasone sodium phosphate	4 mg/mL 10 mg/mL	Large: 7.5–15 mg Intermediate: 2–4 mg Small: 1–3 mg	Soluble, not preferred for joints Better for soft tissue due to lower risk of cutaneous changes
Methylprednisolone acetate	20 mg/mL 40 mg/mL 80 mg/mL	Large: 40–80 mg Intermediate: 10–40 mg Small: 5–10 mg	Slightly soluble
Triamcinolone acetonide	10 mg/mL 40 mg/mL	Large: 20–80 mg Intermediate: 10–40 mg Small: 10–20 mg	Least soluble Longest duration of effect

[a] Large = glenohumeral joint, knee, hip, subacromial bursa; Intermediate = wrist, elbow, ankle, acromioclavicular joint, olecranon bursa; Small = finger, toes.
Data from Refs.[80,82,83]

oral administration but also carry risk of local tissue atrophy, infection, and after-injection steroid flare.[46,47,80]

Local anesthetics

Local anesthetics induce analgesia by inhibiting nerve excitation or conduction.[46] Volumes of anesthetic used vary based on size of joint, most commonly ranging from 0.25 to 4 mL. **Table 9** lists medications and maximum doses. Adverse effects include possible toxicity to cartilage, which increases in the setting of osteoarthritis. Toxicity varies by agent; ropivacaine, 0.25% bupivacaine, and 0.5% lidocaine are the least toxic. Lidocaine at concentrations of 2% or higher is the most toxic of the local anesthetics.[84,85] Formulations with epinephrine also have higher chondrotoxicity.[46] Because of the potential for chondrotoxicity, some providers dilute corticosteroids with saline rather than anesthetic. In addition, systemic toxicity can occur, which can lead to arrhythmias and CV collapse. Lidocaine and ropivacaine are less likely than bupivacaine to cause systemic effects.[46]

Hyaluronic acid

Hyaluronate is a polysaccharide found in synovial fluid and cartilage of synovial joints. It lubricates and absorbs shock in the joint. Available formulations are obtained from animal tissues or synthesized via bacterial fermentation. Injection into joints increases joint lubrication and may increase production of hyaluronate in the joint. There is additional anti-inflammatory and analgesic effect, and benefits may last up to 24 weeks.[86,87] Recommendations regarding use of hyaluronic acid vary, and it has been a controversial topic recently.[68,86] Some guidelines recommend against use of hyaluronic acid injections,[63,67] whereas many others support the use of hyaluronic acid.[64,65,69,70,72] Overall, the literature suggests that younger individuals with less advanced degenerative changes are more likely to benefit.[88] A recent retrospective analysis of 182,022 patients who underwent total knee arthroplasty found that hyaluronic acid injections delayed time to surgery.[89]

Hyaluronic acid is FDA approved as a biological device for knee osteoarthritis, but has also been used off-label for treatment of osteoarthritis in the hip, ankle, and shoulder. Because of recent controversy and limited evidence for their efficacy, some insurance companies are no longer covering these medications. Dosing varies based on manufacturer and is dosed once or once weekly for 3 to 5 weeks. Hyaluronic acid should not be mixed with local anesthetic, and injections can be repeated every 6 months. Adverse effects include pain at the injection site, skin reaction, joint pain/swelling, and joint infection. Pseudoseptic reaction is rare and occurs with repeat injection after initial sensitization.[86]

Table 9 Injectable local anesthetics				
Anesthetic	**Strengths**	**Maximum Dose**	**Onset**	**Duration**
Bupivacaine	0.25%–0.5% (2.5–5 mg/mL)	175 mg or 225 mg with epinephrine	2–10 min	2–6 h
Lidocaine	0.5%–4% (5–40 mg/mL)	300 mg or 500 mg with epinephrine	30–60 s	0.5–2 h
Ropivacaine	0.2%–1% (2–10 mg/mL)	200 mg	5 min	2–4 h

Data from Refs.[46,84,85]

TENDINOPATHY

Tendinopathy is a chronic condition characterized by tendon degeneration and disorganization without significant inflammation; it is associated with an increased risk for tendon rupture.[79] The primary treatment is nonpharmacologic measures including rest and physical therapy. However, if conservative measures fail or the patient requires medications for analgesia, there are pharmacologic treatments available. Medications can be used to reduce pain or to treat the underlying abnormality. For pain, analgesic medications including topical NSAIDs can be used as reviewed in the section, Acute Musculoskeletal Pain. For treatment of the underlying abnormality, some research studies support the use of topical glyceryl trinitrate (GTN) to improve healing. Injectable steroid medications have also been used, and their use in the setting of tendinopathy is discussed in more detail later. Of note, use of fluoroquinolone antibiotics and steroids increases the risk for tendon disorders and rupture and should be used with caution in active individuals.[90]

Topical Glyceryl Trinitrate

For treatment of the underlying abnormality, there is mixed evidence for use of topical GTN patches.[90] In studies, nitric oxide, which is released by GTN patches, has demonstrated a role in tendon healing through its role in blood flow, collagen synthesis, and cellular adhesion.[79,91] Studies have yielded mixed results, but a 2010 meta-analysis[92] of 7 randomized controlled trials evaluating use of GTN patches for chronic tendinopathy demonstrated reduced pain with activity, reduced night pain, and increased peak muscle force compared with placebo. Most studies demonstrate a greater short-term benefit with the exception of Achilles tendinopathy, which may have greater long-term benefit.[79,91] Some recommend the use of GTN patches before proceeding to more invasive treatments, such as injections or tenotomy, if the patient does not respond to eccentric strengthening exercises.[90] In studies, GTN patches have been used over superficial tendons of the shoulder, elbow, knee, and ankle.[79,90–93] Dosing is one-quarter of a 5 mg/24-hour (0.2 mg/h) patch applied over the area of tendinopathy or maximal tenderness. The patch is replaced every 24 hours. Treatment is continued for up to 12 weeks or until pain subsides.[90] The most common adverse effects are headache and contact dermatitis.[92]

Injectable Corticosteroids

Corticosteroid injections are falling out of favor for tendinopathy such as patellar, Achilles, and lateral and medial epicondyle of the elbow because there is potential for increased pain and tendon rupture, especially with intratendinous injection of corticosteroid.[79,80,93,94] In addition, there is no short-term benefit when compared with NSAIDs for treating shoulder and elbow tendonitis.[95]

In contrast to steroids for tendinopathy, research does suggest a possible benefit with the use of subacromial or intra-articular shoulder injections in the setting of rotator cuff abnormality or frozen shoulder for short-term pain relief.[96,97] In addition, tendon sheath corticosteroid injections are considered effective for trigger finger (stenosing tenosynovitis)[98] and DeQuervain tenosynovitis.[99] For mechanism, dosing, and adverse effects, refer to the Osteoarthritis section and **Table 8**.

SUMMARY

MSK conditions causing pain are common. Unfortunately, there is not strong evidence for the use of medications for most of these conditions. Medications that are appropriate and effective for one individual may not work or be contraindicated in another individual. Taking into account an individual's medical comorbidities in addition to chronicity and distribution of symptoms will optimize pharmacologic treatment of their MSK pain. In general, the first-line treatments include acetaminophen and NSAIDs, which can be used in combination. Topical formulations of NSAIDs can be as effective as oral NSAIDs with fewer side effects, but can only be used for more superficial painful structures. For acute pain, tramadol or opioid medications can be used if first-line medications are contraindicated, not tolerated, or ineffective. For acute spine pain, skeletal muscle relaxants can provide additional benefit. All of these medications have adverse effects and potential risks that must be considered before their recommendation. For chronic pain, especially with comorbid depression, SNRIs and TCAs are effective. Anticonvulsants and topical medications can be more effective for neuropathic pain. Injectable medications are generally useful in the setting of osteoarthritis but have no evidence of long-term benefit. Other medications have specific indications such as calcitonin for vertebral compression fracture in osteoporosis and topical GTN for chronic tendinopathy.

REFERENCES

1. Sauver JLS, Warner DO, Yawn BP, et al. Why patients visit their doctors: assessing the most prevalent conditions in a defined american population. Mayo Clin Proc 2013;88(1):56–67.
2. Kean WF, Rainsford KD, Kean IRL. Management of chronic musculoskeletal pain in the elderly: opinions on oral medication use. Inflammopharmacology 2008; 16(2):53–75.
3. Bannuru RR, Vaysbrot EE, Sullivan MC, et al. Relative efficacy of hyaluronic acid in comparison with NSAIDs for knee osteoarthritis: a systematic review and meta-analysis. Semin Arthritis Rheum 2014;43(5):593–9.
4. Sullivan WJ, Panagos A, Foye PM, et al. Industrial medicine and acute musculoskeletal rehabilitation. 2. Medications for the treatment of acute musculoskeletal pain. Arch Phys Med Rehabil 2007;88(3 Suppl 1):10–3.
5. Aminoshariae A, Khan A. Acetaminophen: old drug, new issues. J Endod 2015; 41(5):588–93.
6. Scarpignato C, Lanas A, Blandizzi C, et al. Safe prescribing of non-steroidal anti-inflammatory drugs in patients with osteoarthritis-an expert consensus addressing benefits as well as gastrointestinal and cardiovascular risks. BMC Med 2015; 13:55.
7. Paoloni JA, Milne C, Orchard J, et al. Non-steroidal anti-inflammatory drugs in sports medicine: guidelines for practical but sensible use. Br J Sports Med 2009;43(11):863–5.
8. Chou R. Pharmacological management of low back pain. Drugs 2010;70(4): 387–402.
9. Lee C, Straus WL, Balshaw R, et al. A comparison of the efficacy and safety of nonsteroidal antiinflammatory agents versus acetaminophen in the treatment of osteoarthritis: a meta-analysis. Arthritis Rheum 2004;51(5):746–54.
10. Brewer AR, McCarberg B, Argoff CE. Update on the use of topical NSAIDs for the treatment of soft tissue and musculoskeletal pain: a review of recent data and current treatment options. Phys Sportsmed 2010;38(2):62–70.
11. Malanga GA, Dennis RL. Treatment of acute low back pain: use of medications. J Musculoskelet Med 2005;22:79–89.

12. McGettigan P, Henry D. Cardiovascular risk with non-steroidal anti-inflammatory drugs: systematic review of population-based controlled observational studies. PLoS Med 2011;8(9):e1001098.

13. Ong CKS, Lirk P, Tan CH, et al. An evidence-based update on nonsteroidal anti-inflammatory drugs. Clin Med Res 2007;5(1):19–34.

14. American Geriatrics Society Panel on the Pharmacological Management of Persistent Pain in Older Persons. Pharmacological management of persistent pain in older persons. J Am Geriatr Soc 2009;57(8):1331–46.

15. Bhatt DL, Scheiman J, Abraham NS, et al. ACCF/ACG/AHA 2008 expert consensus document on reducing the gastrointestinal risks of antiplatelet therapy and NSAID use. J Am Coll Cardiol 2008;52(18):1502–17.

16. Derry S, Moore RA, Gaskell H, et al. Topical NSAIDs for acute musculoskeletal pain in adults [review]. Cochrane Database Syst Rev 2015;(6):CD007402.

17. Stanos SP. Topical agents for the management of musculoskeletal pain. J Pain Symptom Manage 2007;33(3):342–55.

18. Holt RJ, Taiwo T, Kent JD. Bioequivalence of diclofenac sodium 2% and 1.5% topical solutions relative to oral diclofenac sodium in healthy volunteers. Postgrad Med 2015;127(6):581–90.

19. Derry S, Moore RA, Rabbie R. Topical NSAIDs for chronic musculoskeletal pain in adults. Cochrane Database Syst Rev 2012;(9):CD007400.

20. Schilling A, Corey R, Leonard M, et al. Acetaminophen: old drug, new warnings. Cleve Clin J Med 2010;77(1):19–27.

21. Grond S, Sablotzki A. Clinical pharmacology of tramadol. Clin Pharmacokinet 2004;43(13):879–923.

22. Reig E. Tramadol in musculoskeletal pain—a survey. Clin Rheumatol 2002; 21(Suppl 1):S9–12.

23. Kroenke K, Krebs EE, Bair MJ. Pharmacotherapy of chronic pain: a synthesis of recommendations from systematic reviews. Gen Hosp Psychiatry 2009;31(3): 206–19.

24. McCarberg BH. Acute back pain: benefits and risks of current treatments. Curr Med Res Opin 2010;26(1):179–90.

25. Ballantyne JC, Mao J. Opioid therapy for chronic pain. N Engl J Med 2003;349: 1943–53.

26. Benyamin R, Trescot AM, Datta S, et al. Opioid complications and side effects. Pain Physician 2008;11:S105–20.

27. Visco CJ, Cheng DS, Kennedy DJ. Pharmaceutical therapy for radiculopathy. Phys Med Rehabil Clin N Am 2011;22(1):127–37.

28. Lee M, Silverman SM, Hansen H, et al. A comprehensive review of opioid-induced hyperalgesia. Pain Physician 2011;14:145–61.

29. Gatti A, Sabato E, Di Paolo AR, et al. Oxycodone/paracetamol. Clin Drug Investig 2010;30(Suppl. 2):3–14.

30. Ruoff GE, Rosenthal N, Jordan D, et al. Tramadol/acetaminophen combination tablets for the treatment of chronic lower back pain: a multicenter, randomized, double-blind, placebo-controlled outpatient study. Clin Ther 2003;25(4):1123–41.

31. Binder AI. Cervical spondylosis and neck pain. BMJ 2007;334(7592):527–31.

32. Hurwitz EL, Carragee EJ, van der Velde G, et al. Treatment of neck pain: noninvasive interventions. J Manipulative Physiol Ther 2009;32(2):S141–75.

33. Balagué F, Mannion AF, Pellisé F, et al. Non-specific low back pain. Lancet 2012; 379(9814):482–91.

34. Koes BW, van Tulder M, Lin C-WC, et al. An updated overview of clinical guidelines for the management of non-specific low back pain in primary care. Eur Spine J 2010;19(12):2075–94.

35. Toth PE, Urtis J. Commonly used muscle relaxant therapies for acute low back pain: a review of carisoprodol, cyclobenzaprine hydrochloride, and metaxalone. Clin Ther 2004;26(9):1355–67.

36. Beebe FA, Barkin RL, Barkin S. A clinical and pharmacologic review of skeletal muscle relaxants for musculoskeletal conditions. Am J Ther 2005;12:151–71.

37. van Tulder MW, Touray T, Furlan AD, et al. Muscle relaxants for non-specific low-back pain. Cochrane Database Syst Rev 2003;(4):CD004252.

38. Goldberg H, Firtch W, Tyburski M, et al. Oral steroids for acute radiculopathy due to a herniated lumbar disk: a randomized clinical trial. J Am Med Assoc 2015; 313(19):1915–23.

39. Pillastrini P, Gardenghi I, Bonetti F, et al. An updated overview of clinical guidelines for chronic low back pain management in primary care. Joint Bone Spine 2012;79(2):176–85.

40. Chou R, Peterson K, Helfand M. Comparative efficacy and safety of skeletal muscle relaxants for spasticity and musculoskeletal conditions: a systematic review. J Pain Symptom Manage 2004;28(2):140–75.

41. Waldman HJ, Waldman SD, Waldman KA. Centrally acting skeletal muscle relaxants and associated drugs. J Pain Symptom Manage 1994;9(7):434–41.

42. Dapas F, Hartman SF, Martinez L, et al. Baclofen for the treatment of acute low-back syndrome: a double-blind comparison with placebo. Spine (Phila Pa 1976) 1985;10(4):345–9.

43. Chouinard G. Issues in the clinical use of benzodiazepines: potency, withdrawal, and rebound. J Clin Psychiatry 2004;65(suppl 5):7–12.

44. Holve RL, Barkan H. Oral steroids in initial treatment of acute sciatica. J Am Board Fam Med 2008;21(5):469–74.

45. Onks CA, Billy G. Evaluation and treatment of cervical radiculopathy. Prim Care 2013;40(4):837–48.

46. MacMahon PJ, Eustace SJ, Kavanagh EC. Injectable corticosteroid and local anesthetic preparations: a review for radiologists. Radiology 2009;252(3):647–61.

47. Habib GS. Systemic effects of intra-articular corticosteroids. Clin Rheumatol 2009;28(7):749–56.

48. Rej SR, Dew MA, Karp JF. Treating concurrent chronic low back pain and depression with low-dose venlafaxine: an initial identification of "easy-to- use" clinical predictors of early response. Pain 2014;15(7):1154–62.

49. Skljarevski V, Zhang S, Desaiah D, et al. Duloxetine versus placebo in patients with chronic low back pain: a 12-week, fixed-dose, randomized, double-blind trial. J Pain 2010;11(12):1–9.

50. O'Connor AB, Dworkin RH. Treatment of neuropathic pain: an overview of recent guidelines. Am J Med 2009;122(10):S22–32.

51. Dworkin RH, O'Connor AB, Audette J, et al. Recommendations for the pharmacological management of neuropathic pain: an overview and literature update. Mayo Clin Proc 2010;85(3):S3–14.

52. Blau LA, Hoehns JD. Analgesic efficacy of calcitonin for vertebral fracture pain. Ann Pharmacother 2003;37(4):564–70.

53. Kim DH, Vaccaro AR. Osteoporotic compression fractures of the spine; current options and considerations for treatment. Spine J 2006;6(5):479–87.

54. Knopp-Sihota JA, Newburn-Cook CV, Homik J, et al. Calcitonin for treating acute and chronic pain of recent and remote osteoporotic vertebral compression fractures: a systematic review and meta-analysis. Osteoporos Int 2012;23(1):17–38.

55. Esses SI, McGuire R, Jenkins J, et al. The treatment of symptomatic osteoporotic spinal compression fractures. J Am Acad Orthop Surg 2011;19:176–82.

56. Foye PM, Shupper P, Wendel I. Coccyx fractures treated with intranasal calcitonin. Pain Physician 2014;17:E229–33.

57. Finnerup NB, Attal N, Haroutounian S, et al. Pharmacotherapy for neuropathic pain in adults: a systematic review and meta-analysis. Lancet Neurol 2015; 14(2):162–73.

58. Attal N, Cruccu G, Baron R, et al. EFNS guidelines on the pharmacological treatment of neuropathic pain: 2010 revision. Eur J Neurol 2010;17(9):1113–1113.e88.

59. Moulin DE, Clark AJ, Gilron I, et al. Pharmacological management of chronic neuropathic pain—consensus statement and guidelines from the Canadian Pain Society. Pain Res Manag 2007;12(1):13–21.

60. Jorge LL, Feres CC, Teles VE. Topical preparations for pain relief: efficacy and patient adherence. J Pain Res 2011;4:11–24.

61. Hayman M, Kam PCA. Capsaicin: a review of its pharmacology and clinical applications. Curr Anaesth Crit Care 2008;19:338–43.

62. Mason L, Moore RA, Derry S, et al. Systematic review of topical capsaicin for the treatment of chronic pain. Br Med J 2004;328(7446):991.

63. Jevsevar DS. Treatment of osteoarthritis of the knee: evidence-based guideline, 2nd edition. J Am Acad Orthop Surg 2013;21:571–6.

64. Sinusas K. Osteoarthritis: diagnosis and treatment. Am Fam Physician 2012; 1(86):49–56.

65. Bruyère O, Cooper C, Pelletier JP, et al. An algorithm recommendation for the management of knee osteoarthritis in Europe and internationally: a report from a task force of the European Society for Clinical and Economic Aspects of Osteoporosis and Osteoarthritis (ESCEO). Semin Arthritis Rheum 2014;44(3):253–63.

66. McAlindon TE, Bannuru RR, Sullivan MC, et al. OARSI guidelines for the non-surgical management of knee osteoarthritis. Osteoarthr Cartil 2014;22(3):363–88.

67. National Institute for Health and Care Excellence. Osteoarthritis: care and management. London: NICE guideline (CG177). 2014.

68. Nelson AE, Allen KD, Golightly YM, et al. A systematic review of recommendations and guidelines for the management of osteoarthritis: the Chronic Osteoarthritis Management Initiative of the U.S. Bone and Joint Initiative. Semin Arthritis Rheum 2014;43(6):701–12.

69. Hochberg MC, Altman RD, April KT, et al. American College of Rheumatology 2012 recommendations for the use of nonpharmacologic and pharmacologic therapies in osteoarthritis of the hand, hip, and knee. Arthritis Care Res 2012; 64(4):465–74.

70. Zhang W, Doherty M, Arden N, et al. EULAR evidence based recommendations for the management of hip osteoarthritis: report of a task force of the EULAR Standing Committee for International Clinical Studies Including Therapeutics (ESCISIT). Ann Rheum Dis 2005;64(5):669–81.

71. Zhang W, Doherty M, Leeb BF, et al. EULAR evidence based recommendations for the management of hand osteoarthritis: report of a Task Force of the EULAR Standing Committee for International Clinical Studies Including Therapeutics (ESCISIT). Ann Rheum Dis 2007;66(3):377–88.

72. Jordan KM, Arden NK, Doherty M, et al. EULAR Recommendations 2003: an evidence based approach to the management of knee osteoarthritis: report of a

Task Force of the Standing Committee for International Clinical Studies Including Therapeutic Trials (ESCISIT). Ann Rheum Dis 2003;62(12):1145–55.

73. Huskisson EC. Glucosamine and chondroitin for osteoarthritis. J Int Med Res 2008;36(6):6.

74. Bruyere O, Reginster J-Y. Glucosamine and chondroitin sulfate as therapeutic agents for knee and hip osteoarthritis. Drugs Aging 2007;24(7):573–80.

75. Ho Y, Woo LJ, Jae S, et al. Effect of glucosamine or chondroitin sulfate on the osteoarthritis progression: a meta-analysis. Rheumatol Int 2010;30(3):357–63.

76. Vangsness CT, Spiker W, Erickson J. A review of evidence-based medicine for glucosamine and chondroitin sulfate use in knee osteoarthritis. Arthroscopy 2009;25(1):86–94.

77. Richy F, Bruyere O, Ethgen O, et al. Structural and symptomatic efficacy of glucosamine and chondroitin in knee osteoarthritis: a comprehensive meta-analysis. Arch Intern Med 2003;163(13):1514–22.

78. Dahmer S, Schiller RM. Glucosamine. Am Fam Physician 2008;78(4):471–6.

79. Kahlenberg CA, Knesek M, Terry MA. New developments in the use of biologics and other modalities in the management of lateral epicondylitis. Biomed Res Int 2015;2015:439309.

80. Cardone DA, Tallia AF. Joint and soft tissue injection. Am Fam Physician 2002; 66(2):283–8.

81. Zhang W, Moskowitz RW, Nuki G, et al. OARSI recommendations for the management of hip and knee osteoarthritis, part II: OARSI evidence-based, expert consensus guidelines. Osteoarthr Cartil 2008;16(2):137–62.

82. Schumacher HR, Chen LX. Injectable corticosteroids in treatment of arthritis of the knee. Am J Med 2005;118(11):1208–14.

83. Skedros JG, Hunt KJ, Pitts TC. Variations in corticosteroid/anesthetic injections for painful shoulder conditions: comparisons among orthopaedic surgeons, rheumatologists, and physical medicine and primary-care physicians. BMC Musculoskelet Disord 2007;8:63.

84. Breu A, Rosenmeier K, Kujat R, et al. The cytotoxicity of bupivacaine, ropivacaine, and mepivacaine on human chondrocytes and cartilage. Anesth Analg 2013;117(2):514–22.

85. Dragoo JL, Braun HJ, Kim HJ, et al. The in vitro chondrotoxicity of single-dose local anesthetics. Am J Sports Med 2012;40(4):794–9.

86. Hunter DJ. Viscosupplementation for osteoarthritis of the knee. N Engl J Med 2015;372(11):1040–7.

87. Axe JM, Snyder-Mackler L, Axe MJ. The role of viscosupplementation. Sports Med Arthrosc 2013;21(1):18–22.

88. Evaniew N, Simunovic N, Karlsson J. Cochrane in CORR®: viscosupplementation for the treatment of osteoarthritis of the knee. Clin Orthop Relat Res 2014;472(7): 2028–34.

89. Altman R, Lim S, Steen R, et al. Intra-articular hyaluronic acid delays total knee replacement in patients with knee osteoarthritis: evidence from a large U.S. health claims database. Osteoarthr Cartil 2015;2015(23):A403–4.

90. Asplund CA, Best TM. Achilles tendon disorders. Br Med J 2013;346:f1262.

91. Bokhari AR, Murrell GAC. The role of nitric oxide in tendon healing. J Shoulder Elbow Surg 2012;21(2):238–44.

92. Gambito ED, Gonzalez-Suarez CB, Oquiñena TI, et al. Evidence on the effectiveness of topical nitroglycerin in the treatment of tendinopathies: a systematic review and meta-analysis. Arch Phys Med Rehabil 2010;91:1291–305.

93. Rosso F, Bonasia DE, Cottino U, et al. Patellar tendon: from tendinopathy to rupture. Asia-Pacific J Sport Med Arthrosc Rehabil Technol 2015;2(4):99–107.

94. Erickson JL, Hall MM. Evidence-based treatment of common extensor tendinopathy. Curr Phys Med Rehabil Rep 2015;3:50–9.

95. Gaujoux-Viala C, Dougados M, Gossec L. Efficacy and safety of steroid injections for shoulder and elbow tendonitis: a meta-analysis of randomised controlled trials. Ann Rheum Dis 2009;68(12):1843–9.

96. Arroll B, Goodyear-Smith F. Corticosteroid injections for painful shoulder: a meta-analysis. Br J Gen Pract 2005;55(512):224–8.

97. Buchbinder R, Green S, Youd JM. Corticosteroid injections for shoulder pain. Cochrane Database Syst Rev 2003;(1):CD004016.

98. Peters-Veluthamaningal C, van der Windt DAWM, Winters JC, et al. Corticosteroid injection for trigger finger in adults. Cochrane Database Syst Rev 2009;(1):CD005617.

99. Earp BE, Han CH, Floyd WE, et al. De Quervain tendinopathy: survivorship and prognostic indicators of recurrence following a single corticosteroid injection. J Hand Surg Am 2015;40(6):1161–5.

Pharmacotherapy for Substance Use Disorders

Jared Wilson Klein, MD, MPH

KEYWORDS

- Substance use disorder • Varenicline • Naltrexone • Methadone • Buprenorphine

KEY POINTS

- There are several very effective pharmacotherapy options for patients with substance use disorders, although prescribers underuse these treatments.
- Combination nicotine replacement therapy (patch plus gum or lozenge) is the first-line treatment of tobacco use.
- Naltrexone is an effective option at reducing harmful drinking, but usually does not promote complete abstinence.
- There is strong evidence that opioid agonist therapy, either with methadone or buprenorphine, improves outcomes in multiple domains.

INTRODUCTION

Substance use can precipitate a broad array of illnesses. These disorders continue to carry significant stigma, both in society at large as well as within the medical community.[1] In the United States, 42 million adults, or 17.8% of the population, use tobacco products.[2] Alcohol use is even more prevalent, with 25% of US adults reporting binge alcohol consumption and 7% (nearly 17 million), diagnosed with alcohol use disorders.[3,4] Although smaller proportions use other substances,[5] these are often responsible for illness,[6,7] increased health care use,[8] more frequent interactions with the criminal justice system,[9] and numerous other adverse outcomes.[10]

Screening

Primary care physicians are often the initial health care providers to encounter many patients with substance use problems and are well positioned to screen for, diagnose, and initiate treatment or referral for patients with addiction. Studies have shown that single-item screens have good sensitivity and specificity for detection of concerning substance use and are easy to implement in primary care settings (Table 1).[11]

Disclosures: The author has nothing to disclose.
Division of General Internal Medicine, Department of Medicine, Harborview Medical Center, University of Washington, 325 Ninth Avenue, Box 359780, Seattle, WA 98104, USA
E-mail address: jaredwk@uw.edu

Med Clin N Am 100 (2016) 891–910
http://dx.doi.org/10.1016/j.mcna.2016.03.011
0025-7125/16/$ – see front matter © 2016 Elsevier Inc. All rights reserved.

Table 1
Screening for substance use disorders

Substance	Screening Questions	Positive Screen	Sensitivity (%)	Specificity (%)
Tobacco	In the past year have you used tobacco products?	Any	95	97
Alcohol	In the past year have you had 5 or more (4 or more for women) drinks in a day?	For men >5 drinks/d For women >4 drinks/d	82	79
Other substances	In the past year have you used illegal drugs or prescription drugs for nonmedical reasons?	Any	100	73.5

Diagnosis

With the publication of the Diagnostic and Statistical Manual, Version 5 (DSM-5), the terminology and criteria for addictive disorders has been substantially clarified.[12] Confusing and vague semantics such as "abuse" and "dependence" have been replaced by the more universal "substance use disorder," which is stratified into mild, moderate, and severe forms of disease (**Table 2**). Diagnostic criteria are fairly uniform across various drugs of abuse and include common-sense symptoms such as craving, tolerance, withdrawal, failure to fulfill social obligations, and use despite harms. Although use of specific DSM-5 criteria is often unnecessary in primary care settings, physicians should be familiar with the overarching principles in order to confidently identify and diagnose patients with addiction.

Treatment Principles

In considering pharmacotherapy for substance use disorders, it is important to determine the goals of the patient and the physician. Although complete abstinence from substance use is often the best option from a medical perspective, this may or may not be compatible with the patient's goals. A frank, nonjudgmental discussion is important to ensure clear communication and maintain the therapeutic alliance.

Once the patient has agreed to address the substance use problem, treatment options should be discussed. Patients or providers might have strong feelings about the

Table 2
DSM-5 criteria for substance use disorders (SUDs)

Criteria	Severity
Using larger amounts than intended	0–1 criteria = no SUD
Persistent desire to cut down or quit	2–3 criteria = mild SUD
Significant time spent taking or obtaining substance	4–5 criteria = moderate SUD
Craving or urge to use substance	>5 criteria = severe SUD
Failure to fulfill obligations	
Continued use despite negative interpersonal consequences	
Reduced social or recreational activities	
Use in physically hazardous situations	
Use despite knowledge of harms	
Tolerance (excludes prescription medication)	
Withdrawal (excludes prescription medication)	

use of medication-assisted treatment versus behavioral treatments for addiction. Often, outcomes are best when these approaches are combined.[13] If pharmacotherapy is used, some patients prefer to undergo detoxification only. However, for some substances, there is strong evidence that ongoing treatment (either with agonists or antagonists) leads to better outcomes.[14,15] Several studies have suggested that pharmacotherapy is considerably underused in the treatment of substance use disorders.[16,17]

TOBACCO USE DISORDERS
Pharmacology of Nicotine

Nicotine, the primary addictive component of tobacco products, is a stimulant that exerts its effects via nicotinic acetylcholine receptors. These ligand-gated ion channels are located diffusely throughout the brain and interact with multiple other neural pathways to exert nicotine's diffuse effects: increased blood pressure, accelerated heart rate, heightened arousal, and reward. When smoked, nicotine is rapidly delivered to the central nervous system (CNS) and is subsequently metabolized by the brain, liver, and lung via cytochrome P 26A into cotinine, the primary metabolite.

Epidemiology of Tobacco Use

Although smoking rates in the United States have decreased dramatically over the past few decades, nearly 18% of Americans (or 42 million) currently smoke cigarettes.[2] An additional 3.6% use smokeless tobacco and there are increasing numbers of adolescents and young adults using electronic cigarettes.[18,19] Despite restrictive smoking laws, secondhand smoke continues to affect millions of Americans and has been associated with cardiovascular disease and lung cancer.[20,21]

First-line Agents

Nicotine replacement therapy
Nicotine that is delivered via noninhaled routes can alleviate withdrawal symptoms typically associated with abstinence, allowing patients to disrupt the behaviors associated with tobacco use. Nicotine replacement therapy, the cornerstone of assisting patients in quitting smoking, is US Food and Drug Administration (FDA) approved for the treatment of tobacco use disorders and is available in a variety of delivery systems (**Table 3**). Multiple studies have shown that nicotine replacement therapy approximately doubles the success rate of patients attempting to quit smoking versus placebo alone (from 10% to 20%).[22] The efficacy is even higher when nicotine patches are combined with a short-acting form of nicotine replacement, therefore this is the recommended approach for most patients.[23] Adverse effects are uncommon and unique to the delivery system used (see **Table 3**). General side effects of excess nicotine exposure include nausea, vomiting, gastrointestinal upset, and headaches.

Varenicline
Varenicline (**Table 4**), a high-affinity partial agonist at the nicotinic acetylcholine receptor, blocks the binding of nicotine to the receptor while alleviating the withdrawal symptoms associated with abstinence from tobacco use. Studies have shown that varenicline increases smoking cessation success rates by 2-fold to 3-fold and is equally efficacious as combination nicotine replacement therapy.[23] Varenicline is uptitrated the week before a patient's quit date as follows: 0.5 mg daily for 3 days, then 0.5 mg twice daily for 4 days, then 1 mg twice daily (on the quit date). The drug is renally excreted, so dosing must be adjusted in patients with renal insufficiency. Treatment is usually continued for at least 12 weeks, but can be extended to improve the

Table 3
Nicotine replacement therapy

Route	Dosing	Route-specific Adverse Effects	Approximate Cost of 30-d Supply ($)
Patch	• 21 mg transdermal daily (>1 pack/d) • 14 mg transdermal daily (0.5 pack/d) • 7 mg transdermal daily (<1/2 pack/d)	Skin irritation, insomnia	70
Gum	2–4 mg chew and park in mucosa every 1–2 h PRN for cravings	Mouth/throat irritation, aphthous ulcers	50
Lozenge	2–4 mg dissolve orally every 1–2 h PRN for cravings	Mouth/throat irritation, aphthous ulcers	50
Inhaler	6–16 cartridges/d PRN for cravings	Mouth/throat irritation	200
Nasal spray	1–2 sprays per hour, do not exceed 10 sprays per hour or 80 sprays/d	Nasal irritation, rhinitis, sneezing	120

Abbreviation: PRN, as needed.

success of the quit attempt.[24] One randomized study suggests that combining varenicline with nicotine replacement can improve success rates.[25] Some evidence also supports the use of varenicline to promote smoking cessation among patients not currently contemplating a quit attempt.[26] Many patients report insomnia and vivid

Table 4
Prescription pharmacotherapy for tobacco use

Drug	Dosing (Usually Continued for 3–6 mo)	Adverse Effects	Contraindications/ Precautions	Cost	Efficacy at 6 mo[a] (%)
Varenicline	• 0.5 mg daily for 3 d, then • 0.5 mg BID for 4 d, then • 1 mg twice daily on quit date	Nausea, insomnia, vivid dreams	Reduce dose with renal insufficiency, caution with psychiatric disease	$$$	33
Bupropion	• 150 mg daily for 3 d, then • 150 mg BID by quit date	Dry mouth, headaches, insomnia	Do not use if seizure disorder, caution with psychiatric disease	$	20
Nortriptyline	• Start at 25 mg daily • Titrate up to 100 mg daily over 2–3 wk before quit date	Dry mouth, sedation, constipation, urinary retention	Caution with cardiovascular or psychiatric disease	$	20

Abbreviations: $, least expensive; $$$, most expensive; BID, twice a day.
[a] Approximate rate of smoking abstinence at 6 months (placebo rate of 10%).

(sometimes disturbing) dreams, but the association with depression or suicidal idea-tion is less clear.[27] As a precaution, many physicians avoid prescribing varenicline to patients with unstable or significant psychiatric comorbidities. Although trials have failed to associate varenicline use with adverse cardiovascular events, there is concern that these studies have been underpowered to identify differences.[28] There-fore, caution is advised when recommending varenicline to patients at high risk for acute coronary events. Although costly, most commercial insurers cover varenicline and the manufacturer provides assistance to limit patients' out of pocket costs.[29]

Bupropion

Bupropion is a norepinephrine and dopamine reuptake inhibitor frequently used as an antidepressant. It has been FDA approved to aid in smoking cessation among pa-tients, irrespective of comorbid depression. Although this medication is primarily thought to alter the brain's reward pathways via dopaminergic effects, bupropion also has some activity at the nicotinic acetylcholine receptors. The sustained-release formulation of bupropion is started 1 week before the planned quit date, which allows drug levels to reach steady state. Dosing is 150 mg daily for 3 days, then 150 mg twice daily. Bupropion approximately doubles the chance of successfully quit-ting smoking compared with placebo, and adding nicotine replacement therapy might further improve the success rate.[30] Bupropion lowers the seizure threshold, so is con-traindicated for patients with seizure disorders or at risk for seizures. Although an elegant therapy for smokers with depression, bupropion has been associated with a slight increase in suicidal behaviors so patients should be warned about neuropsychi-atric side effects.[31] More common side effects include insomnia, xerostomia, and headaches. Bupropion is associated with weight loss in some patients and may atten-uate the usual weight gain seen after quitting smoking.[32] Bupropion is generally less costly than varenicline and widely available in generic formulations.

Second-line Agents

Nortriptyline

Nortriptyline, a tricyclic antidepressant, is the best-studied non–FDA-approved medi-cation for smoking cessation. A meta-analysis has showed nortriptyline to have similar efficacy to bupropion, with approximate doubling of the successful quit rate at 3 months.[30] Because of the risk of inducing serotonin syndrome, nortriptyline should not be combined with other serotonergic medications, including selective serotonin reuptake inhibitors, monoamine oxidase inhibitors, or linezolid. Its use is also limited by significant side effects, including sedation, xerostomia, constipation, and urinary retention. Dosing is fairly straightforward (see **Table 4**). As with bupropion, nortripty-line is widely available as a generic medication, limiting cost concerns.

Combination Therapy

There are limited data to support combining medications to support patients attempt-ing to quit smoking. As mentioned earlier, combination nicotine replacement therapy and the addition of bupropion to nicotine replacement therapy are reasonable strate-gies. Preliminary studies also support the addition of varenicline to nicotine replace-ment therapy, although this approach deserves additional research.

Special Circumstances

Pregnancy and lactation

Given the known adverse effect of tobacco exposure on the fetus (including low birth weight, miscarriage, and prematurity) and newborn (decreased breast milk production, increased risk of sudden infant death syndrome), smoking cessation should be strongly advised to all pregnant and lactating women. Although evidence is limited, first-line medications include nicotine replacement therapy and bupropion.[33] Given the paucity of data, varenicline and nortriptyline are often avoided as an initial approach in treating pregnant or lactating women.

Older adults
Although the rate of tobacco use is lower among older adults, the therapeutic approach is similar to what is described earlier.[2] Caution should be used when titrating the doses of medications for smoking cessation, particularly in patients at risk for polypharmacy and those with comorbidities that could alter the pharmacokinetics. Tricyclic antidepressants, such as nortriptyline, should be avoided in older adults.

Relapsed smokers
When patients have failed a particular pharmacologic smoking cessation aid, a conversation should take place with the clinician to explore the underlying reasons. It is often appropriate to try again with the same medication, but with changes to the patients' support systems. In general, nicotine replacement therapy is used as the initial pharmacologic approach, whereas varenicline and bupropion are reserved for treatment failures.

ALCOHOL USE DISORDERS
Pharmacology of Alcohol

Ethanol, the primary active compound in most alcohol products, exerts widespread effects throughout the body, including the CNS. In the CNS, ethanol activates gamma-aminobutyric acid (GABA)-A receptors and antagonizes N-methyl-d-aspartate–glutamate receptors, resulting in overall depression of CNS activity. Multiple other neuroreceptors have been implicated in alcohol's physiologic effects, including opioid, serotonin, and nicotinic acetylcholine receptors, but the precise mechanisms are not as clearly delineated.

Epidemiology of Alcohol Use

Most Americans consume alcohol at least occasionally.[34] More than 30% use alcohol in a risky manner, such as exceeding the recommended frequency or quantity of alcoholic drinks or binge drinking.[35] Although genuine alcohol use disorders are less frequent, they are the most common substance use disorders in the United States, with an annual prevalence of about 7% (17 million people).[36]

Detoxification

Unlike most other substance use disorders, withdrawal from alcohol is potentially fatal and should be managed thoughtfully by physicians. Mild withdrawal can start within hours of the last drink and manifests as headache, diaphoresis, agitation, and tremor. More severe symptoms include seizures, hallucinations, and delirium tremens, which usually occur within a few days of abstinence. The Clinical Institute Withdrawal Assessment for Alcohol (CIWA-A) can be used to monitor the severity of alcohol withdrawal and titrate medications (**Table 5**). There are multiple online and mobile resources that can be used to calculate patients' CIWA-A scores. Standard of care for the treatment of alcohol detoxification are benzodiazepines, although barbiturates can also be used (**Table 6**). Evidence suggests that symptom-driven protocols are just as effective as scheduled-dose regimens, but expose the patient to lower total doses of benzodiazepine and result in decreased lengths of stay in the hospital.[37]

Table 5
Components of the CIWA-alcohol withdrawal scale

Item	Scale
Nausea/vomiting	1–7
Diaphoresis	1–7
Anxiety	1–7
Agitation	1–7
Tremor	1–7
Headache	1–7
Auditory disturbances	1–7
Visual disturbances	1–7
Tactile disturbances	1–7
Orientation	0–4

Total Score		Potential Management Options
Very mild	<10	Monitor closely
Mild	10–15	Consider PRN benzodiazepines
Moderate	16–20	Consider scheduled benzodiazepines
Severe	>20	Consider ICU transfer

Abbreviation: ICU, intensive care unit.
Adapted from Sullivan JT, Skyora K, Schneiderman J, et al. Assessment of alcohol withdrawal: the revised Clinical Institute Withdrawal Assessment for Alcohol scale (CIWA-Ar). Br J Addict 1989;84(11):1354; with permission.

Maintenance Therapy: First-line Agents

Naltrexone

Naltrexone is an opioid receptor antagonist that is FDA approved for the treatment of alcohol use disorders. Blockade of mu-opioid receptors reduces the reinforcing effects of alcohol, allowing naltrexone to moderate the intake of heavy alcohol users. Studies have shown that naltrexone can reduce heavy drinking days by 17% to 25%, but there is little evidence that naltrexone can boost the rate of complete alcohol abstinence.[15] Naltrexone has straightforward dosing, with once-a-day oral formulations and 4-weekly intramuscular formulations (the latter being preferred for patients at risk of poor compliance) (**Table 7**). Most trials have examined dosing for 3 to 6 months, but clinicians can consider extending the duration of treatment depending on the patient's response to treatment and the severity of the diagnosis. Although generally well tolerated, naltrexone can cause nausea, fatigue, headaches, and other nonspecific symptoms. There has been concern for using naltrexone in patients with

Table 6
Dosing regimens for alcohol detoxification

Medication	Oral Dose (mg)	IV Dose (mg)	Frequency (h)
Diazepam	5–10	5–10	Every 1–2 PRN
Lorazepam	2–4	2–4	Every 1–2 PRN
Chlordiazepoxide	50–100	NA	Every 2–4 PRN
Phenobarbital	NA	130–260	Every 0.5–1 PRN

Abbreviations: IV, intravenous; NA, not applicable.

Table 7
Naltrexone oral versus intramuscular comparison

Formulation	Dose (mg)	Frequency	Side Effects
Oral	50	Daily	Nausea, headache, mild transaminitis
Intramuscular	380	Every 4 wk	Injection-site reactions, nausea, fatigue

underlying liver disease because of the risk of transaminitis (particularly with the oral formulation). Unless the patient has decompensated cirrhosis or acute hepatitis, naltrexone can likely be safely used, although regular monitoring of liver function tests is recommended. As an opioid receptor antagonist, naltrexone use is contraindicated in patients on opioid therapy; however, it can be used if patients are still consuming alcohol.

Acamprosate

Acamprosate has a poorly understood mechanism of action, but is thought to affect the brain's glutamate receptors, providing a means of reducing cravings for alcohol. The primary limitation of acamprosate is the dosing regimen of 666 mg 3 times per day. Lower doses should be used in patients with renal impairment or low body weight, but acamprosate can safely be used in patients with liver disease. Studies have shown that acamprosate increases the abstinence rate by about 10% (number needed to treat of 10 patients for 6 months to prevent 1 relapse).[38] The medication can be started in patients who are still drinking and clinical trials have studied durations of 3 to 6 months. As with naltrexone, continued use beyond this time point should be at the discretion of the physician and patient. The primary side effect of acamprosate is gastrointestinal upset, specifically diarrhea.

Maintenance Therapy: Second-line Agents

Disulfiram

Although FDA approved for the treatment of alcohol use disorders, disulfiram should not be considered a first-line agent. Disulfiram is an aversive agent that blocks the metabolism of ethanol, leading to the accumulation of acetaldehyde and resulting in headache, flushing, and other unpleasant physiologic effects (**Fig. 1**). The efficacy of disulfiram is best among highly motivated patients who are participating in highly structured treatment programs (methadone maintenance clinics with daily observed dosing or residential alcohol treatment programs).[39] When used in primary care settings, disulfiram is not more effective than placebo.[38] If prescribed, disulfiram should be initiated at 500 mg daily for 1 to 2 weeks, then reduced to 250 mg daily (the higher dose can be continued for significant cravings, whereas a lower dose of 125 mg can be used if there are significant side effects). Patients should not take disulfiram if they are actively drinking, because this could precipitate an aversive reaction. Patients should be warned about hidden alcohols in other products, such as cough syrup

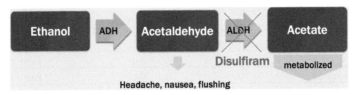

Fig. 1. Mechanism of disulfiram in the metabolism of ethanol. ADH, alcohol dehydrogenase; ALDH, aldehyde dehydrogenase.

and mouthwash, and counseled that the medication can persist in the body for up to 14 days after the last dose. Other serious side effects are rare, but caution should be used in patients with significant liver disease.

Other agents
There are several non–FDA-approved medications that have shown potential in the treatment of alcohol use disorders. Topiramate, an antiepileptic medication that modulates glutamate and GABA receptors, has been shown to reduce alcohol consumption in several randomized controlled trials.[40,41] If prescribed, topiramate should be initiated at 50 mg daily and slowly uptitrated over several weeks to a maximum dose of 150 mg twice a day. A recent study showed a dose-response relationship between gabapentin and reduced alcohol consumption, but the effect was not statistically significant.[42] Additional evidence is necessary before gabapentin can be recommended for routine treatment of alcohol use disorders. Baclofen has been proposed as a treatment of alcohol use disorder, but studies have shown mixed results.[43,44] When dosed at 30 mg/d baclofen is generally well tolerated, although sedation and nausea can occur. Selective serotonin reuptake inhibitors have been proved ineffective for the treatment of alcohol use disorders in the absence of a co-occurring mood disorder.[45]

Combination Therapy

There is limited evidence to support the use of combinations of medications to treat alcohol use disorders, so this approach cannot be recommended at this time.[46,47]

Special Circumstances

Pregnancy and lactation
Despite the known harms of alcohol to the fetus (**Box 1**), there is a notable dearth of evidence regarding pharmacotherapy for pregnant women with alcohol use disorders. Naltrexone is generally considered safe and is the most frequently prescribed medication for pregnant or lactating women with alcohol problems. Acamprosate is teratogenic in animal models and disulfiram can lead to the accumulation of acetaldehyde in the fetus, so these agents are usually avoided.

Box 1
Features of fetal alcohol spectrum disorders

Growth deficiency

- Low birth weight

- Small for age

Abnormal facial features

- Smooth philtrum

- Thin vermillion

- Small palpebral fissures

Central nervous system problems

- Developmental delay

- Learning disabilities

- Seizures

Older adults

Because of comorbidities, health risks, and medication interactions, recommended alcohol consumption limits are lower for adults more than 65 years old (**Table 8**).[48] Alcohol use disorders are often unrecognized among older adults.[49] Pharmacotherapy options for older adults with alcohol use disorders are identical to those for younger adults, but care should be taken to dose medications appropriately for patients' renal and hepatic functions.

OPIOID USE DISORDERS
Pharmacology of Opioids

Opioid receptors are G protein–coupled receptors located throughout the brain and spinal cord, as well as the digestive tract. Endogenous opioids act via these receptors to mediate emotional and pain responses (**Fig. 2**, **Table 9**). Most exogenous opioids, both licit and illicit, exert their plethora of effects via the mu subset of opioid receptors (**Table 10**). Tolerance to opioids develops rapidly, exacerbating the abuse potential of these substances. Opioids have widely disparate half-lives (from morphine at about 2 hours to methadone at >24 hours) and many metabolites remain active. Hepatic or renal impairment can further extend the effects of opioids.

Epidemiology of Opioid Use

The lifetime prevalence of heroin use in the United States is nearly 5 million adults and adolescents, or almost 2% of the population, and the incidence seems to be increasing.[50,51] Rates of prescription opioid misuse are more difficult to estimate, but the number of patients seeking treatment of nonheroin opioid use disorders is increasing.[52] This phenomenon could represent a consequence of recent restrictions in the prescribing of opioids, particularly for chronic, noncancer pain.[53,54] Prescription opioid misuse is pervasive across racial, geographic, and socioeconomic boundaries, although some risk factors have been consistently identified (**Table 11**).

Detoxification Versus Maintenance

Because dependence reliably develops among patients on opioids, withdrawal is inevitable among chronic users. Continued use is largely a means of self-treatment to stave off withdrawal symptoms (**Table 12**). Although detoxification (with or without opioid antagonist therapy) has not been directly compared with opioid maintenance therapy, the latter is generally considered preferable. Opioid agonist therapy evens out peaks and troughs, permitting patients to stabilize in other domains, such as housing and employment (**Fig. 3**).

Table 8	
Low-risk alcohol consumption levels	
Group	**Low-risk Consumption Level**
Women	<2 drinks/d
Men	<3 drinks/d
Adults ≥65 y old	<2 drinks/d

Standard alcoholic drink contains 15 mL (0.5 fluid ounces) of ethanol and is typically equivalent to: (1) 355 mL (12 ounces) of beer; (2) 148 mL (5 ounces) of wine; (3) 45 mL (1.5 ounces) of 80-proof liquor.

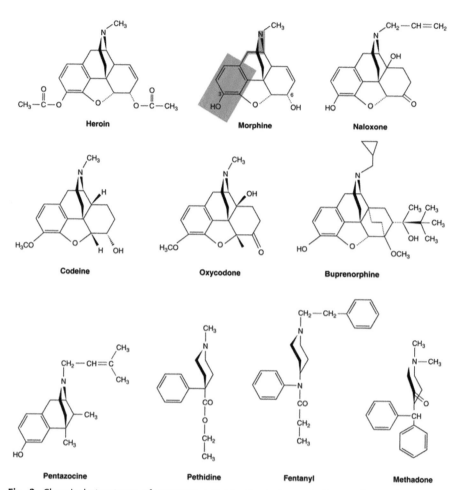

Fig. 2. Chemical structures of common opioids. Shaded area indicates chemical structure that mimics endogenous endorphins. (*From* Rang HP, Ritter JM, Flower RJ, et al. Rang & Dale's pharmacology. 8th edition. Elsevier; 2015; with permission.)

Table 9		
Common endogenous, licit, and illicit opioid receptor agonists		
Endogenous Opioids	**Licit Opioids**	**Illicit Opioids**
Dynorphins	• Natural	Heroin
Enkephalins	○ Morphine	Etorphine
Endorphins	○ Codeine	
Endomorphins	• Semisynthetic	
Nociceptin	○ Oxycodone	
	○ Hydrocodone	
	○ Hydromorphone	
	• Synthetic	
	○ Methadone	
	○ Fentanyl	
	○ Tramadol	

Table 10	
Common effects of opioid agonists	
Therapeutic Effects	**Adverse Effects**
Sedation	Somnolence
Analgesia	Respiratory depression
Respiratory depression (palliation)	Constipation
Euphoria (illicit use)	Nausea
	Pruritus
	Hyperalgesia (chronic use)
	Hypogonadism (chronic use)

First-line Agents

Methadone

Methadone is a long-acting full mu agonist that has been used for more than 40 years in the treatment of opioid addiction. At sufficiently high dosages, methadone blocks the ability of other opioids to bind mu receptors (so-called narcotic blockade) and suppresses opioid cravings. Typical doses are in the range of 80 to 120 mg/d to attain therapeutic effect. Federal law mandates that methadone can only be dispensed for addiction treatment via tightly regulated methadone maintenance programs. In addition to directly observed dosing and urine toxicology monitoring, these programs offer chemical dependency counseling and, often, mental health services. In such settings, methadone is highly effective in preventing a diverse array of undesirable outcomes (**Box 2**).[55] Although methadone is generally well tolerated, side effects such as constipation, respiratory depression, and corrected QT interval prolongation can occur. A complete listing of US methadone maintenance programs by state can be found at http://dpt2.samhsa.gov/treatment/directory.aspx.

Table 11		
Opioid risk tool to identify risk factors for prescription opioid misuse		
	Score	
Domain	**Female**	**Male**
Family History of Substance Abuse		
Alcohol	1	3
Illegal drugs	2	3
Prescription drugs	4	4
Personal History of Substance Abuse		
Alcohol	3	3
Illegal drugs	4	4
Prescription drugs	5	5
Age ≤45 y	1	1
History of preadolescent sexual abuse	3	0
Psychiatric Disease		
Depression	1	1
Attention deficit disorder, obsessive-compulsive disorder, bipolar disorder, schizophrenia	2	2

Risk levels: 0 to 3, low risk; 4 to 7, moderate risk; ≥8, high risk.
From Webster LR, Webster R. Predicting aberrant behaviors in Opioid–treated patients: preliminary validation of the opioid risk tool. Pain Med 2005;6(6):432; with permission.

Table 12	
Opioid withdrawal symptoms	
Early Symptoms	**Later Symptoms**
Anxiety	Vomiting
Cravings	Diarrhea
Restlessness	Tremor
Yawning	Tachycardia
Insomnia	Piloerection
Abdominal cramping	Hypertension
Rhinorrhea	Fever
Lacrimation	

Buprenorphine

Buprenorphine is an opioid partial agonist with very high affinity for mu receptors, thereby providing adequate opioid effect while reducing the risk of respiratory depression. Buprenorphine is often coformulated with naloxone as an abuse deterrent (naloxone blocks any opioid agonist effect if the buprenorphine is illicitly injected, but passes through the gastrointestinal tract without being absorbed if the medication is taken as instructed). Doses start between 4 and 8 mg sublingually daily for several days, with dose escalation up to 16 to 24 mg daily for maintenance. Although typically dosed once a day, the dose can be split if needed to control cravings. Extreme care must be taken when starting buprenorphine in patients currently taking opioids, particularly long-acting opioids such as methadone. Because of the partial agonist activity, buprenorphine can displace full agonists from opioid receptors and precipitate withdrawal. Common opioid side effects, including sedation, constipation, and nausea, can be seen with buprenorphine; however, respiratory depression is uncommon. Evidence shows that outcomes for patients treated with buprenorphine are similar to those for patients on methadone maintenance (**Table 13**).[56] Unlike methadone used for addiction treatment, buprenorphine has been classified as Schedule III by the US Drug Enforcement Administration.[57] Providers who have obtained additional training can be prescribed buprenorphine for addiction treatment in the outpatient setting. More information about buprenorphine, including a searchable listing of prescribers and details about how to become a buprenorphine prescriber, is available at http://www.samhsa.gov/medication-assisted-treatment.

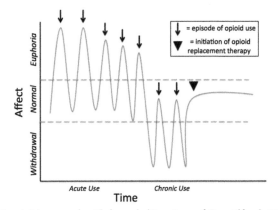

Fig. 3. Pattern of opioid use and withdrawal. (*Courtesy of* Dan Alford, MD, Boston, MA.)

Box 2
Outcomes of methadone maintenance

Increased retention in treatment

Decreased illicit opioid use

Decreased transmission of hepatitis C virus and human immunodeficiency virus

Reduced rates of incarceration

Increased employment

Increased survival

Second-line Agents

Naltrexone

Naltrexone, an opioid receptor antagonist, can be used for the treatment of opioid use disorder. The efficacy of naltrexone has not been directly compared with opioid agonist therapy, but antagonist therapy is more effective than placebo when adherence can be assured.[58,59] Naltrexone might be particularly useful in certain subsets of patients (Box 3). Dosing is identical to that used in alcohol use disorders (50 mg by mouth daily or 380 mg intramuscularly monthly). It is critical that patients be completely detoxified from all opioids lest withdrawal be precipitated.

Other agents

Various combinations of supportive medications have been suggested to manage opioid detoxification. These combinations are primarily targeted to specific withdrawal symptoms (Table 14). Although commonly used in clinical practice, this approach is empiric. As discussed previously, detoxification alone is an inadequate approach for most patients.[60]

Table 13
Buprenorphine versus methadone for opioid use disorder

Domain	Methadone	Buprenorphine
Mechanism of action	Full mu-receptor opioid agonist	Partial mu-receptor opioid agonist
Typical dosing regimen	80–120 mg daily	16–24 mg daily
Retention	Gold standard (approximately 50% retention)	Similar to methadone at adequate doses ($\geq$16 mg/d)
Abuse potential	Low because of directly observed dosing	Low because of coformulation with naloxone as abuse deterrent
Common side effects	Respiratory depression most common	Respiratory depression uncommon
Legal status	DEA Schedule II	DEA Schedule III
Clinical setting	Can only be dispensed by strictly regulated treatment programs	May be prescribed in outpatient setting by specially trained physicians

Abbreviation: DEA, US Drug Enforcement Administration.

Box 3
Potential candidates for naltrexone therapy to treat opioid use disorder

- Structured treatment settings
- Highly motivated patients
- Patients with occupational contraindications to opioid agonist therapy:
  - Health care workers
  - Law enforcement officers
  - Commercial drivers/pilots

Special Circumstances

Pregnancy and lactation

Methadone is the treatment of choice for pregnant women with opioid use disorders. Evidence shows that treatment improves connection with prenatal care, engagement with addiction treatment, and fetal outcomes such as birth weight and full-term delivery.[61] Methadone doses must often be increased during pregnancy, particularly during the third trimester, because of expanded plasma volume and increased drug metabolism. Split dosing (twice a day) is also sometimes necessary because of increased methadone clearance. Buprenorphine is also an acceptable option for the treatment of opioid use disorders in pregnant women, but the monotherapy form (buprenorphine alone) should be used given a small association between naloxone exposure and congenital abnormalities.[62] Newborns delivered by women on methadone or buprenorphine should be monitored closely by experienced providers for neonatal abstinence syndrome.[63] Although drug levels of both methadone and buprenorphine are detectable in breast milk, most experts think that the benefit of continued treatment outweighs any potential harm to the newborn.[64]

Older adults

Although opioid use disorders are less common among older adults, treatment recommendations are no different among this subset of patients. Some evidence shows that, compared with younger counterparts, older adults are more successful in methadone maintenance programs.[65]

Table 14
Symptomatic treatment of opioid withdrawal

Agents	Symptoms Addressed
Benzodiazepines	Anxiety, restlessness, insomnia
Clonidine	Tachycardia, hypertension
Loperamide	Diarrhea
Octreotide	Diarrhea
Promethazine	Nausea
Baclofen	Muscle cramping
Acetaminophen, NSAIDs	Pain

Abbreviation: NSAIDs, nonsteroidal antiinflammatory drugs.

OTHER SUBSTANCE USE DISORDERS

Despite urgent clinical need and extensive research, to date there are no efficacious pharmacotherapies for other addictive substances, including stimulants (cocaine, methamphetamines), marijuana or synthetic cannabinoids (also known as spice or K2), hallucinogens (ketamine, LSD [D-lysergic acid diethylamide], PCP [phencyclidine]) or so-called club drugs (MDMA [methylenedioxymethamphetamine; ecstasy, Molly]).

SUMMARY

Thanks to better understanding of the neurobiological mechanisms of addiction, the past few decades have seen extensive advances in the availability of medication options to treat substance use disorders. Ongoing efforts need to be focused on the development of treatment options for more substances (particularly stimulants such as cocaine and methamphetamines) as well as on the dissemination of best practices in addiction medicine to a wider audience of health care providers. For patients, societal stigma remains a barrier to treatment and the medical system should work to overcome such obstacles.

REFERENCES

1. Ahern J, Stuber J, Galea S. Stigma, discrimination and the health of illicit drug users. Drug Alcohol Depend 2007;88:188–96.
2. Centers for Disease Control and Prevention. Current cigarette smoking among adults—United States, 2005–2013. MMWR Morb Mortal Wkly Rep 2014;63(47): 1108–12.
3. Substance Abuse and Mental Health Services Administration (SAMHSA). 2013 National Survey on Drug Use and Health (NSDUH). Table 2.41B—Alcohol use in lifetime, past year, and past month among persons aged 18 or older, by demographic characteristics: percentages, 2012 and 2013. Available at: http://www. samhsa.gov/data/sites/default/files/NSDUH-DetTabsPDFWHTML2013/Web/HTML/ NSDUH-DetTabsSect2peTabs1to42-2013.htm#tab2.41b. Accessed November 7, 2015.
4. SAMHSA. 2013 National Survey on Drug Use and Health (NSDUH). Table 2.46B— alcohol use, binge alcohol use, and heavy alcohol use in the past month among persons aged 18 or older, by demographic characteristics: percentages, 2012 and 2013. Available at: http://www.samhsa.gov/data/sites/default/files/NSDUH-DetTabsPDFWHTML2013/Web/HTML/NSDUH-DetTabsSect2peTabs43to84-2013. htm#tab2.46b. Accessed November 7, 2015.
5. Center for Behavioral Health Statistics and Quality. Behavioral health trends in the United States: results from the 2014 National Survey on Drug Use and Health (HHS publication no. SMA 15-4927, NSDUH Series H-50). 2015. Available at: http://www.samhsa.gov/data/. Accessed November 7, 2015.
6. US Department of Health and Human Services. The health consequences of smoking: a report of the Surgeon General. Atlanta (GA); Washington, DC: Centers for Disease Control and Prevention, National Center for Chronic Disease Prevention and Health Promotion; Office on Smoking and Health; 2004.
7. Rehm J, Mathers C, Popova S, et al. Global burden of disease and injury and economic cost attributable to alcohol use and alcohol-use disorders. Lancet 2009;373(9682):2223–33.
8. French MT, McGeary KA, Chitwood DD, et al. Chronic illicit drug use, health services utilization and the cost of medical care. Soc Sci Med 2000;50(12):1703–13.

9. Mumola CJ, Karberg JC. Drug use and dependence, state and federal prisoners, 2004. Bureau of Justice Statistics Special Report. 2006. NJC 213530. Available at: http://www.bjs.gov/index.cfm?ty=pbdetail&iid=778. Accessed November 7, 2015.

10. US Department of Justice, National Drug Intelligence Center. Impact of drugs on society in national drug threat assessment 2010. 2010. Available at: http://www.justice.gov/archive/ndic/pubs38/38661/drugImpact.htm#foot6. Accessed November 7, 2015.

11. Madras B, Compton W, Avula D, et al. Screening, brief intervention, referral to treatment (SBIRT) for illicit drug and alcohol use at multiple healthcare sites: Comparison at intake and 6 months later. Drug Alcohol Depend 2009;99(1–3): 280–95.

12. American Psychiatric Association. Diagnostic and statistical manual of mental disorders: DSM-5. Washington, DC: American Psychiatric Association; 2013.

13. National Institute on Drug Abuse. Treatment approaches for drug addiction. Available at: http://www.drugabuse.gov/publications/drugfacts/treatment-approaches-drug-addiction. Accessed November 7, 2015.

14. Sees KL, Delucchi KL, Masson C, et al. Methadone maintenance vs 180-day psychosocially enriched detoxification for treatment of opioid dependence: a randomized controlled trial. JAMA 2000;283(10):1303–10.

15. Rösner S, Hackl-Herrwerth A, Leucht S, et al. Opioid antagonists for alcohol dependence. Cochrane Database Syst Rev 2010;(12):CD001867.

16. Knudsen HK, Abraham AJ, Roman PM. Adoption and implementation of medications in addiction treatment programs. J Addict Med 2011;5(1):21–7.

17. Mark TL, Kranzler HR, Poole VH, et al. Alcohol and opioid dependence medications: prescription trends, overall and by physician specialty. Drug Alcohol Depend 2009;99(1–3):345–9.

18. Centers for Disease Control and Prevention. State-specific prevalence of current cigarette smoking and smokeless tobacco use among adults aged ≥18 years—United States 2011–2013. MMWR Morb Mortal Wkly Rep 2015;64(19):532–6.

19. Centers for Disease Control and Prevention. Tobacco Use among middle and high school students—United States, 2011–2014. MMWR Morb Mortal Wkly Rep 2015;64(14):381–5.

20. Centers for Disease Control and Prevention. Vital signs: disparities in non-smokers' exposure to secondhand smoke—United States, 1999–2012. MMWR Morb Mortal Wkly Rep 2015;64(4):103–8.

21. US Department of Health and Human Services. The health consequences of involuntary exposure to tobacco smoke: a report of the Surgeon General. Atlanta (GA): US Department of Health and Human Services, Centers for Disease Control and Prevention, National Center for Chronic Disease Prevention and Health Promotion, Office on Smoking and Health; 2006.

22. Stead LF, Perera R, Bullen C, et al. Nicotine replacement therapy for smoking cessation. Cochrane Database Syst Rev 2012;(11):CD000146.

23. Cahill K, Stevens S, Perera R, et al. Pharmacological interventions for smoking cessation: an overview and network meta-analysis. Cochrane Database Syst Rev 2013;(5):CD009329.

24. Tonstad S, Tønnesen P, Hajek P, et al. Effect of maintenance therapy with varenicline on smoking cessation: a randomized controlled trial. JAMA 2006;296(1):64.

25. Koegelenberg CF, Noor F, Bateman ED, et al. Efficacy of varenicline combined with nicotine replacement therapy vs varenicline alone for smoking cessation: a randomized clinical trial. JAMA 2014;312(2):155–61.

26. Ebbert JO, Hughes JR, West RJ, et al. Effect of varenicline on smoking cessation through smoking reduction: a randomized clinical trial. JAMA 2015;313(7):687.

27. Thomas KH, Martin RM, Knipe DW, et al. Risk of neuropsychiatric adverse events associated with varenicline: systematic review and meta-analysis. BMJ 2015;350: h1109.

28. Rigotti NA, Pipe AL, Benowitz NL, et al. Efficacy and safety of varenicline for smoking cessation in patients with cardiovascular disease: a randomized trial. Circulation 2010;121(2):221.

29. Available at: https://www.chantix.com/how-to-get#chantix-cost. Accessed February 9, 2016.

30. Hughes JR, Stead LF, Hartmann-Boyce J, et al. Antidepressants for smoking cessation. Cochrane Database Syst Rev 2014;(1):CD000031.

31. Moore TJ, Furberg CD, Glenmullen J, et al. Suicidal behavior and depression in smoking cessation treatments. PLoS One 2011;6(11):e27016.

32. Parsons AC, Shraim M, Inglis J, et al. Interventions for preventing weight gain after smoking cessation. Cochrane Database Syst Rev 2009;(1):CD006219.

33. Chan B, Einarson A, Koren G. Effectiveness of bupropion for smoking cessation during pregnancy. J Addict Dis 2005;24(2):19.

34. Centers for Disease Control and Prevention, National Center for Chronic Disease Prevention and Health Promotion, Division of Population Health. BRFSS prevalence & trends data [online]. 2015. Available at: http://www.cdc.gov/brfss/brfssprevalence/. Accessed November 27, 2015.

35. Saitz R. Unhealthy alcohol use. N Engl J Med 2005;352:596–607.

36. National Institute on Alcohol Abuse and Alcoholism. Alcohol use disorder. Available at: http://www.niaaa.nih.gov/alcohol-health/overview-alcohol-consumption/alcohol-use-disorders. Accessed November 27, 2015.

37. Daeppen JB, Gache P, Landry U, et al. Symptom-triggered vs fixed-schedule doses of benzodiazepine for alcohol withdrawal: a randomized treatment trial. Arch Intern Med 2002;162(10):1117.

38. Jonas DE, Amick HR, Feltner C, et al. Pharmacotherapy for adults with alcohol use disorders in outpatient settings: a systematic review and meta-analysis. JAMA 2014;311(18):1889–900.

39. Laaksonen E, Koski-Jännes A, Salaspuro M, et al. A randomized, multicentre, open-label, comparative trial of disulfiram, naltrexone and acamprosate in the treatment of alcohol dependence. Alcohol Alcohol 2008;43(1):53–61.

40. Johnson BA, Ait-Daoud N, Bowden CL, et al. Oral topiramate for treatment of alcohol dependence: a randomised controlled trial. Lancet 2003;361(9370):1677.

41. Johnson BA, Rosenthal N, Capece JA, et al. Topiramate for treating alcohol dependence: a randomized controlled trial. JAMA 2007;298(14):1641.

42. Mason BJ, Quello S, Goodell V, et al. Gabapentin treatment for alcohol dependence: a randomized clinical trial. JAMA Intern Med 2014;174(1):70–7.

43. Addolorato G, Leggio L, Ferrulli A, et al. Effectiveness and safety of baclofen for maintenance of alcohol abstinence in alcohol-dependent patients with liver cirrhosis: randomised, double-blind controlled study. Lancet 2007;370(9603): 1915.

44. Garbutt JC, Kampov-Polevoy AB, Gallop R, et al. Efficacy and safety of baclofen for alcohol dependence: a randomized, double-blind, placebo-controlled trial. Alcohol Clin Exp Res 2010;34(11):1849–57.

45. Torrens M, Fonseca F, Mateu G, et al. Efficacy of antidepressants in substance use disorders with and without comorbid depression. A systematic review and meta-analysis. Drug Alcohol Depend 2005;78(1):1.

46. Kiefer F, Jahn H, Tarnaske T, et al. Comparing and combining naltrexone and acamprosate in relapse prevention of alcoholism: a double-blind, placebo-controlled study. Arch Gen Psychiatry 2003;60(1):92.

47. Anton RF, O'Malley SS, Ciraulo DA, et al. Combined pharmacotherapies and behavioral interventions for alcohol dependence: the COMBINE study: a randomized controlled trial. JAMA 2006;295(17):2003.

48. National Institute on Alcohol Abuse and Alcoholism. The physicians' guide to helping patients with alcohol problems. Washington, DC: Government Printing Office; 1995.

49. Mirand AL, Welte JW. Alcohol consumption among the elderly in a general population, Erie County, New York. Am J Public Health 1996;86:978–84.

50. 2013 National survey on drug use and health: detailed tables. Rockville (MD): Center for Behavioral Health Statistics and Quality; Substance Abuse and Mental Health Administration; 2014. Available at: http://www.samhsa.gov/data/sites/default/files/2013MHDetTabs/NSDUH-MHDetTabs2013.pdf. Accessed November 29, 2015.

51. Jones CM, Logan J, Gladden RM, et al. Vital signs: demographic and substance use trends among heroin users - United States, 2002-2013. MMWR Morb Mortal Wkly Rep 2015;64(26):719–25.

52. Substance Abuse and Mental Health Services Administration, Center for Behavioral Health Statistics and Quality. The TEDS report: 2001-2011 national admissions to substance abuse treatment services. Rockville (MD): 2013. Available at: http://www.samhsa.gov/data/sites/default/files/TEDS2011St_Web/TEDS2011St_Web/TEDS2011St_Web.pdf. Accessed November 29, 2015.

53. Pollini RA, Banta-Green CJ, Cuevas-Mota J, et al. Problematic use of prescription-type opioids prior to heroin use among young heroin injectors. Subst Abuse Rehabil 2011;2(1):173–80.

54. Lankenau SE, Teti M, Silva K, et al. Initiation into prescription opioid misuse amongst young injection drug users. Int J Drug Policy 2012;23(1):37–44.

55. Mattick RP, Breen C, Kimber J, et al. Methadone maintenance therapy versus no opioid replacement therapy for opioid dependence. Cochrane Database Syst Rev 2009;(3):CD002209.

56. Mattick RP, Breen C, Kimber J, et al. Buprenorphine maintenance versus placebo or methadone maintenance for opioid dependence. Cochrane Database Syst Rev 2014;(2):CD002207.

57. Office of Diversion Control. Buprenorphine. Springfield, VA: Drug Enforcement Administration; 2013. Available at: http://www.deadiversion.usdoj.gov/drug_chem_info/buprenorphine.pdf. Accessed November 30, 2015.

58. Minozzi S, Amato L, Vecchi S, et al. Oral naltrexone maintenance treatment for opioid dependence. Cochrane Database Syst Rev 2011;(4):CD001333.

59. Krupitsky E, Nunes EV, Ling W, et al. Injectable extended-release naltrexone for opioid dependence: a double-blind, placebo-controlled, multicentre randomised trial. Lancet 2011;377(9776):1506.

60. O'Connor PG. Methods of detoxification and their role in treating patients with opioid dependence. JAMA 2005;294(8):961–3.

61. Burns L, Mattick RP, Lim K, et al. Methadone in pregnancy: treatment retention and neonatal outcomes. Addiction 2007;102(2):264.

62. Johnson RE, Jones HE, Fisher G. Use of buprenorphine in pregnancy: patient management and effects on the neonate. Drug Alcohol Depend 2003;70: S87–101.

63. Jones HE, Kaltenbach K, Heil SH, et al. Neonatal abstinence syndrome after methadone or buprenorphine exposure. N Engl J Med 2010;363:2320–31.

64. American Academy of Pediatrics Committee on Drugs. The transfer of drugs and other chemicals into human milk. Pediatrics 2001;108(3):776–89.

65. Firoz S, Carlson G. Characteristics and treatment outcome of older methadone-maintenance patients. Am J Geriatr Psychiatry 2004;12(5):539–41.

New Approaches to Antibiotic Use and Review of Recently Approved Antimicrobial Agents

 CrossMark

Andrew W. Hahn, MD[a],*, Rupali Jain, PharmD[b],
David H. Spach, MD[a]

KEYWORDS

- Antimicrobial resistance • Soft tissue abscess • Intraabdominal abscess
- Dalbavancin • Oritavancin • Ceftaroline fosamil • Ceftolozane-tazobactam
- Ceftazidime-avibactam

KEY POINTS

- The White House National Action Plan for Combating Antibiotic Resistant Bacteria outlines a multidisciplinary approach to address the urgent and serious drug-resistant bacterial threats in the United States.
- New evidence supports a lesser role with shorter-course antimicrobial therapy in the setting of adequate source control for the management of both soft tissue abscesses and complicated intraabdominal abscesses.
- The novel approach of displaying poster-sized letters of commitment to guideline-concordant antibiotic usage seems to increase clinicians' concordance with evidence-based prescribing guidelines related to antibiotic usage.
- In recent years, 5 new antimicrobials have been approved by the US Food and Drug Administration that have the potential to be used for drug-resistant bacteria: dalbavancin, oritavancin, ceftaroline, ceftolozane-tazobactam, and ceftazidime-avibactam.
- Although each of these agents has appealing properties for off-label use, the authors encourage caution because high-quality clinical data for these off-label practices are limited.

Disclosure Statement: The authors have nothing to disclose.
[a] Division of Infectious Diseases, University of Washington School of Medicine, 1959 Northeast Pacific Street, Seattle, WA 98195, USA; [b] University of Washington School of Pharmacy, 1959 Northeast Pacific Street, Seattle, WA 98195, USA
* Corresponding author. 1959 Northeast Pacific Street, Box 356423, Seattle, WA 98195-6423.
E-mail address: ahahn47@uw.edu

Med Clin N Am 100 (2016) 911–926
http://dx.doi.org/10.1016/j.mcna.2016.03.012
0025-7125/16/$ – see front matter © 2016 Elsevier Inc. All rights reserved.

medical.theclinics.com

INTRODUCTION

According to the U S Centers for Disease Control and Prevention, approximately 2 million people become infected with a pathogen that is resistant to antimicrobials each year, contributing to at least 23,000 deaths annually.[1] The Infectious Diseases Society of America (IDSA), with support from the federal government, has proposed legislative, regulatory, and funding incentives to address this crisis.[2]

Strategies to address this crisis have included efforts to reduce unnecessary antimicrobial use as well as to support development of new antibiotics targeting drug-resistant pathogens. To this end, recent research has revealed several areas in which fewer and shorter courses of antimicrobials may be appropriate. In addition, as evidence and clinical practice guidelines continue to evolve and embrace judicious prescribing practices, educational efforts, and systems to help implement practice in concordance with newer guidelines have become increasingly important. This article reviews a new federal action plan to combat antibiotic-resistant bacteria, new data related to shorter-course antimicrobial therapy for skin and soft tissue abscesses as well as intraabdominal infections, and 5 antibiotics recently approved by the US Food and Drug Administration (FDA) that expand options for the management of infections caused by drug-resistant bacteria.

WHITE HOUSE STEWARDSHIP INITIATIVE

In the past decade, the emergence of antimicrobial drug resistance has partially reversed the antibiotic advancements that have occurred during the last 80 years. In 2015, the US White House unveiled the National Action Plan for Combating Antibiotic-Resistant Bacteria, a document that provides a roadmap for combating antimicrobial resistance.[3] The goal of this federal document is to guide action by public health, health care, and veterinary partners in the common effort to address the urgent and serious drug-resistant threats that affect people in the United States. This includes efforts to strengthen national surveillance of resistant bacteria, advance development of innovative diagnostic tests for resistant bacteria, and accelerate research and development for new antibiotics. Specifically, the national plan recommends implementing health care policies and antibiotic stewardship programs that will improve patient outcomes and minimize development of resistance by ensuring each patient receives the appropriate antibiotic at the right time, at the correct dose, and for the appropriate duration.

THE DIMINISHED ROLE OF ANTIBIOTICS IN SKIN AND SOFT TISSUE ABSCESSES

The decision whether or not to treat skin and soft tissue abscesses with adjunctive antibiotics is important and has undergone inquiry for decades.[4] The nomenclature has changed during the past several decades with most earlier studies mixing in subjects with abscesses of various sizes and complexity. Subsequent studies contrasted the term simple cutaneous abscess to complicated skin and soft tissue infection, the later referring to larger, more complex abscesses. In 2013, the FDA encouraged use of the nomenclature acute bacterial skin and skin structure infection (ABSSSI) for infections with greater lesion size, presence of leukocytosis, fever, and systemic inflammatory response syndrome. They further differentiated between minor cutaneous abscess (smaller than approximately 75 cm^2) and major cutaneous abscess (greater than approximately 75 cm^2).[5]

Recent randomized controlled trials (RCTs) and observational studies have had fairly wide disagreement as to the importance of antibiotic therapy in preventing treatment failure following source control with incision and drainage.[6,7] Several recent meta-analyses have reviewed the available literature and failed to show a statistically significant reduction in treatment failure when adjunctive antibiotics are used.[8,9] Importantly, these meta-analyses grouped major and minor cutaneous abscesses (ie, all sizes) because that nomenclature was not in common use before 2013. The interpretation of more recent studies is further complicated by the transition from a before to after period of methicillin-resistant *Staphylococcus aureus* (MRSA). Critique of these studies centered on low numbers of subjects and inability to demonstrate smaller differences, as well as the possibility of different outcomes for MRSA infections. Several earlier RCTs had a significant percentage of MRSA isolates but treatment arms consisted of agents not active against MRSA.[7]

More recently, 2 large RCTs have demonstrated the lack of efficacy of systemic antibiotics following incision and drainage of a simple abscess.[6,10] These study protocols specifically included appropriate treatment of MRSA in the study design. One very recent meta-analysis attempted to clarify differences in MRSA-era and MRSA-only studies. This meta-analysis excluded MRSA-containing studies that used non-MRSA antibiotics and found no significant reduction in treatment failure when adjunctive antibiotics were used.

Very recently, a large multicenter, double-blind, randomized control trial named "Strategies Using Off-Patent Antibiotics for Methicillin Resistant *S Aureus* (STOP MRSA)" found trimethoprim-sulfamethoxazole treatment improved clinical cure rates of drained, uncomplicated abscesses in emergency department patients older than 12 years.[11] This study used trimethoprim-sulfamethoxazole versus placebo in a total of 1265 patients who underwent drainage of a cutaneous abscess. Notably, 45.3% of the participants had wound cultures that were positive for MRSA. Clinical failure was defined as occurrence of any of the following: "fever attributable to the infection), an increase in the maximal dimension of erythema by >25% from baseline, or worsening of wound swelling and tenderness by the visit during the treatment period (day 3 or 4); fever, no decrease in the maximal dimension of erythema from baseline, or no decrease in swelling or tenderness by the visit at the end of the treatment period (day 8–10); and fever or more than minimal erythema, swelling, or tenderness by the test-of-cure visit (day 14–21)."[11] In the modified intention-to-treat population, clinical cure occurred in 507 of 630 participants (80.5%) in the trimethoprim–sulfamethoxazole group versus 454 of 617 participants (73.6%) in the placebo group revealing an effect size of 6.9% (95% confidence interval [CI], 2.1–11.7; P = .005). In addition, trimethoprim–sulfamethoxazole treatment yielded better results for secondary outcomes, including significantly lower rates of subsequent surgical drainage procedures (3.4% vs 8.6%), skin infections at new sites (3.1% vs 10.3%), and infections in household members (1.7% vs 4.1%). There was no significant difference in invasive infections between the two groups. Trimethoprim–sulfamethoxazole was associated with slightly more gastrointestinal side effects (mostly mild) than placebo. The trial's authors attempted to reconcile their findings with the results of prior negative studies by pointing out that other recent trials were not sufficiently powered to detect a smaller effect size. Other authors have indeed pointed out that prior trials were underpowered to detect an effect size of 5 to 10 percent.[12] Overall, this trial provides strong evidence that adjunctive trimethoprim–sulfamethoxazole does provide a small increase in cure rates for drained, uncomplicated abscesses.

Notably, on the basis of these studies (though before the STOP MRSA trial results), the 2014 Infectious Diseases Society of America (IDSA) guidelines concluded "the addition of systemic antibiotics to incision and drainage of cutaneous abscesses does not improve cure rates, even in those due to MRSA, but did have a modest effect on the time to recurrence of other abscesses."[13] The guidelines thus suggest use of MRSA-active antibiotics as an "adjunct to incision and drainage should be made based on the presence or absence of systemic inflammatory response syndrome (SIRS)." There are less-common scenarios where the IDSA guidelines suggest using antibiotics following incision and drainage: severe or extensive disease (eg, multiple sites of infection), rapid disease progression and associated cellulitis, systemic illness, immunosuppression, extremes of age, and difficult to drain locations (eg, face, hands, or genitalia).[8] The emergency medicine practice guidelines do not address the simple cutaneous abscess (which could be treated on an outpatient basis), but confirm the IDSA guidelines' emphasis on antibiotic treatment for complex cases in addition to surgical incision and drainage, possible admission, and comorbidity management for patients with ABSSSI.[14]

Applicability of these studies to the ambulatory setting is somewhat unclear as many abscesses included in the trials were surgically incised (or addressed in the emergency department) where extensive incisions are more frequently performed than in ambulatory clinic settings. The authors of the STOP MRSA study noted that their enrolled patients "had typical skin abscesses, which were generally small (most only 2 to 3 cm). Most participants, however, had a total lesion size, including associated erythema, of more than 5 cm, and many met other guideline criteria for antibiotic treatment."[11] Thus, although evidence for or against the use of adjunctive antibiotics in simple cutaneous abscesses remains controversial, available studies and practice guidelines all support the notions that (1) definitive incision and drainage is the most important element of therapy for patients with simple or complex cutaneous abscesses and (2) more complex abscesses or high-risk patients will likely benefit from adjunctive antibiotics.

SHORT-COURSE THERAPY FOR COMPLICATED INTRAABDOMINAL INFECTION

Another recent example of a shift towards a supporting role for antimicrobials comes from the general surgery literature on complicated intraabdominal infection (cIAI). For several years the IDSA and Surgical Infection Society's guidelines, "Diagnosis and Management of Complicated Intraabdominal Infection in Adults and Children," has recommended relatively shorter courses of antimicrobials assuming that a reasonable degree of source control can be obtained.[15] Specifically, the 2010 guidelines state the antimicrobials "should be limited to 4 to 7 days, unless it is difficult to achieve adequate source control."[14]

A recent study pushed this trend farther by comparing standard duration to a shorter course in patients with cIAI. Sawyer and colleagues[16] randomly assigned 518 subjects with cIAI and adequate source control to receive antibiotics until 2 days after the resolution of fever, leukocytosis, and ileus (maximum of 10 days); or to receive a fixed course of antibiotics for 4 plus or minus 1 days. They found that their composite endpoint of surgical-site infection, recurrent intraabdominal infection, or death occurred in 21.8% of subjects in the experimental, short-course group versus 22.5% of subjects in the control group. This study clearly supports recent guidelines for shorter-course antibiotic therapy for cIAI with adequate source control.

GUIDELINE-CONCORDANT ANTIBIOTIC PRESCRIBING

The issue of excessive antibiotic use has been pervasive in clinical care for many years. With the advent and increasing use of evidence-based clinical practice guidelines, it has become more feasible to track and address the discordance between guideline recommendations and clinical practice patterns. One group recently performed an RCT that examined modifying antimicrobial-prescribing behavior through use of environmental influences.[17] The study was conducted at 5 outpatient primary care clinics and included 954 subject visits. The investigators randomized clinicians into 2 groups, balanced with respect to prior antibiotic prescribing patterns based on retrospective chart review. Subsequently, baseline data were collected for both groups comparing antibiotic prescriptions with the International Classification of Diseases (ICD)-9 billing codes for 9 months (May through January). Starting in February (peak cold and flu season in the study area), the study group placed poster-sized letters of commitment to consistent use of guidelines for appropriate antibiotic prescribing with a signed photograph of the clinician in each examination room and the control group continued standard practice. The poster emphasized to the patient the importance of the clinician in determining whether or not antibiotics were appropriate for a given illness. The investigators reported that, during the 3-month implementation period, the simple intervention nudged the providers towards better adherence to guideline-based antibiotic prescription use. Clinicians in the intervention group shifted their average rate of inappropriate antibiotic use from 43.5% to 33.7% during the implementation period, whereas those randomized to the control group shifted from 43.8% inappropriate use to 52.7%. The increase in the control group's inappropriate antibiotic prescribing was attributed by the investigators to the onset of peak respiratory infection season. Overall, the study found a 19.7% absolute reduction in inappropriate antibiotic prescribing with the simple intervention.

This study is a significant advancement because it is the first to apply the concept of commitment and consistency without implementation of an intensive educational intervention in the area of clinician prescribing behavior. The principle of commitment and consistency is that the individuals will change behavior based on a "desire to remain consistent with a prior public commitment."[17] Earlier efforts to curb inappropriate prescribing have focused on models of audit with feedback and pay for performance.[18] Prior studies have suggested that these later models had a tendency to shift providers' coding practice without showing sustained effect on the desired outcome.[19] This new trial suggests an approach that has minimal implementation cost, minimal time investment by providers, and yet may have substantial impact in nudging prescribing practices in line with evidence-based guidelines.

NOVEL ANTIMICROBIALS

Although new approaches to antimicrobial therapy have been used in recent years, the problem of infections with drug-resistant organisms remains pervasive and challenging. In recent years, 5 new antimicrobials have been FDA-approved that have the potential to be used for drug-resistant bacteria: dalbavancin, oritavancin, ceftaroline, ceftolozane-tazobactam, and ceftazidime-avibactam (**Table 1**). In hopes of familiarizing the reader with these agents, this article describes each new antimicrobial in terms of mechanism and spectrum, then explores the data behind their indications and their potential role in the expanding antimicrobial armamentarium.

DALBAVANCIN AND ORITAVANCIN

Dalbavancin and oritavancin are semisynthetic lipoglycopeptide antimicrobials with broad gram-positive activity. They share the FDA-indication (both approved in 2014) for ABSSSI caused by susceptible isolates of *Staphylococcus aureus*

Table 1
Key points for 5 new antimicrobial agents

Drug, Dose	FDA-Approved Indications	Average Wholesale Price Per Day	Precautions
Ceftaroline, 600 mg IV q12	ABSSSI, community-acquired pneumonia	$333.25	No major adverse events No pseudomonas or anaerobic activity
Ceftazidime-avibactam, 2.5 g IV q8h	cIAI, cUTI when no other option available	$684	Dose adjustment required for renal dysfunction
Ceftolozane-tazobactam, 1.5 g IV q8h	cIAI, cUTI	$298	Dose adjustment required for renal dysfunction
Dalbavancin, 1500 mg IV once Or 1000 mg IV, 500 mg IV 1 wk later	ABSSSI	$383 (averaged from $5364 per 14-d course)	Red man syndrome Unable to remove exposure in the event of adverse reaction
Oritavancin, 1200 mg IV once	ABSSSI	$244 (averaged from $3420 per 14-d course)	Avoid in likely osteomyelitis Artificial elevation of activated partial thromboplastin time Unable to remove exposure in the event of adverse reaction

Abbreviations: IV, intravenous; q, every.

(both methicillin-susceptible [MSSA] and MRSA), *Streptococcus pyogenes, Streptococcus agalactiae, Streptococcus anginosus* group, and vancomycin-susceptible *Enterococcus faecalis.*[20,21]

These newer agents share several features with the glycopeptide vancomycin. Similar to vancomycin, these drugs bind to the terminal D-Ala-D-Ala peptidoglycan chain and thereby inhibit polymerization and cross-linkage in bacterial cell wall synthesis.[22] The primary added value in these agents lies in their prolonged half-life, enabling dalbavancin dosing using either a once weekly, 2-dose regimen or a high-dose single-dose option and oritavancin as a single-dose regimen.

Clinical Efficacy

Two randomized, double-blind, noninferiority trials (DISCOVER 1 and 2) assessed the safety and efficacy of dalbavancin for the treatment of subjects with ABSSI and at least 1 systemic sign of illness.[23] These studies used the same enrollment criteria and treatment protocol; a total of 659 (DISCOVER 1) and 653 (DISCOVER 2) subjects were randomized to receive treatment with either a 2-dose regimen of dalbavancin (1000 mg intravenous [IV] initially followed by 500 mg IV 1 week later) or vancomycin (15 mg/kg IV every 12 hours) for 2 weeks. Physicians blinded to the regimen could switch to oral medications—oral placebo in the dalbavancin arm and oral linezolid 600 mg orally every 12 hours in the vancomycin arm. The primary endpoint (no increase in infection area and no temperature>37.6 C) was achieved in 79.7%

of subjects in the dalbavancin arm and in 79.8% of those in the vancomycin arm. Serious adverse events were reported in 2.6% of the dalbavancin group and in 4.0% of the vancomycin group.

In an open-label, RCT of 75 subjects with catheter-related bloodstream infection, investigators compared 2 doses of dalbavancin (given 1 week apart) with a 14-day course of vancomycin.[24] A clinical or microbiologic response was observed in 87% of subjects receiving dalbavancin compared with only 50% in those treated with vancomycin. Unfortunately, the marked difference in the rate of catheter removal (93.3% in dalbavancin subjects and only 55.6% in vancomycin subjects) confounded the analysis.

In a recently completed study, 698 subjects with ABSSSI were randomized to receive either a single dose of dalbavancin (1500 mg IV) or the standard 2-dose dalbavancin regimen (1000 mg IV on day 1 followed 1 week later by 500 mg IV).[25] The primary endpoint was a greater than or equal to 20% reduction in the area of erythema at 48 to 72 hours. This endpoint was met in 81.4% of subjects treated with single-dose dalbavancin and in 84.2% of subjects treated with a standard dose. Although the study was limited by an unequal proportion of MRSA isolates (considerably more in the 2-dose arm), it was able to establish noninferiority of the single dose regimen, leading to the recent approval of a 1500 mg single-dose option.

Oritavancin was evaluated in the SOLO I and SOLO II trials, which compared a single dose of oritavancin to 7 to 10 days of vancomycin for the treatment of subjects with cellulitis (40%), wound infection (29%), or major cutaneous abscess (31%), in a total of 954 (SOLO I) and 1005 (SOLO II) subjects.[26,27] Subjects received either a single 1200-mg intravenous dose of oritavancin followed by intravenous placebo (every 12 hours) or intravenous vancomycin (1 g or 15 mg/kg, every 12 hours). Both groups received therapy (or placebo infusions) for 7 to 10 days. Aztreonam and metronidazole were permitted for gram-negative and anaerobic coverage, respectively, when deemed appropriate by the clinician. The SOLO I and II trials showed no differences in the primary clinical response endpoint (no increase in lesion size, no fever, and no initiation of rescue antimicrobials) between the 2 treatment groups.

The encouraging results of the SOLO I and II trials led the approval of oritavancin for the treatment of ABSSSI caused by susceptible bacteria, including *Staphylococcus aureus* (methicillin-susceptible and methicillin-resistant strains), various *Streptococcus* species, and vancomycin-susceptible strains of *E faecalis*.

Both dalbavancin and oritavancin have been reported to cause anaphylaxis and serious skin reactions, though insufficient data exist to establish incidence relative to other antimicrobials. In a patient experiencing an adverse reaction to 1 of these agents, the very long half-life of these agents could be problematic. There are no data available regarding the cross-sensitivity of these agents with vancomycin.[28] Both drugs are reported to cause infusion-related rash, pruritus, and flush consistent with the red man syndrome, as seen with vancomycin. Slower infusion reduces the risk and intensity of these reactions.

Oritavancin is known to artificially elevate activated partial thromboplastin time levels; therefore, unfractionated heparin is contraindicated for 48 hours after administering oritavancin.[27] In phase 3 ABSSSI clinical trials, more cases of osteomyelitis were reported in the oritavancin-treated arm than in the vancomycin-treated arm.[20] Because the study enrolled only subjects with ABSSSI, it is unclear whether there were simply more unrecognized cases of osteomyelitis in the oritavancin-treated arm or if osteomyelitis emerged on therapy as a result of treatment failure. The oritavancin package insert recommends selecting an alternative regimen if osteomyelitis is considered likely.[20]

Currently, neither dalbavancin nor oritavancin have clinically available methods for determining minimum inhibitory concentration (MIC) values. Based on available study data, dalbavancin and oritavancin MICs correlate well with vancomycin susceptibility.[29,30] Thus, until new antimicrobial susceptibility tests become approved, it is reasonable to infer susceptibility from vancomycin MIC cut-offs.

Place in Therapy

At present, the authors recommend that the lipoglycopeptides be reserved for their FDA indication of ABSSSI in adult patients. Because of the similar efficacy of established therapy, relative lack of experience, and high drug cost, these agents are best reserved for special circumstances wherein adherence, IV access, and drug allergy make other regimens challenging or problematic. Avoiding the use of an indwelling catheter in hospitalized patients could have several potential advantages, including reducing the risk of catheter-related infections, decreasing hospital stay, and reducing complications that can potentially arise with placement of longer-term catheters.

Off-label use of these agents in the treatment of catheter-related blood-stream infections should be avoided (or used with caution) until more clinical data are available. Because there is little experience with prolonged half-life drugs for antimicrobial therapy, the impact on resistance or repeated courses is yet to be elucidated.

CEFTAROLINE

Ceftaroline is unique as the only FDA-approved cephalosporin with activity against MRSA. In addition, ceftaroline demonstrates excellent broad-spectrum activity against a wide range of gram-positive and gram-negative pathogens. Ceftaroline has received FDA approval for the treatment of ABSSSI and community-acquired bacterial pneumonia.[31] It is bactericidal by way of binding and inhibiting penicillin-binding proteins (PBPs), including a high affinity for PBP-2a (the altered PBP protein that confers beta-lactam resistance in MRSA).[32] In vitro susceptibility studies have demonstrated ceftaroline's activity against a broad range of gram-positive organisms, including MRSA, MSSA, vancomycin-resistant *Staphylococcus aureus*, daptomycin and linezolid nonsusceptible *Staphylococcus aureus*, *Streptococcus pyogenes*, *Streptococcus agalactiae*, and *Streptococcus pneumoniae*. In addition, ceftaroline has efficacy against many gram-negative pathogens, including *Escherichia coli*, *Klebsiella pneumoniae*, *K oxytoca*, and *Haemophilus influenzae*.[16] Ceftaroline does not have good activity against *Pseudomonas* species, nor is it thought to adequately cover predominantly anaerobic pathogens.

Clinical Efficacy

The safety and efficacy of ceftaroline in subjects with ABSSSI was evaluated in the CANVAS 1 and 2 trials.[33–35] These, noninferiority RCTs enrolled 1394 subjects in total and compared ceftaroline 600 mg IV every 12 hours versus the combination of vancomycin 1 g IV every 12 hours plus aztreonam 1 g IV every 12 hours; therapy in both arms was administered for 5 to 14 days. The most common pathogen isolated was *Staphylococcus aureus* (with MRSA representing about 35% of the staphylococcal isolates in both trials).[34] The primary endpoint was defined as resolution of all signs and symptoms of the infection. The study met the definition for noninferiority with clinical response seen in 74.0% of ceftaroline subjects versus 66.2% of subjects treated with vancomycin and aztreonam. No major safety concerns were noted with ceftaroline and adverse events rates (most commonly nausea and headache) were similar in both treatment groups.

Investigators subsequently evaluated ceftaroline for the treatment of subjects with community-acquired pneumonia (CAP) in the FOCUS 1 and FOCUS 2 trials.[36,37] A total of 1240 subjects were randomized to receive ceftaroline 600 mg IV every 12 hours or ceftriaxone 1 g IV every 24 hours.[38] In FOCUS 1, subjects in both arms also received adjunctive therapy with 2 doses of clarithromycin given on day 1, whereas in FOCUS 2 they did not. Given this irregularity in design, the investigators performed a subset analysis confirming that clarithromycin was unlikely to have an effect outside of subjects with atypical pathogens (total of 129 subjects in both trials). Both trials were limited to nonintensive care unit pneumonia subjects, all of whom had a Pneumonia Outcome Research Team (PORT) risk class of III or IV. The primary outcome (resolution of all CAP-related signs and symptoms) was met in 86.6% of clinically evaluable cases in the ceftaroline arm compared with 78.2% in the with ceftriaxone arm. FOCUS 2 had similar findings supportive of noninferiority.

Place in Therapy

Ceftaroline fosamil is a well-tolerated beta-lactam with a very broad spectrum of activity. It is a reasonable alternative for ABSSSI and CAP caused by pathogens that include suspected or proven MRSA. Although this drug is an attractive option for MRSA and many gram-negative pathogens, it is ineffective against *Pseudomonas* species and anaerobes, which precludes use as single-agent empiric therapy for ventilator-associated pneumonia or suspected aspiration pneumonia.

CEFTOLOZANE-TAZOBACTAM

Ceftolozane-tazobactam received FDA approval in December 2014 for the treatment of cIAI (used in combination with metronidazole) and complicated urinary tract infection (cUTI), including pyelonephritis.[39] Ceftolozane is a novel, broad-spectrum cephalosporin with activity against *Pseudomonas* and *Enterobacteriaceae* species, including *E coli* and *Klebsiella* species. The coformulation with the beta-lactamase inhibitor tazobactam extends the spectrum of activity against the *Enterobacteriaceae* group that harbor extended spectrum beta-lactamases (ESBLs) and some AmpC beta-lactamases; however, it is not active against *Enterobacteriaceae* species that produce carbapenemases.[40]

In a multicenter, surveillance study that included multidrug-resistant (defined as nonsusceptible to $\geq$ 1 agent in $\geq$ 3 antimicrobial classes) *Pseudomonas* and *Enterobacteriaceae* isolates, ceftolozane-tazobactam remained active in 79% and 44% of the isolates, respectively.[41] Among gram-positive organisms, ceftolozane-tazobactam is active against *Streptococcus* species, but has limited activity against *Staphylococcus* species and minimal activity against *Enterococcus* species.[40] Ceftolozane-tazobactam has limited activity against gram-negative anaerobes and does not adequately cover *Bacteroides fragilis*, the most commonly encountered anaerobe in intra-abdominal infections. When specific anaerobic coverage is required, an additional agent is recommended.

Clinical Efficacy

The clinical efficacy of ceftolozane-tazobactam was evaluated in 2 phase III trials involving subjects with cIAI and cUTI. The ASPECT-cIAI was a double-blind, noninferiority RCT that compared ceftolozane-tazobactam (1.5 g IV every 8 hours) plus metronidazole (500 mg IV every 8 hours) versus meropenem (1g IV every 8 hours) for the treatment of hospitalized subjects with cIAIs.[42] The primary efficacy endpoint was eradication of isolated pathogen at the test-of-cure (TOC) visit (day 24–32 of therapy). In total, 806 subjects qualified for the microbiological intent-to-treat (MITT) analysis and approximately 50% of the subjects in each group received therapy for up to 7 days. Overall, the ceftolozane-tazobactam was noninferior to meropenem (83% vs 87.3%, respectively) in the MITT population. Among subjects with ESBL-producing *Enterobacteriaceae*, the clinical cure rate was 95.8% (23/24) in the ceftolozane-tazobactam plus metronidazole group and 88.5% (23/26) in the meropenem group. The incidence of any adverse effects and the rate of discontinuation were similar in the 2 arms.

The ASPECT-cUTI was a randomized, double-blind, double-dummy, noninferiority trial evaluating ceftolozane-tazobactam versus levofloxacin for cUTI or pyelonephritis in 1968 hospitalized subjects.[43] The primary efficacy endpoint was defined as complete resolution or marked improvement of clinical symptoms and microbiological eradication at the test of cure visit (7 days after last dose) in the microbiological modified MITT (mMITT) population, which included subjects who received medication and had at least 1 pathogen in the urine. The mMITT population consisted of 800 subjects with cUTI, including 82% with pyelonephritis. In the mMITT population, the clinical cure rate was 76.9% with ceftolozane-tazobactam and 68.4% with levofloxacin. The statistically significant lower response rate in the levofloxacin group was attributed to the 26.5% of the pathogens that had baseline resistance to levofloxacin. In a subgroup analysis of subjects with ESBL-producing uropathogens, the clinical cure rate was 90.2% in the ceftolozane-tazobactam group and 73.7% in the levofloxacin group. The incidence of adverse events was similar with the ceftolozane-tazobactam and levofloxacin groups; the most common side effect in both groups was headache and gastrointestinal symptoms.

In both phase III trials, cure rates were lower in the ceftolozane-tazobactam subject groups with baseline renal impairment.[41,42] In the cIAI and cUTI trials, the subjects in all treatment arms who had moderate renal insufficiency (creatinine clearance [CrCL] >30 to<50 mL/min) showed a lower response compared with subjects with normal renal function when evaluated by the MITT analysis.[44] This was true for both the ceftolozane-tazobactam arms and the comparator-drug arms (meropenem and levofloxacin, respectively). The difference in outcomes between subjects with moderate renal insufficiency and normal renal function was more marked in the ceftolozane-tazobactam arms of each trials but this was due a higher number of indeterminate outcomes (missing data or protocol deviation) that were considered treatment failure in the MITT analysis. When these indeterminate results were removed in the analysis of microbiologically evaluable subjects, the disproportionate increase in failure rate of subjects with moderate renal insufficiency was no longer apparent.

Place in Therapy

Ceftolozane-tazobactam provides an alternative option for cUTI and intra-abdominal infections when other options are unsuitable, such as when avoidance of carbapenem use for cIAI is required for allergy or other considerations. Caution is advised in patients with renal impairment in which clinical cure rates were found to be lower than in patients with normal renal function. Ceftolozane-tazobactam demonstrates in vitro activity beyond its currently FDA-approved indications, including ESBL-producing *Enterobacteriaceae* and drug-resistant *Pseudomonas*; however, current clinical data are insufficient to support its routine clinical use in patients infected with these organisms. Future studies will clarify the efficacy of ceftolozane-tazobactam in patients with ventilator-associated pneumonia.

CEFTAZIDIME-AVIBACTAM

Ceftazidime-avibactam was approved in February 2015 for the treatment of cIAI (used in combination with metronidazole) and cUTI, including pyelonephritis, in patients with few or no other treatment options.[45] As of February 2016, the clinical phase III data for ceftazidime-avibactam had not yet been published.

Spectrum of Activity

Ceftazidime-avibactam is a combination of cephalosporin and beta-lactamase inhibitor. The beta-lactamase inhibitor, avibactam, improves the spectrum of activity of ceftazidime against resistant *Enterobacteriaceae* (*E coli* and *Klebsiella* species) and *Pseudomonas* species.[46] For example, ceftazidime-avibactam can inhibit a very high percentage and broader range of *Enterobacteriaceae* that harbor ESBLs, including some carbapenemases. Among all *Pseudomonas* isolates, ceftazidime-avibactam was effective against 96.9% of them. In isolates with meropenem resistance or ceftazidime resistance, the susceptibility rates of ceftazidime-avibactam were reduced to 87.3% and 82.1%, respectively.[47] Among multidrug-resistant and extremely drug-resistant *Pseudomonas* isolates, susceptibility rates drop to 81% and 74%, respectively.[48] Ceftazidime-avibactam has minimal activity against *Acinetobacter* species, gram-negative bacteria that harbor metallo-beta-lactamases, anaerobic bacteria, and gram-positive organisms.[29,30]

Clinical Efficacy

Two phase II trials were completed to evaluate the safety and efficacy of ceftazidime-avibactam in cIAI and cUTI.[43] Neither trial was powered to conclude noninferiority to their comparator drugs but both were able to estimate efficacy and safety of ceftazidime-avibactam. Phase III trials have been completed but the results have not yet been published. Information related to the phase III cIAI trial contained in the ceftazidime-avibactam full prescribing information state that ceftazidime-avibactam plus metronidazole had increased mortality compared with meropenem (2.5% vs 1.5%, respectively).[43] Among a subgroup of subjects with baseline CrCl 30 to 50 mL/min, death occurred in 25.8% of subjects who received ceftazidime-avibactam compared with only 8.6% of subjects who received meropenem. Within this subgroup, subjects treated with ceftazidime-avibactam received a 33% lower daily dose than is currently recommended. In subjects with normal renal function or mild renal impairment (baseline CrCl>50 ml/min), death occurred in 1% of subjects who received ceftazidime-avibactam and 1% of subjects who received meropenem. The causes of death varied. Contributing factors included progression of underlying infections, baseline pathogens isolated that were unlikely to respond to the study drug, and delayed surgical intervention.

In a phase II, prospective, double-blind active RCT, subjects with cIAI were randomized to the combination of ceftazidime-avibactam (2.0–0.5 g IV every 8 hours) plus metronidazole (500 mg IV every 8 hours) versus meropenem (1 g every 8 hours) plus placebo infusions.[49] Treatment duration ranged from 5 to 14 days depending on clinical response. The primary efficacy endpoint was clinical response after 2 weeks evaluated at the TOC visit in the microbiologically evaluable population. The microbiologically evaluable population consisted of subjects who had at least 1 pathogen susceptible to ceftazidime-avibactam and meropenem. In the microbiologically evaluable population, favorable clinical response was 91.2% and 93.4% in the ceftazidime-avibactam plus metronidazole and meropenem groups, respectively. Observed adverse effects were 64.4% and 57.8% in the ceftazidime-avibactam plus metronidazole group and meropenem group, respectively. Nausea, vomiting, and abdominal pain were common in the ceftazidime-avibactam plus metronidazole group, whereas there were more cases of elevated liver enzymes in the meropenem group. Significant adverse effects and deaths were similar in the 2 groups.

Ceftazidime-avibactam was compared with imipenem for treatment of cUTI in a phase II, prospective, multicenter, double-blinded comparative study.[50] Subjects were randomized to either ceftazidime-avibactam (0.5 g–0.125 g IV every 8 hours) or imipenem (0.5 g IV every 6 hours). The dose of ceftazidime-avibactam in this trial was lower than the current FDA-approved dose. The primary endpoint was evaluated in the microbiologic evaluable population for favorable microbiological response at the TOC visit, which was 5 to 9 days after completion of antibiotics. The microbiologically evaluable population consisted of subjects with positive urine culture with bacteria susceptible to either antibiotic at enrollment ($\geq 10^5$ colony-forming unit [CFU]/mL or$>10^4$ CFU/mL if bacteremia present). Clinical and microbiological evaluation was done at TOC visit and the subjects received at least 7 days of antibiotics or treatment failures after 48 hours of IV therapy. Overall, 135 subjects received the study medications of which 62 were included in the microbiologically evaluable population. Favorable microbiological response in the microbiologically evaluable population was 70.4% in the ceftazidime-avibactam and 71.4% in the imipenem group. All 63 organisms isolated were susceptible to imipenem but 20 organisms were found to be resistant to ceftazidime alone. Among the subjects with the ceftazidime-resistant uropathogens, favorable microbiological response was achieved in 85.7% and 81.8% subjects in the ceftazidime-avibactam and imipenem groups, respectively. Adverse effects reported were 67.6% and 76.1% in the ceftazidime-avibactam and imipenem-cilastatin groups, respectively.[34] Treatment-emergent serious adverse effects were reported in 8.8% in the ceftazidime-avibactam and 3.0% imipenem-cilastatin groups. For ceftazidime-avibactam, the drug-related significant adverse effects were renal failure, diarrhea, and unintentional overdose.

Place in Therapy

Despite the lack of phase III data, ceftazidime-avibactam is a promising new antimicrobial for resistance gram-negative infections when other antimicrobials are anticipated to be ineffective. Therefore, ceftazidime-avibactam should only be used in consultation with an infectious diseases clinician. The phase III data reporting increased mortality with ceftazidime-avibactam are concerning but details regarding these findings remain unpublished.[43]

SUMMARY

After many years with very few new antimicrobials despite increasing prevalence of multidrug-resistant organisms, it is encouraging to see new efforts to address this problem. The White House initiative gives a roadmap for the many players involved in combating antimicrobial resistance. New research highlights the pivotal importance of drainage in the management of cutaneous abscesses. Treatment of abdominal abscesses has new evidence supporting a shorter course of antimicrobials. The new approach of posting letters of commitment seems to nudge clinicians towards great concordance with evidence-based guidelines.

Several recently approved antimicrobials will expand the options for management of antimicrobial resistance. Dalbavancin and oritavancin have the potential to greatly simplify dosing for several gram-positive infections (especially MRSA). Ceftaroline is an attractive new beta-lactam alternative for treatment of skin and skin structure infections, as well as for pneumonia. The 2 new agents for resistant, gram-negative organisms, ceftolozane-tazobactam and ceftazidime-avibactam, have broad antimicrobial spectra against resistant organisms. Taken together, these new antimicrobials significantly add to the clinician's options for treating infections caused by resistant bacterial pathogens.

REFERENCES

1. CDC. Antibiotic resistance threats in the United States. 2013. Available at: http://www.cdc.gov/drugresistance/threat-report-2013/index.html. Accessed December 13, 2015.
2. Boucher HW, Talbot GH, Benjamin DK Jr, et al. Infectious Diseases Society of America. 10 x '20 Progress–development of new drugs active against gram-negative bacilli: an update from the Infectious Diseases Society of America. Clin Infect Dis 2013;56(12):1685–94.
3. National action pan for combating antimicroial-resistant bacteria. Available at: https://www.whitehouse.gov/sites/default/files/docs/national_action_plan_for_combating_antibotic-resistant_bacteria.pdf. Accessed February 19, 2016.
4. Macfie J, Harvey J. The treatment of acute superficial abscesses: a prospective clinical trial. Br J Surg 1977;64(4):264–6.
5. FDA Guideline ABSSSI 2013. Available at: http://www.fda.gov/downloads/Drugs/.../Guidances/ucm071185.pdf. Accessed February 20, 2016.
6. Singer AJ, Talan DA. Management of skin abscesses in the era of methicillin-resistant Staphylococcus aureus. N Engl J Med 2014;370:1039–47.
7. Duong M, Markwell S, Peter J, et al. Randomized, controlled trial of antibiotics in the management of community-acquired skin abscesses in the pediatric patient. Ann Emerg Med 2010;55:401–7.
8. Fahimi J, Singh A, Frazee BW. The role of adjunctive antibiotics in the treatment of skin and soft tissue abscesses: a systematic review and meta-analysis. CJEM 2015;17(4):420–32.
9. Singer AJ, Thode HC Jr. Systemic antibiotics after incision and drainage of simple abscesses: a meta-analysis. Emerg Med J 2014;31:576–8.
10. Schmitz GR, Bruner D, Pitotti R, et al. Randomized controlled trial of trimethoprim-sulfamethoxazole for uncomplicated skin abscesses in patients at risk for community-associated methicillin-resistant Staphylococcus aureus infection. Ann Emerg Med 2010;56:283–7 [Erratum appears in Ann Emerg Med 2010;56:588].
11. Talan DA, Mower WR, Krishnadasan A, et al. Trimethoprim–Sulfamethoxazole versus Placebo for Uncomplicated Skin Abscess. N Engl J Med 2016;374:823–32.
12. Spellberg B, Boucher H, Bradley J, et al. To treat or not to treat: adjunctive antibiotics for uncomplicated abscesses. Ann Emerg Med 2011;57:183–5.
13. Stevens DL, Bisno AL, Chambers HF, et al. Practice guidelines for the diagnosis and management of skin and soft tissue infections: 2014 update by the Infectious Diseases Society of America. Clin Infect Dis 2014;59(2):e10–52.
14. Pollack CV Jr, Amin A, Ford WT Jr, et al. Acute bacterial skin and skin structure infections (ABSSSI): practice guidelines for management and care transitions in the emergency department and hospital. J Emerg Med 2015;48(4):508–19.

15. Solomkin JS, Mazuski JE, Bradley JS, et al. Diagnosis and management of complicated intra-abdominal infection in adults and children: guidelines by the Surgical Infection Society and the Infectious Diseases Society of America. Surg Infect (Larchmt) 2010;11(1):79–109.

16. Sawyer RG, Claridge JA, Nathens AB, et al. Trial of short-course antimicrobial therapy for intraabdominal infection. N Engl J Med 2015;372(21):1996–2005.

17. Meeker D, Knight TK, Friedberg MW, et al. Nudging guideline-concordant antibiotic prescribing: a randomized clinical trial. JAMA Intern Med 2014;174(3): 425–31.

18. Blumenthal D, Epstein AM. Quality of health care. Part 6: The role of physicians in the future of quality management. N Engl J Med 1996;335(17):1328–31.

19. Roth S, Gonzales R, Harding-Anderer T, et al. Unintended consequences of a quality measure for acute bronchitis. Am J Manag Care 2012;18(6):e217–24.

20. Dalvance [package insert]. Chicago, IL: Durata Therapeutics; 2016. [initial approval: 2014].

21. Orbactiv [package insert]. Parsippany, NJ: The Medicines Company; 2014.

22. Zhanel GG, Calic D, Schweizer F, et al. New lipoglycopeptides: a comparative review of dalbavancin, oritavancin and telavancin [review]. Drugs 2010;70(7): 859–86 [Erratum appears in Drugs 2011;71(5):526].

23. Boucher HW, Wilcox M, Talbot GH, et al. Once-weekly dalbavancin versus daily conventional therapy for skin infection. N Engl J Med 2014;370(23):2169–79.

24. Raad I, Darouiche R, Vazquez J, et al. Efficacy and safety of weekly dalbavancin therapy for catheter-related bloodstream infection caused by gram-positive pathogens. Clin Infect Dis 2005;40(3):374–80.

25. Dunne MW, Puttagunta S, Giordano P, et al. A Randomized Clinical Trial of Single Dose vs. Weekly Dalbavancin for Treatment of Acute Bacterial Skin and Skin Structure Infection. Clin Infect Dis 2015;62(5):545–51.

26. Corey GR, Kabler H, Mehra P, et al. Single-dose oritavancin in the treatment of acute bacterial skin infections. N Engl J Med 2014;370(23):2180–90.

27. Corey GR, Good S, Jiang H, et al. Single-dose oritavancin versus 7-10 days of vancomycin in the treatment of gram-positive acute bacterial skin and skin structure infections: the SOLO II noninferiority study. Clin Infect Dis 2015;60(2):254–62.

28. Roberts KD, Sulaiman RM, Rybak MJ. Dalbavancin and Oritavancin: an innovative approach to the treatment of gram-positive infections. Pharmacotherapy 2015;35(10):935–48 [review].

29. Jones RN, Farrell DJ, Flamm RK, et al. Surrogate analysis of vancomycin to predict susceptible categorization of dalbavancin. Diagn Microbiol Infect Dis 2015; 82(1):73–7.

30. Jones RN, Turnidge JD, Moeck G, et al. Use of in vitro vancomycin testing results to predict susceptibility to oritavancin, a new long-acting lipoglycopeptide. Antimicrob Agents Chemother 2015;59(4):2405–9.

31. Teflaro [package insert]. Parsippany, NJ: Actavis; 2010.

32. Kiang TK, Wilby KJ, Ensom MH. A critical review on the clinical pharmacokinetics, pharmacodynamics, and clinical trials of ceftaroline. Clin Pharmacokinet 2015;54(9):915–31.

33. Corey GR, Wilcox MH, Talbot GH, et al. CANVAS 1: the first Phase III, randomized, double-blind study evaluating ceftaroline fosamil for the treatment of patients with complicated skin and skin structure infections. J Antimicrob Chemother 2010;65(Suppl 4):iv41–51.

34. Wilcox MH, Corey GR, Talbot GH, et al. CANVAS 2: the second Phase III, randomized, double-blind study evaluating ceftaroline fosamil for the treatment

of patients with complicated skin and skin structure infections. J Antimicrob Chemother 2010;65(Suppl 4):iv53–65.

35. Corey GR, Wilcox M, Talbot GH, et al. Integrated analysis of CANVAS 1 and 2: phase 3, multicenter, randomized, double-blind studies to evaluate the safety and efficacy of ceftaroline versus vancomycin plus aztreonam in complicated skin and skin-structure infection. Clin Infect Dis 2010;51(6):641–50.

36. File TM Jr, Low DE, Eckburg PB, et al. FOCUS 1: a randomized, double-blinded, multicentre, Phase III trial of the efficacy and safety of ceftaroline fosamil versus ceftriaxone in community-acquired pneumonia. J Antimicrob Chemother 2011; 66(Suppl 3):iii19–32.

37. Low DE, File TM Jr, Eckburg PB, et al. FOCUS 2: a randomized, double-blinded, multicentre, Phase III trial of the efficacy and safety of ceftaroline fosamil versus ceftriaxone in community-acquired pneumonia. J Antimicrob Chemother 2011; 66(Suppl 3):iii33–44.

38. File TM Jr, Low DE, Eckburg PB, et al. Integrated analysis of FOCUS 1 and FOCUS 2: randomized, doubled-blinded, multicenter phase 3 trials of the efficacy and safety of ceftaroline fosamil versus ceftriaxone in patients with community-acquired pneumonia. Clin Infect Dis 2010;51(12):1395–405 [Erratum appears in Clin Infect Dis 2011;52(7):967].

39. Zerbaxa [package insert]. Syracuse, NY: Merck; 2015.

40. Zhanel GG, Chung P, Adam H, et al. Ceftolozane/tazobactam: a novel cephalosporin/β-lactamase inhibitor combination with activity against multidrug-resistant gram-negative bacilli. Drugs 2014;74(1):31–51.

41. Farrell DJ, Flamm RK, Sader HS, et al. Antimicrobial activity of ceftolozane-tazobactam tested against Enterobacteriaceae and Pseudomonas aeruginosa with various resistance patterns isolated in U.S. Hospitals (2011-2012). Antimicrob Agents Chemother 2013;57(12):6305–10.

42. Solomkin J, Hershberger E, Miller B, et al. Ceftolozane/Tazobactam Plus Metronidazole for Complicated Intra-abdominal Infections in an Era of Multidrug Resistance: results from a randomized, double-blind, phase 3 Trial (ASPECT-cIAI). Clin Infect Dis 2015;60(10):1462–71.

43. Wagenlehner FM, Umeh O, Steenbergen J, et al. Ceftolozane-tazobactam compared with levofloxacin in the treatment of complicated urinary-tract infections, including pyelonephritis: a randomised, double-blind, phase 3 trial (ASPECT-cUTI). Lancet 2015;385(9981):1949–56.

44. Palchak M, Popejoy M, Miller B, et al. Poster 901. Outcomes of Ceftolozane/Tazobactam (C/T) in Patients with Moderate Renal Impairment in Two Phase 3 Trials for the Treatment of Complicated Intra-abdominal Infection (cIAI) and Complicated Urinary Tract Infection (cUTI) ID Week poster 901. Abstract Open Forum Infect Dis 2015;2(Suppl 1):S235. http://www.ofid.oxfordjournals.org/content/2/suppl_1/S263.3.short.

45. Avycaz [package insert] Parsippany, NJ: Actavis; 2015.

46. Zhanel GG, Lawson CD, Adam H, et al. Ceftazidime-avibactam: a novel cephalosporin/β-lactamase inhibitor combination. Drugs 2013;73(2):159–77.

47. Sader HS, Castanheira M, Flamm RK, et al. Antimicrobial activity of ceftazidime-avibactam against Gram-negative organisms collected from U.S. medical centers in 2012. Antimicrob Agents Chemother 2014;58(3):1684–92.

48. Sader HS, Castanheira M, Mendes RE, et al. Ceftazidime-avibactam activity against multidrug-resistant Pseudomonas aeruginosa isolated in U.S. medical centers in 2012 and 2013. Antimicrob Agents Chemother 2015;59(6):3656–9.

49. Lucasti C, Popescu I, Ramesh MK, et al. Comparative study of the efficacy and safety of ceftazidime/avibactam plus metronidazole versus meropenem in the treatment of complicated intra-abdominal infections in hospitalized adults: results of a randomized, double-blind, Phase II trial. J Antimicrob Chemother 2013;68(5): 1183–92.
50. Vazquez JA, González Patzán LD, Stricklin D, et al. Efficacy and safety of ceftazidime-avibactam versus imipenem-cilastatin in the treatment of complicated urinary tract infections, including acute pyelonephritis, in hospitalized adults: results of a prospective, investigator-blinded, randomized study. Curr Med Res Opin 2012;28(12):1921–31.

Antiretroviral Therapy for Prevention of Human Immunodeficiency Virus Infection

CrossMark

Aley G. Kalapila, MD, PhD[a],*, Jeanne Marrazzo, MD, MPH[b]

KEYWORDS

- Human immunodeficiency virus (HIV) infection • Antiretroviral therapy (ART)
- HIV prevention • HIV treatment as prevention • Pre-exposure prophylaxis (PrEP)
- Postexposure prophylaxis (PEP)
- Non-occupational postexposure prophylaxis (nPEP)
- Prevention of mother-to-child transmission (PMTCT)

KEY POINTS

- Human immunodeficiency virus (HIV) is now a chronic medical illness.
- All patients with HIV should be considered for treatment initiation with combination antiretroviral therapy (cART).
- cART serves a critical public health role in the prevention of HIV transmission in high-risk individuals.
- A comprehensive understanding of the pharmacotherapy of HIV drugs will be beneficial to primary care physicians to optimize chance of HIV treatment success and for HIV prevention.

INTRODUCTION

The evolution of combination antiretroviral therapy (cART) as human immunodeficiency virus (HIV) treatment is one of the great biomedical advancements of the twenty-first century. Since the discovery of zidovudine (AZT) in the 1980s, the armamentarium of drugs active against HIV has grown rapidly and the concept of a combination drug treatment of HIV has turned the tide of the epidemic. What was once a uniformly fatal disease has now become a chronic medical illness because cART has led to a remarkable reduction in overall morbidity and mortality.[1,2] As a result, life expectancy of the

[a] Division of Infectious Diseases, Department of Medicine, Emory University School of Medicine, Atlanta, GA, USA; [b] Division of Infectious Diseases, University of Alabama at Birmingham, Birmingham, AL, USA
* Corresponding author. Grady Infectious Diseases Program, 341 Ponce De Leon Avenue Northeast, Atlanta, GA 30308.
E-mail address: akalapi@emory.edu

Med Clin N Am 100 (2016) 927–950
http://dx.doi.org/10.1016/j.mcna.2016.03.013
0025-7125/16/$ – see front matter © 2016 Elsevier Inc. All rights reserved.

medical.theclinics.com

HIV-infected population has caught up with that of the general public, requiring that primary care physicians become well grounded in the care of these individuals. This becomes especially important in the context of treating the widely acknowledged, non-infectious complications of HIV, including cardiovascular disease, malignancies not defined by acquired immunodeficiency syndrome (AIDS), bone disease, and metabolic syndrome. Furthermore, the use of antiretroviral therapy (ART) as chemoprophylaxis against HIV acquisition (pre-exposure prophylaxis [PrEP]) is now supported by data from large multicenter randomized trials. Consequently, primary care physicians also have a unique opportunity to advocate for and implement risk-reduction strategies, including PrEP, in patients at high risk for acquiring the infection. This article provides an overview of the most commonly used HIV therapeutic agents as they are prescribed for HIV infection in treatment-naïve individuals and for prevention of HIV transmission.

ANTIRETROVIRAL THERAPY FOR PREVENTION

The last decade has seen a marked paradigm shift in the public health discourse around HIV with the emergence of the concept of using ART for HIV prevention. This field can be divided into 4 main categories: treatment as prevention; prevention of mother-to-child transmission (PMTCT); postexposure prophylaxis (PEP), including non-occupational exposures (nPEP), and most recently, PrEP.

TREATMENT AS PREVENTION

The hypothesis of HIV treatment as prevention as a public health approach is rooted in the principle that treating HIV-infected individuals with cART decreases their viral load, making them less infectious to their sexual partners.[3] Several persuasive observational studies in HIV serodiscordant couples and ecological studies in community populations have supported this theory, culminating with the landmark HPTN052 study, a randomized multicenter clinical trial that followed 1763 HIV-serodiscordant couples, 98% of whom were heterosexual.[3–11] Half the subjects were randomized to receive cART early, whereas the rest started cART when the HIV-infected partner had a CD4 count lower than or equal to 350 cells/mm^3 or an AIDS-defining illness. The primary endpoint was genetically linked HIV transmission to the uninfected partner. Four years after enrollment began in 2007, 39 HIV transmission events had been recorded, only 4 in the early therapy cohort. Of these 4, only 1 was genetically linked to the infected partner, representing a 96% reduction in risk of transmission. Furthermore, the single linked transmission in the early therapy group likely occurred in the first 3 months of treatment initiation, when the viral load was probably not suppressed. In 2011, the data safety monitoring board (DSMB) discontinued the study early when it became apparent that the individuals on cART were 20 times less likely to infect their partners than those left untreated.[5] The European PARTNER study in both heterosexual and men who have sex with men (MSM) serodiscordant couples has also reported similarly low rates of HIV transmission when the HIV-infected partner is taking cART and has an HIV viral load less than 200 copies per milliliter. As of 2014, no linked transmission events had been reported.[12] These studies lend credence to the scientific validity of HIV treatment as prevention while endorsing its applicability to heterosexual, MSM, and injection drug use groups at risk.

WHEN TO START HUMAN IMMUNODEFICIENCY VIRUS TREATMENT

The timing for cART initiation has evolved considerably as observational studies established marked benefits in AIDS and non-AIDS related morbidity and mortality with earlier treatment. The arsenal of safe and tolerable HIV therapeutics has also grown, with reduced pill burdens and toxicity profiles.[5,13–16] In March 2012, the Department of Health and Human Services (DHHS) guidelines recommended treatment of all HIV-infected patients, regardless of CD4 count.[17] The most convincing proof of principle came with results from the INSIGHT-START study group, a randomized, controlled multicenter, multinational clinical trial with a primary goal to determine the optimal time to initiate cART. Approximately 4600 treatment-naïve, asymptomatic HIV-infected adults with CD4 count greater than 500 cells/mm³ were enrolled in 2011. They were randomized to start cART immediately or defer treatment until the CD4 was less than 350. The primary endpoint was any serious AIDS-related or non-AIDS–related disease (eg, cardiovascular, renal, liver disease, or cancers not defined by AIDS) or death from any cause. The DSMB terminated the study early when the results confirmed that early cART initiation dramatically reduced rates of serious AIDS-related illnesses and non-AIDS–related disease and death compared with the deferred treatment group. Primary end points occurred in 42 subjects in the early treatment group, compared with 96 subjects in the deferred-treatment group. More than two-thirds of the primary end points were in subjects who had a CD4 greater than 500. These results confirmed that starting cART soon after HIV diagnosis provides significant protective health benefits.[18]

COMMONLY USED ANTIRETROVIRAL DRUGS

The life cycle of the HIV virus consists of multiple steps in order for successful replication and subsequent viral propagation to occur. Experiences with the nucleoside or nucleoside reverse transcriptase inhibitors (NRTIs) at the start of the HIV epidemic led to the observation that regimens targeting a single step in the viral replication process eventually failed due to rapid resistance and rebound viremia.[19] Defined as use of 3 or more active agents, cART uses drugs that act on different stages in the viral life cycle and allows for sustained antiviral effect while preventing the selection of resistant mutants. Thus, cART is now standard clinical practice for treatment of the HIV-infected individual.

Available HIV treatments are distributed among 5 drug classes, with varying mechanisms of action (**Fig. 1**). These include NRTIs, non-NRTIs (nNRTIs), protease inhibitors (PIs), entry inhibitors, and integrase inhibitors (INSTIs). Furthermore, there are now multiple fixed-dose-combination (FDC) tablets, which have simplified treatment options for patients while reducing pill burdens and facilitating adherence. **Table 1** summarizes the commonly recommended and frequently used ART drugs, including their mechanisms of action and **Table 2** lists the FDCs that are available at this time.[19] Many drug copay programs and patient assistant programs exist to help with the often prohibitive cost of these medications, particularly for individuals with little or no health insurance. Further details can be found at http://www.aidsmeds.com/articles/PAPs_Copays_19740.shtml or by going directly to the drug manufacturer web site.

TREATMENT INITIATION AND LABORATORY MONITORING

HIV therapy is a life-long commitment. To that end, a provider must tailor cART selection to minimize toxicity and optimize adherence. Selection of an initial cART regimen may need to be individualized to each patient based on several factors, including baseline HIV RNA level, CD4 count, comorbid conditions (eg, renal or liver disease), hepatitis B or C coinfection, concurrent medications, and pregnancy.

According to the most up-to-date DHHS guidelines, from November 2015, the cART regimens recommended for treatment-naïve individuals consist of a 2 NRTI backbone

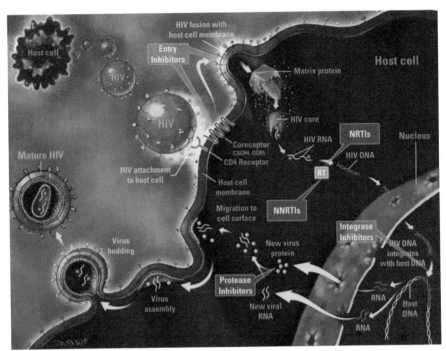

Fig. 1. Potential points of intervention of antiretroviral agents in HIV life-cycle. (*Courtesy of David H. Spach, MD, University of Washington, Harborview Medical Center, Seattle, WA.*)

with either a PI or INSTI, some of which are available as FDC tablets (**Table 3**).[17] Entry inhibitors are not considered first-line agents for treatment of HIV infection and are typically used in salvage settings when extensive HIV resistance and treatment experience exists. These latter drugs should be prescribed after discussion with an infectious disease specialist.

Before treatment initiation, baseline labs must be obtained as shown in **Table 4**.[17,20] Opportunistic infections and/or AIDS-defining illness that warrant concomitant therapy or prophylaxis, as well as other chronic medical conditions and medicines, should be taken into consideration when tailoring cART regimens to an individual patient.

Once a cART regimen has been initiated, longitudinal monitoring is necessary (see **Table 4**). The primary goal of cART is to suppress the serum HIV viral load below the limit of detection, with secondary objectives that include immune reconstitution (as demonstrated by increases in CD4 count), prolonged survival, maintaining quality of life by reducing morbidity associated with chronic HIV infection, and preventing the transmission of HIV. Persistent viremia (>200 copies/ml) can indicate several problems, including nonadherence, resistance (from archived mutations), inadequate drug absorption, or drug interactions with concomitant medications. Immune reconstitution, as manifested by a rise in CD4 count, although highly desirable, is not the main objective of cART, nor is it a requirement for successful therapy. Several contributing factors can lead to discordant CD4 counts, despite an undetectable viral load, including length of time a patient has been infected and off cART, active opportunistic infections, or other bone marrow–suppressive drugs. Consequently, major changes should not be made to cART regimens because of inadequate immune reconstitution, provided viral suppression has been achieved.[21]

Table 1 Commonly prescribed ART drugs by class		
Generic Name	**Brand Name**	**Mechanism of Action**
Nucleoside/nucleotide reverse transcriptase inhibitor (NRTI)		
Zidovudine (AZT)	Retrovir	First class of antiretrovirals approved in the US. They
Lamivudine (3TC)	Epivir	interfere with the reverse transcriptase enzyme
Abacavir (ABC)	Ziagen	preventing transcription of viral RNA to DNA.
Tenofovir (TDF)	Viread	
Emtricitabine (FTC)	Emtriva	
Non-nucleoside reverse transcriptase inhibitor (nNRTI)		
Efavirenz (EFV)	Sustiva	These drugs bind to the reverse transcriptase
Rilpivirine (RPV)	Edurant	enzyme near the catalytic site, resulting in a
Etravirine (ETR)	Intelence	conformational change in protein structure which
		decreases its enzymatic ability.
Protease inhibitors (PIs)		
Darunavir (DRV)	Prezista	Potent drug class with high genetic barrier to
Atazanavir (ATV)	Reyataz	resistance, so multiple mutations must be accrued
		for clinically significant resistance. They bind to
		the HIV protease enzyme and block production of
		functional virions. These drugs must always be
		prescribed with a pharmacologic enhancer
		(Ritonavir or Cobicistat), which inhibits the
		cytochrome P450 enzyme pathway, allowing for
		therapeutic levels of the PIs and thus, also account
		for several drug interactions associated with this
		class.
Integrase Inhibitors (INSTI)		
Raltegravir (RAL)	Isentress	Most recently discovered group that exert their
Elvitegravir (EVG)	Vitekta	antiviral effect by binding to the HIV integrase
Dolutegravir (DTG)	Tivicay	enzyme, thwarting integration of proviral DNA
		into the host cell genome. There are no human
		homologs of HIV integrase, allowing for minimal
		side effects and/or interactions.
Entry Inhibitors		
CCR5 Antagonist: Maraviroc (MVC)	Selzentry	CCR5 antagonists bind to the CCR5 co-receptor to block HIV binding to the CD4 cell and inhibit fusion of the virion with host cell. However, virions binding to a CD4 cell can utilize CCR5 and/or another HIV co-receptor, CXCR4. Hence, this drug can work only if an individual is infected with HIV that solely binds to the CCR5 co-receptor.
Fusion Inhibitor: Enfuvirtide (ENF, T-20)	Fuzeon	This drug prevents HIV fusion with a CD4 cell by binding to viral envelope protein, gp4.
Pharmacokinetic Enhancers		
Cobicistat (COBI)	Tybost	By inhibiting the cytochrome P450 3A enzymes,
Ritonavir (RTV)	Norvir	these drugs boost serum levels of the co-administered ART medications. RTV is co-administered only with PIs. Whereas, COBI must always be prescribed with a PI or INSTI, Elvitegravir (as part of FDCs, Stribild or Genvoya[a]).

This table does not list all available ART drugs. It only includes those that are most commonly pre-scribed for treatment naïve individuals.

[a] On November 5th, 2015, the US Food and Drug Administration approved Gilead's single tablet regimen Genvoya, which is similar to Stribild except that it contains Tenofovir Alafenamide, a novel prodrug of the NRTI drug, Tenofovir.

Table 2
Commonly used fixed dose combination ART regimens

Generic Name	Brand Name
NRTI Combinations	
TDF/FTC	Truvada
3TC/ABC	Epzicom
3TC/AZT	Combivir
Tenofovir Alafenamide (TAF)/FTC[a]	Descovy
PI Combinations	
DRV/COBI	Prezcobix
ATV/COBI	Evotaz
Single Tablet cART Combinations	
TDF/FTC/EFV	Atripla
TDF/FTC/RPV	Complera
TDF/FTC/EVG/COBI	Stribild
3TC/ABC/DTG	Triumeq
TAF/FTC/EVG/COBI[b]	Genvoya
TAF/FTC/RPV[c]	Odefsey

[a] On April 4th, 2016, the US Food and Drug Administration (FDA) approved a new FDC from Gilead, Odefsey, which is similar to Tenofovir except that it contains Tenofovir Alafenamide (TAF), a novel prodrug of the NRTI drug, Tenofovir.
[b] On November 5th, 2015, the US FDA approved Gilead's single tablet regimen Genvoya, which is similar to Stribild except that it contains TAF.
[c] On March 1st, 2016, the US FDA approved Gilead's single tablet regimen Odefsey, which is similar to Complera except that it contains TAF.

Table 3
Department of Health and Human Services Guidelines: Recommended combined antiretroviral therapy regimens for treatment-naïve individuals as of November, 2015

INSTI-based regimens	3TC/ABC/DTG (available as FDC Triumeq)[a]
	TDF/FTC (available as FDC Truvada) + DTG
	TDF/FTC/EVG/COBI (available as FDC Stribild)
	Tenofovir alafenamide (TAF)/FTC/EVG/COBI (available as FDC Genvoya)
	TDF/FTC + RAL[b]
PI-based regimens	TDF/FTC + DRV + RTV[b]
DHHS Guidelines: Alternative cART regimens	
nNRTI-based regimens	TDF/FTC/EFV (available as FDC Atripla)
	TDF/FTC/RPV (available as FDC Complera)[c]
PI-based regimens	TDF/FTC + ATV + RTV[b]
	TDF/FTC + ATV/COBI (available as FDC Evotaz)
	TDF/FTC + DRV/COBI (available as FDC Prezcobix)
	3TC/ABC (available as FDC Epzicom) + DRV/COBI[a]
	3TC/ABC + DRV + RTV[a]

[a] Regimen recommended only for patients who are human leukocyte antigen B57*01-negative.
[b] Recommended for use in treatment-naïve pregnant patients.
[c] Only for patients whose pretreatment HIV RNA is <100,000 copies/ml and CD4 cell count greater than 200/mm.^{3}.
Data from Panel on Antiretroviral Guidelines for Adults and Adolescents. Guidelines for the use of antiretroviral agents in HIV-1 infected adults and adolescents. Department of Health and Human Services. Available at: https://aidsinfo.nih.gov/contentfiles/lvguidelines/adultandadolescentgl.pdf. Accessed November 22, 2015.

Table 4
Laboratory monitoring before and after combined antiretroviral therapy initiation[a]

Labs	Before cART	At cART Initiation	Every 2–8 wk After cART Initiation	Every 3–6 mo	Every 6 mo
HIV viral load	X	X	X[b] Expect ~1.0log$_{10}$ decrease from baseline viral load	X	X Only for patients with viral suppression for ≥2 y
CD4 count	X	X		X Can be done annually if viral suppression for ≥2 y and CD4 >300 cells/mm^3	X
Resistance testing	X				
Human leukocyte antigen B57*01 Antigen	X[c] If considering use of Abacavir				
Hepatitis B serologies[d]	X	X If clinically indicated			
Comprehensive metabolic panel[e]	X	X	X	X	
Complete blood count with differential	X	X	X	X	
Urinalysis	X	X			X If on tenofovir
Pregnancy test	X	X			

[a] Tests should be ordered at more frequent intervals if clinically indicated.

[b] If the HIV viral load is detectable up to 8 weeks post-cART initiation, repeat the laboratory tests every 4 to 8 weeks until viral load is suppressed to less than 200 copies/mL and, thereafter, every 3 to 6 months.

[c] Avoid Abacavir use in patients who are human leukocyte antigen B57*01-positive because of the risk of a potentially fatal hypersensitivity reaction.

[d] If patient has evidence of chronic hepatitis B infection, then tenofovir plus either emtricitabine or lamivudine should be used as part of the cART regimen to treat both the hepatitis B and HIV infections.

[e] Includes basic chemistry, alanine aminotransferase, aspartate aminotransferase, and total bilirubin.

Adapted from Panel on Antiretroviral Guidelines for Adults and Adolescents. Guidelines for the use of antiretroviral agents in HIV-1 infected adults and adolescents. Department of Health and Human Services. Available at: https://aidsinfo.nih.gov/contentfiles/lvguidelines/adultandadolescentgl.pdf. Accessed November 22, 2015.

PREVENTION OF MOTHER-TO-CHILD TRANSMISSION

PMTCT plays an important role within the paradigm of ART for prevention, especially in settings when there is a delay in linking an HIV-infected woman to care before pregnancy. Ideally, perinatal counseling should begin at preconception for HIV-infected women. Women, who are considering conception, should be started on cART as soon as possible with a goal for viral suppression before pregnancy. Studies have demonstrated marked reduction in risk of perinatal transmission of HIV when the viral load of HIV-infected women remains suppressed to less than 50 copies per milliliter throughout pregnancy.[22,23] Accordingly, current DHHS guidelines recommend that cART should be started in all pregnant women with HIV, regardless of stage of pregnancy, taking into consideration the same factors one would consider in nonpregnant individuals, as well as careful examination of potential drug toxicities to the developing fetus and mother.

Due to the urgency of treatment initiation in this population, waiting for resistance testing results is not recommended. Hence the regimen choice should be one with a low prevalence of clinically significant resistance in the population. A cART regimen based on PI or INSTI is primarily recommended, anchored by a 2 NRTI backbone, given available data on toxicities to mother and fetus, favorable adverse effect profile, and pharmacokinetic data in pregnancy, as well as potency, efficacy, and persistence of viral suppression (see **Table 3**). Additionally, women who become pregnant on an effective cART regimen are usually kept on the same regimen throughout their pregnancy. Further details on PMTCT guidelines are found at https://aidsinfo.nih.gov/contentfiles/lvguidelines/perinatalgl.pdf.

OCCUPATIONAL AND NONOCCUPATIONAL POSTEXPOSURE PROPHYLAXIS

PEP is the administration of ART to decrease the risk of HIV transmission following possible exposure to HIV, be it in an occupational or nonoccupational PEP (nPEP) setting. It is another core strategy underlying the paradigm of ART for HIV prevention. The efficacy of PEP was validated in 1997, when a case control study evaluating HIV seroconversion of health care workers after a percutaneous exposure demonstrated that prophylaxis with AZT alone conferred an 81% reduction of odds of infection after an HIV exposure.[24,25] Ethical concerns of further investigations into PEP in human subjects led to much of the subsequent work being conducted in primate models. A recent meta-analysis regarding the efficacy of PEP evaluated 25 studies with most data favoring its use, especially in light of the highly potent cART regimens, with minimal toxicity, available in the United States today.[25] These data support the theory that ART chemoprophylaxis soon after exposure stunts the viral replication cycle, diminishing the productive infection of T cells, particularly in regional lymph nodes. This is hypothesized to abort the establishment of a latent reservoir by the virus. Furthermore, by inhibiting systemic infection, PEP is also thought to enhance cellular immunity, thereby reducing risk of persistent HIV infection.[26] **Fig. 2** indicates the risk of HIV transmission from exposure to an infected source.[27]

Occupational transmission of HIV is exceedingly rare with only 57 documented transmission events in the United States and none since 1999. The guiding principle behind PEP is that the time between potential exposure and ART initiation should be minimized as much as possible, ideally less than 72 hours. In the event of an occupational exposure to blood or potentially infectious body fluid, baseline laboratory testing on the health care worker must be done, including HIV and hepatitis B and C, as well as a complete blood count (CBC) and comprehensive metabolic

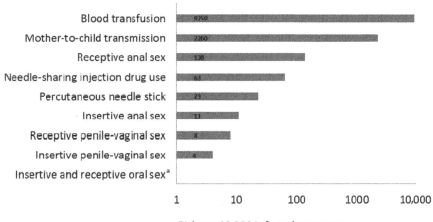

Fig. 2. Estimated probability of HIV transmission from an infected source, by exposure route. [a] Low risk, relative to other sexual exposures, but not zero. (*Data from* Patel P, Borkowf CB, Brooks JT, et al. Estimating per-act HIV transmission risk: a systematic review. AIDS 2014;28(10):1509–19.)

panel (CMP) to evaluate renal and liver function. PEP should be initiated immediately (and within 72 hours) while attempts to perform HIV testing of the source are underway.[28]

The preferred cART regimen for occupational PEP is shown in **Table 5**. It is tenofovir-emtricitabine (TDF/FTC; Truvada) along with the INSTI Raltegravir, based on tolerability and a favorable toxicity profile that includes minimal drug interactions.[28] Alternative regimens include the use of TDF/FTC and a boosted PI. If the source patient is found to be HIV-negative, PEP can be discontinued. Otherwise, PEP should be taken for 28 days following exposure. Subsequent evaluation should include adherence monitoring, contraception and sexual behavior counseling, and

Table 5
Recommendations for HIV PEP regimens from the 2013 US Public Health Service Guidelines

Preferred Regimen	
TDF/FTC (Truvada) + RAL[a]	
Alternative Regimens	
Use a 2 NRTI drug combination from the left column with drug(s) from the right column	
TDF/FTC	RAL
TDF + 3TC	DRV + RTV
AZT/3TC (Combivir)	ETR
AZT + FTC	RPV
	ATV + RTV
TDF/FTC/EVG/COBI (Administered as Stribild, without additional drugs)	

[a] Also recommended as one of the first line regimens for non-occupational PEP along with TDF/FTC + DTG

Adapted from Kuhar DT, Henderson DK, Struble KA, et al. Updated US Public Health Service Guidelines for the management of occupational exposures to human immunodeficiency virus and recommendations for postexposure prophylaxis. Infect Control Hosp Epi 2013;34(9):875–92.

monitoring for drug toxicities. Follow-up HIV testing is to be done at 6 weeks, 12 weeks, and 6 months. If the more sensitive fourth-generation HIV assay is used, follow-up testing can end at 4 months.[28] However, signs or symptoms consistent with acute HIV infection must prompt testing much sooner than the timelines previously delineated.[28]

The treatment of individuals exposed to blood or bodily fluids from known, or suspected, HIV-positive individuals is nPEP. Patients presenting for nPEP afford a unique opportunity for primary care providers to discuss multiple issues, including risk-reduction education and counseling, as well as serving as a gateway to PrEP. In high-risk individuals, PrEP is the preferred modality of HIV prevention, rather than repeated courses of nPEP, provided the patient has remained HIV-negative. Aside from HIV testing of the exposed individual, simultaneous screening for other conditions relevant to the exposure, including pregnancy, hepatitis B and C and other sexually transmitted diseases (STDs), as well as monitoring basic CBC and CMP must be done.

An algorithm for determining need for nPEP is shown in **Fig. 3**. If nPEP is warranted, as with occupational exposures, a 28-day course of a 3-drug cART regimen is recommended. A new iteration of the guidelines is anticipated. The CDC, as well as the New York State Department of Health and US Public Health Service guidelines recommend similar regimens and follow-up testing as that for occupational PEP. TDF/FTC in combination with an INSTI, either Raltegravir or Dolutegravir, is the first-line nPEP cART regimen due to a tolerable side effect profile and the idea that this drug combination acts at an earlier stage of the viral replication cycle, preventing integration into the host genome.[28–32]

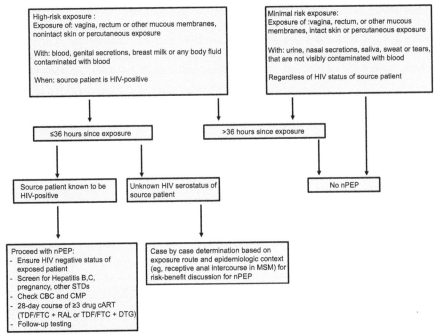

Fig. 3. nPEP algorithm. CMP includes chemistries and renal and liver functions tests. DTG, dolutegravir; RAL, raltegravir.

PRE-EXPOSURE PROPHYLAXIS

The scientific plausibility for PrEP is extended from the well-established observation in PEP that minimizing the time between HIV exposure and postexposure ART administration increases the efficacy of PEP. It then follows that having adequate levels of ART in blood and genital tissue before HIV exposure should attenuate the risk of HIV transmission.[33] Such a prophylactic approach, analogous to current malaria prevention methods, represents a significant advancement in HIV prevention.

There have been and continue to be multiple preclinical and early clinical studies with varied drugs, dosing schedules, and drug delivery systems for PrEP, including oral pills, intramuscular injectable agents, vaginal and rectal microbicides, and long-acting vaginal rings. However, at present, the most significant evidence favoring PrEP is with the drug TDF/FTC. It is currently the only available FDA-approved regimen for PrEP. **Table 6** summarizes results from some of the most prominent studies in the PrEP arena that have played an instrumental role in defining this key public health measure to prevent HIV transmission in high-risk groups.[33–40]

The FEM-PrEP and VOICE studies occurring in heterosexual women demonstrated disappointing results compared with the overwhelming evidence favoring TDF/FTC for PrEP. However, these discrepancies can largely be explained by variability in adherence, which directly correlates with the degree of protection against HIV acquisition.[38,41–43] Moreover, concentrations of the active form of tenofovir (TDF) are 100 times higher in rectal tissue than in cervicovaginal tissue.[44] Hence, poor adherence to PrEP may have a greater negative implication in women than in men. Further investigation is needed into the level of adherence to PrEP required for therapeutic efficacy for HIV prevention.

Concerns regarding the effectiveness of PrEP as it pertains to adherence, risk compensation, toxicity, cost or reimbursement, and drug resistance are some of the impediments to widespread implementation. Despite this, recent evidence suggests that PrEP uptake is increasing, particularly in MSM. PrEP is likely cost-effective in certain settings, and patient assistance programs can help with expensive copays or deductibles from insurances or, in many cases, even pay for the drug outright.[45,46] Many state-based programs also exist for financial assistance to expand access to PrEP.[33] Data on so-called risk compensation—namely, adoption of or increase in unprotected sex as a consequence of PrEP use—is currently mixed, with conflicting results from various large PrEP studies.[33,43,47,48] With regard to concerns for emergence of resistant virus, results from several phase III trials suggest that HIV seroconversion with resistant virus is a rare event. It is also clear that resistance mutations and virus are highly associated with administration of PrEP in the presence of occult primary HIV infection.[34,36,38,39,49–51] For the practicing clinician, it is imperative to avoid starting PrEP if the patient manifests any symptoms suggestive of a viral illness that may masquerade for unrecognized primary HIV infection. The latter must be excluded with adequate testing before PrEP initiation.

Table 7 is a summary of the most current CDC guidelines for PrEP administration. For now, PrEP is to be taken on a daily basis. However, ongoing large cohort studies and randomized clinical trials have results demonstrating considerable efficacy with intermittent dosing of TDF/FTC in the MSM population. Pharmacokinetic studies, as well as demonstration projects, indicate that intermittent pericoital oral PrEP, at least among MSM, are effective.[52,53] It is evident that PrEP is a rapidly

Table 6
Important human immunodeficiency virus pre-exposure prophylaxis studies evidence summary

Study	Drugs	Population	Results
iPREX[36]	Oral TDF/FTC	MSM in United States and countries in Southeast Asia, Africa, and South America	44% efficacy (92% in those with detectable drug levels)
Conclusion: Once-daily TDF/FTC (Truvada) is a recommended and effective PrEP option for HIV prevention in MSM who are at high risk for HIV acquisition, particularly when there is medication adherence.			
FEM-PrEP[40]	Oral TDF/FTC	Women in Africa	Terminated because of lack of efficacy Low adherence noted in the trial
TDF-2[39]	Oral TDF/FTC	Heterosexual men and women in Botswana	62% efficacy
PARTNERS PrEP[34]	Oral TDF/FTC, oral TDF	Heterosexual, serodiscordant couples in Kenya and Uganda	67% efficacy with oral TDF (86% in those with detectable drug levels) 75% efficacy with oral TDF/FTC (90% in those with detectable drug levels)
VOICE[38]	Oral TDF/FTC, oral TDF, topical tenofovir gel	Women in Africa	Terminated because of lack of efficacy Low adherence noted in trial
Conclusion: Once-daily TDF/FTC is a recommended and effective PrEP option for HIV prevention in heterosexual men and women who are at high risk of HIV acquisition, particularly when there is medication adherence.			
BTS[35]	Oral TDF	Injection drug users in Thailand	49% efficacy
Conclusion: Once-daily TDF/FTC (or TDF alone) is a recommended and effective PrEP option for HIV prevention in injection drug users who are at high risk for HIV acquisition, particularly when there is medication adherence.			

Adapted from US Public Health Service. PreExposure prophylaxis for the prevention of HIV infection in the United States–2014 clinical practice guideline. Available at: http://www.cdc.gov/hiv/pdf/prepguidelines2014.pdf. Accessed March 4, 2016; and Marrazzo JM, del Rio C, Holtgrave DR, et al. HIV Prevention in Clinical Care Settings: 2014 recommendations of the International Antiviral Society – USA Panel. JAMA 2014;312(4):390–409.

Table 7
Administering human immunodeficiency virus pre-exposure prophylaxis (Centers for Disease Control and Prevention and US Public Health Service, May 2014)

	MSM	Heterosexual Men and Women	Injection Drug Users
Defining high risk for HIV acquisition	HIV-positive partner without viral suppression Recent bacterial sexually transmitted disease Inconsistent condom use Multiple sexual partners		HIV-positive injection partner Sharing needles Active injection drug use
Eligibility criteria	HIV-negative test result *must* be documented before prescribing PrEP No active symptoms consistent with acute HIV infection Normal renal function No contraindicated medication Documentation of hepatitis B virus infection and/or vaccination status		
Prescription	≤90 d supply of once daily TDF/FTC (Truvada)[a]		
Follow-up visits every 3 mo[a]	Continued HIV testing Medication adherence Counseling on behavioral risk-reduction strategies Monitoring renal function and side effects Symptom screening and testing for other sexually transmitted diseases (oral, rectal, cervicovaginal sites)[a] Pregnancy testing and intent Access to drug treatment programs Access to clean injection drug equipment		

[a] Timing of follow-up appointments may need to be more frequent than 3 months, and should be tailored by need for more intensive risk assessment and HIV/STD screening.
Data from US Public Health Service, PreExposure prophylaxis for the prevention of HIV infection in the United States–2014 Clinical Practice Guideline. Available at: http://www.cdc.gov/hiv/pdf/prepguidelines2014.pdf. Accessed March 4, 2016.

evolving field in HIV prevention as such new data comes to light, including dosing and frequency of TDF/FTC, as well as alternative therapeutic options for potential PrEP agents.

ANTIRETROVIRAL THERAPY SIDE EFFECTS AND DRUG INTERACTIONS

With the improved life expectancy of persons living with HIV, primary care providers now routinely confront issues pertaining to chronic disease management. Under the circumstances, having a basic understanding of the toxicity profile of cART regimens and their potential for drug interactions, especially with other comorbid conditions, is critical. These factors play a significant role in ensuring therapeutic levels of drugs and optimizing adherence to cART. Fortunately, several resources exist to help clinicians with up-to-date information regarding ART adverse effects and drug interactions.

Although the current roster of ART agents has markedly improved safety and tolerability, there are specific adverse effects that physicians should be aware of. **Table 8** reviews toxicities frequently encountered with the most commonly used ART agents.[54] For the primary care provider, some of the common issues that may arise include nephrotoxicity associated with TDF use, the gastrointestinal side effects and drug interactions of PIs, and neuropsychiatric problems from efavirenz. There are some mixed data regarding reduction in bone mineral density associated with cART. TDF-containing regimens, once started, can cause some modest bone loss, which later levels off.[55–57] Boosted PIs have also been shown to decrease bone mineral

Table 8
Common adverse effects with frequently prescribed antiretroviral therapy drugs

Drug Class	Adverse Effects	Comments
NRTI (TDF, 3TC, ABC, AZT, FTC, Didanosine [ddl][a])	Nephrotoxicity	Commonly associated with TDF. All NRTIs must be renally dose-adjusted
	Hypersensitivity reaction	Seen with ABC in human leukocyte antigen B57*01-positive individuals
	Lactic acidosis	Rare, but more common with AZT
	Lipoatrophy	Associated with AZT
	Decreased bone mineralization density	Prolonged TDF use
	Bone marrow suppression, macrocytic anemia	Associated with AZT
	Fanconi syndrome	Rare condition associated with TDF. Manifests as glycosuria, proteinuria, and hypophosphatemia
	Myopathy	Associated with AZT
	Increased risk of cardiovascular events	Associated with ABC, but considered controversial
	Diarrhea, pancreatitis, neuropathy	Associated with ddl
	Noncirrhotic portal hypertension	Associated with ddl. Can occur months to years after starting ddl
NNRTI (EFV, RPV, ETR)	Several drug interactions	NNRTIs generally induce the CYP450 enzymatic pathway. Most interactions noted with EFV
	Rash	Can treat through this provided it is not severe
	Neuropsychiatric side effects	Mostly associated with EFV, including vivid dreams, exacerbation of depression, headache
	Teratogenicity	EFV is classified as Pregnancy Category D agent by the United States Food and Drug administration after animal studies and retrospective case reports indicated that use of the drug in the first trimester of pregnancy may be associated with neural tube defects

(continued on next page)

Table 8
(continued)

Drug Class	Adverse Effects	Comments
PI (ATV, DRV, RTV)	Several drug interactions	PIs are potent inhibitors of the CYP450 enzymatic pathway
	Gastrointestinal symptoms (nausea, vomiting, diarrhea)	—
	Diabetes, insulin resistance	Less with new PIs (ATV, DRV)
	Dyslipidemia	Less with new PIs (ATV, DRV)
	Hepatotoxicity	Usually with viral hepatitis coinfection
	Lipohypertrophy	Mostly with older PIs
	Nephrolithiasis	Associated with ATV
	Indirect hyperbilirubinemia	Similar to Gilbert syndrome and associated with ATV
	Rash	Associated with DRV, which has a sulfa moiety. There have been rare reports of Stevens-Johnson syndrome.
	Decreased Bone density	—
INSTI (RAL, EVG, DTG)	Insomnia	Associated with DTG
	Headache	Associated with DTG
	Nonpathologic increase in creatinine	Decreased tubular secretion of creatinine that is associated with DTG and cobicistat.
	Rhabdomyolysis	Rare. Associated with RAL
	Depression	Rare. Associated with RAL

[a] ddI is an older NRTI that is rarely used currently, but may be seen with older cART regimens. It has a notable side effect profile.

Data from Panel on Antiretroviral Guidelines for Adults and Adolescents. Guidelines for the use of antiretroviral agents in HIV-1 infected adults and adolescents. Department of Health and Human Services. Available at: https://aidsinfo.nih.gov/contentfiles/lvguidelines/adultandadolescentgl.pdf. Accessed November 22, 2015.

density in the spine and hip, in certain studies, although longitudinal studies have not supported this concern.[58–61] Despite these data, the effect on rates of fractures are unclear, especially when accounting for traditional osteoporosis risk factors, HIV infection itself as a risk factor for bone loss, as well as concomitant hepatitis C infection.[62–65] Regardless, these findings have led to several expert groups recommending bone mineral density screening using dual-energy X-ray absorptiometry (DEXA) scans in HIV-infected postmenopausal women and men over the age of 50.[2,66] Of note, tenofovir alafenamide (TAF), a prodrug of TDF that is expected to be FDA-approved in the near future, achieves greater intracellular concentrations of TDF with decreased plasma exposure, allowing for reductions in dosing with equivalent antiviral efficacy and, hence, less renal and bone toxicity.[67,68] In general, as a drug class, the INSTIs tend to be the best tolerated with the fewest side effects.

Although drug interactions occur via several mechanisms, the cytochrome (CYP)-450 enzymatic pathway is probably the most significant in day-to-day practice.[69]

Table 9
Important drug interactions between newer antiretroviral therapy drugs and frequently used drugs

Coadministered Drug Class	ART Drugs	Drug Interaction Effect	Comments
Gastric Acid Reducers			
H2-receptor antagonists (H2RA)	ATV + RTV, ATV/COBI	Decreases ATV levels by reducing absorption at higher gastric pH	Dose adjustments of H2RA may be necessary Give ART simultaneously with or ≥10 h after H2RA
	RPV	Decreased RPV levels by reducing absorption	Give H2RA ≥12 h before or ≥4 h after RPV
Proton pump inhibitors (PPI)	ATV + RTV, ATV/COBI	—	PPIs to be given ≥12 h before ART. Do not exceed PPI dose equivalent of omeprazole 20 mg daily
	RPV	Decreased RPV levels	*Coadministration is contraindicated*
Corticosteroids			
Inhaled Budesonide, Fluticasone, Mometasone	All RTV and COBI-boosted PI regimens, TDF/FTC/EVG/COBI	Increased glucocorticoid levels	Coadministration can lead to adrenal insufficiency or Cushing's syndrome Avoid coadministration Consider use of inhaled beclomethasone as an alternative
3-Hydroxy-3-methyl-glutaryl (HMG)-CoA reductase inhibitors			
Lovastatin Simvastatin	All RTV and COBI boosted PI regimens, TDF/FTC/EVG/COBI	Significant increase in statin levels	*Coadministration is contraindicated*
Atorvastatin Pravastatin Rosuvastatin	All RTV and COBI boosted PI regimens, TDF/FTC/EVG/COBI	Increase in statin levels	Use lowest starting dose of statin and titrate cautiously Maximum dose not to exceed atorvastatin 20 mg daily and rosuvastatin 10 mg daily
All statins	All nNRTIs	Decrease in statin levels	Adjust statin dose to clinical response Do not exceed maximum recommended statin dose
Narcotics			
Methadone	All RTV and COBI boosted PI regimens, EFV, ETR, RPV, TDF/FTC/EVG/COBI	Decreased methadone levels	Monitor for opioid withdrawal and dose adjust methadone to clinical response

(continued on next page)

Table 9
(continued)

Coadministered Drug Class	ART Drugs	Drug Interaction Effect	Comments
Oral Antihyperglycemics			
Metformin	DTG	Increased metformin levels	Start at lowest metformin dose and titrate to achieve glycemic control while minimizing GI symptoms
Hormonal Contraceptives			
Oral contraceptive pills (OCP)	All RTV and COBI boosted PI regimens, EFV	Decreased OCP levels	Recommend alternative or additional contraceptive method or alternative ART
Levonorgestrel emergency contraception	EFV	Decreased levonorgestrel levels	*Possible decreased efficacy of emergency contraception*
Etonorgesterel subdermal implant (ENG)	EFV	Decreased ENG levels released from implant	Coadminister with caution, consider alternative contraception or alternative cART[70]

Data from Panel on Antiretroviral Guidelines for Adults and Adolescents. Guidelines for the use of antiretroviral agents in HIV-1 infected adults and adolescents. Department of Health and Human Services. Available at: https://aidsinfo.nih.gov/contentfiles/lvguidelines/adultandadolescentgl.pdf. Accessed November 22, 2015; and Refs.[69,70]

PIs (particularly ritonavir) as well as the pharmacologic enhancer, cobicistat, inhibit CYP3A4, an enzyme in the CYP450 family, leading to supratherapeutic levels of drugs that are metabolized by this pathway. In contrast, the nNRTI class of ART agents, with efavirenz being the biggest offender, induces CYP450 enzymes, resulting in subtherapeutic levels of coadministered medicines that are metabolized by this system. **Table 9** summarizes interactions between the commonly prescribed ART agents and other medicines frequently encountered in a primary care scope of practice. A more extensive list of drug interactions and side effects relevant to the internist is shown in **Table 10**. A detailed and comprehensive list can be found at https://aidsinfo.nih.gov/contentfiles/lvguidelines/AA_Tables.pdf and at http://www.hiv-druginteractions.org/.

FUTURE DIRECTIONS AND SUMMARY

HIV treatment and prevention has advanced dramatically during the last few decades. Practitioners are privileged to have a broad array of safe, effective drugs for HIV-infected individuals. Fortunately, there are more medicines in the pipeline that should improve on existing therapies. For instance, TAF, a prodrug of TDF, will soon be approved by the FDA, followed by FDC ART regimens that contain TAF. Other investigational agents, including long-acting injectable agents in the nNRTI and INSTI class, are in development as well, which would permit monthly dosing as well as improved efficacy compared with current therapeutics.[54]

Table 10
Drug interactions between antiretroviral therapy agents and other drugs

Coadministered Drug Class	ART Drugs	Drug Interaction Effect	Comments
Gastric Acid Reducers			
Antacids	ATV + RTV, ATV/COBI	Decreased ATV levels with concomitant use	Give ART ≥2 h before or after antacids
	RPV	Decreased RPV levels with concomitant use	Give antacids ≥2 h before or ≥4 h after RPV
	DTG	Decreased DTG levels with polyvalent cation antacids due to chelation	Give DTG ≥2 h before or ≥6 h after antacids
	TDF/FTC/EVG/COBI	Decreased EVG levels due to chelation	Separate administration of antacids and ART by ≥2 h
	RAL	Decreased RAL levels when administered with Aluminum-Magnesium hydroxide antacids	*Contraindicated* *Do not coadminister RAL with Al-Mg hydroxide antacids*
Anticoagulants and Antiplatelet Therapies			
Coumadin	All RTV and COBI boosted PI regimens, EFV, ETR, TDF/FTC/EVG/COBI	Variable warfarin levels	Need close monitoring of INR with appropriate warfarin dose adjustments especially when initiating or discontinuing ART
Clopidogrel	ETR, EFV	Decreased activation of clopidogrel	Avoid coadministration as ART may prevent metabolism of clopidogrel to its active metabolite
Apixaban Rivaroxaban Ticagrelor Vorapaxar	All RTV and COBI-boosted PI regimens, TDF/FTC/EVG/COBI	Increased levels of anticoagulant	Avoid coadministration
Dabigatran	All RTV and COBI boosted PI regimens, TDF/FTC/EVG/COBI	Increased levels of dabigatran	No dose adjustment if CrCl >50 mL/min Avoid use if CrCl <50 ml/min
Antidepressants, Anxiolytics, Sleep Aids			
Selective serotonin reuptake inhibitors (SSRI)	All RTV and COBI boosted PI regimens, TDF/FTC/EVG/COBI	Increased SSRI levels	Start at lowest SSRI dose and titrate to clinical response
	EFV	Decreased sertraline levels	Titrate sertraline dose based on clinical response

(continued on next page)

Table 10
(continued)

Coadministered Drug Class	ART Drugs	Drug Interaction Effect	Comments
Alprazolam	All RTV and COBI boosted PI regimens, TDF/FTC/EVG/COBI	Increased alprazolam levels	*Coadministration is contraindicated* *Consider alternative benzos including temazepam, lorazepam and oxazepam, which are metabolized by a non-CYP450 pathway*
Zolpidem, Trazodone	All RTV and COBI boosted PI regimens, TDF/FTC/EVG/COBI	Increased zolpidem or trazodone levels	Start with lowest dose of sleep aid and titrate to clinical response
Cardiac Drugs			
Amiodarone	All RTV and COBI boosted PI regimens, TDF/FTC/EVG/COBI	Increased amiodarone or PI levels	Monitor amiodarone levels and for amiodarone drug toxicity Monitor electrocardiogram (EKG)
Beta-blockers (BB) (metoprolol)	All RTV and COBI boosted PI regimens, TDF/FTC/EVG/COBI	Increased beta-blocker levels	Dose adjustment of BB may be necessary. Consider using beta-blockers not metabolized by CYP450 system (Eg: atenolol, labetalol)
Calcium channel blockers (CCB)	All RTV and COBI boosted PI regimens, TDF/FTC/EVG/COBI	Increased CCB levels	Dose adjust CCB and monitor EKG
	EFV	Decreased CCB levels	Dose adjust CCB, titrate dose based on clinical response
Digoxin	All RTV and COBI boosted PI regimens	Increased digoxin levels	Dose adjust and monitor digoxin levels, monitor EKG
Corticosteroids			
Prednisone	All RTV and COBI boosted PI regimens	Increased prednisone levels	Coadministration can lead to adrenal insufficiency or Cushing syndrome
Dexamethasone	All RTV and COBI boosted PI regimens, TDF/FTC/EVG/COBI, EFV, ETR	Decreased ART levels	Use dexamethasone with caution Closely monitor HIV viral load
	RPV	Significantly decreased RPV levels	*Coadministration is contraindicated*

(continued on next page)

Table 10
(continued)

Coadministered Drug Class	ART Drugs	Drug Interaction Effect	Comments
Narcotics			
Fentanyl	All RTV and COBI boosted PI regimens, TDF/FTC/EVG/COBI	Increased fentanyl levels	Monitor closely for side effects, particularly respiratory depression
Phosphodiesterase Type 5 inhibitors			
Sildenafil Tadalafil Vardenafil (PDE5)	All RTV and COBI boosted PI regimens, TDF/FTC/EVG/COBI	Increased PDE5 inhibitor levels	For erectile dysfunction, start with lowest PDE5 dose Significant dose adjustments and decreased dose frequency are needed to avoid toxicities *Coadministration is contraindicated for pulmonary hypertension*
	EFV, ETR, RPV	Decreased PDE5 inhibitor levels	May need to increase PDE5 dose based on clinical response
Herbal products			
St John's Wort	All RTV and COBI boosted PI regimens All NNRTIs All INSTI	Possible decreased levels of ART	*Coadministration is contraindicated*
Miscellaneous			
Salmeterol	All RTV and COBI boosted PI regimens, TDF/FTC/EVG/COBI	Increased salmeterol levels	Contraindicated Do not *coadminister* due to risk of cardiovascular events due to salmeterol toxicity

Adapted from Panel on Antiretroviral Guidelines for Adults and Adolescents. Guidelines for the use of antiretroviral agents in HIV-1 infected adults and adolescents. Department of Health and Human Services. Available at: https://aidsinfo.nih.gov/contentfiles/lvguidelines/adultandadolescentgl.pdf. Accessed November 22, 2015.

A fundamental understanding of the basics of ART is essential to a primary care provider's knowledge base in this time when HIV has become a chronic medical condition. This will both enhance the ability to care for persons living with HIV, and contribute to curtailing the epidemic through informed use of ART for HIV prevention.

REFERENCES

1. Palella FJ Jr, Delaney KM, Moorman AC, et al. Declining morbidity and mortality among patients with advanced human immunodeficiency virus infection. HIV Outpatient Study Investigators. N Engl J Med 1998;338(13):853–60.
2. Aberg JA, Gallant JE, Ghanem KG, et al. Primary care guidelines for the management of persons infected with HIV: 2013 update by the HIV Medicine

Association of the Infectious Diseases Society of America. Clin Infect Dis 2014; 58(1):1–10.

3. Quinn TC, Wawer MJ, Sewankambo N, et al. Viral load and heterosexual transmission of human immunodeficiency virus type 1. Rakai Project Study Group. N Engl J Med 2000;342(13):921–9.

4. Castilla J, Del Romero J, Hernando V, et al. Effectiveness of highly active antiretroviral therapy in reducing heterosexual transmission of HIV. J Acquir Immune Defic Syndr 2005;40(1):96–101.

5. Cohen MS, Chen YQ, McCauley M, et al. Prevention of HIV-1 infection with early antiretroviral therapy. N Engl J Med 2011;365(6):493–505.

6. Del Romero J, Castilla J, Hernando V, et al. Combined antiretroviral treatment and heterosexual transmission of HIV-1: cross sectional and prospective cohort study. BMJ 2010;340:c2205.

7. Donnell D, Baeten JM, Kiarie J, et al. Heterosexual HIV-1 transmission after initiation of antiretroviral therapy: a prospective cohort analysis. Lancet 2010; 375(9731):2092–8.

8. Operskalski EA, Stram DO, Busch MP, et al. Role of viral load in heterosexual transmission of human immunodeficiency virus type 1 by blood transfusion recipients. Transfusion Safety Study Group. Am J Epidemiol 1997;146(8):655–61.

9. Pedraza MA, del Romero J, Roldan F, et al. Heterosexual transmission of HIV-1 is associated with high plasma viral load levels and a positive viral isolation in the infected partner. J Acquir Immune Defic Syndr 1999;21(2):120–5.

10. Reynolds SJ, Makumbi F, Nakigozi G, et al. HIV-1 transmission among HIV-1 discordant couples before and after the introduction of antiretroviral therapy. AIDS 2011;25(4):473–7.

11. Tovanabutra S, Robison V, Wongtrakul J, et al. Male viral load and heterosexual transmission of HIV-1 subtype E in northern Thailand. J Acquir Immune Defic Syndr 2002;29(3):275–83.

12. Rodger V, Bruun T, Cambiano V, et al. HIV transmission risk through condomless sex if HIV+ partner on suppressive ART: PARTNER Study. Conference on Retroviruses and Opportunistic Infections (CROI 2014). Boston, MA, USA, March 3–6, 2014. [Abstract: 153LB].

13. Charlebois ED, Das M, Porco TC, et al. The effect of expanded antiretroviral treatment strategies on the HIV epidemic among men who have sex with men in San Francisco. Clin Infect Dis 2011;52(8):1046–9.

14. Das M, Chu PL, Santos GM, et al. Decreases in community viral load are accompanied by reductions in new HIV infections in San Francisco. PLoS One 2010; 5(6):e11068.

15. Granich RM, Gilks CF, Dye C, et al. Universal voluntary HIV testing with immediate antiretroviral therapy as a strategy for elimination of HIV transmission: a mathematical model. Lancet 2009;373(9657):48–57.

16. Powers KA, Ghani AC, Miller WC, et al. The role of acute and early HIV infection in the spread of HIV and implications for transmission prevention strategies in Lilongwe, Malawi: a modelling study. Lancet 2011;378(9787):256–68.

17. Panel on Antiretroviral Guidelines for Adults and Adolescents. Guidelines for the use of antiretroviral agents in HIV-1 infected adults and adolescents. Department of Health and Human Services. Available at: https://aidsinfo.nih.gov/contentfiles/lvguidelines/adultandadolescentgl.pdf. Accessed November 22, 2015.

18. Group ISS, Lundgren JD, Babiker AG, et al. Initiation of antiretroviral therapy in early asymptomatic HIV infection. N Engl J Med 2015;373(9):795–807.

19. Pau AK, George JM. Antiretroviral therapy: current drugs. Infect Dis Clin North Am 2014;28(3):371–402.
20. Buckhold FR 3rd. Primary care of the human immunodeficiency virus patient. Med Clin North Am 2015;99(5):1105–22.
21. Sell JK. Management of human immunodeficiency virus in primary care. Prim Care 2013;40(3):589–617.
22. Forbes JC, Alimenti AM, Singer J, et al. A national review of vertical HIV transmission. AIDS 2012;26(6):757–63.
23. Townsend CL, Byrne L, Cortina-Borja M, et al. Earlier initiation of ART and further decline in mother-to-child HIV transmission rates, 2000-2011. AIDS 2014;28(7): 1049–57.
24. Cardo DM, Culver DH, Ciesielski CA, et al. A case-control study of HIV seroconversion in health care workers after percutaneous exposure. Centers for Disease Control and Prevention Needlestick Surveillance Group. N Engl J Med 1997; 337(21):1485–90.
25. Irvine C, Egan KJ, Shubber Z, et al. Efficacy of HIV Postexposure Prophylaxis: Systematic Review and Meta-analysis of Nonhuman Primate Studies. Clin Infect Dis 2015;60(Suppl 3):S165–9.
26. Beekmann SE, Henderson DK. Prevention of human immunodeficiency virus and AIDS: postexposure prophylaxis (including health care workers). Infect Dis Clin North Am 2014;28(4):601–13.
27. Patel P, Borkowf CB, Brooks JT, et al. Estimating per-act HIV transmission risk: a systematic review. AIDS 2014;28(10):1509–19.
28. Kuhar DT, Henderson DK, Struble KA, et al. Updated US Public Health Service guidelines for the management of occupational exposures to human immunodeficiency virus and recommendations for postexposure prophylaxis. Infect Control Hosp Epidemiol 2013;34(9):875–92.
29. Ford N, Shubber Z, Calmy A, et al. Choice of antiretroviral drugs for postexposure prophylaxis for adults and adolescents: a systematic review. Clin Infect Dis 2015; 60(Suppl 3):S170–6.
30. Jain S, Mayer KH. Practical guidance for nonoccupational postexposure prophylaxis to prevent HIV infection: an editorial review. AIDS 2014;28(11):1545–54.
31. Mayer KH, Mimiaga MJ, Gelman M, et al. Raltegravir, tenofovir DF, and emtricitabine for postexposure prophylaxis to prevent the sexual transmission of HIV: safety, tolerability, and adherence. J Acquir Immune Defic Syndr 2012;59(4): 354–9.
32. Updated Guidelines for Antiretroviral Postexposure Prophylaxis After Sexual, Injection Drug Use, or Other Nonoccupational Exposure to HIV—United States, 2016. Available at: https://stacks.cdc.gov/view/cdc/38856. Accessed May 12, 2016.
33. Landovitz RJ. Preexposure prophylaxis for HIV prevention: what we know and what we still need to know for implementation. Top Antivir Med 2015;23(2):85–90.
34. Baeten JM, Donnell D, Ndase P, et al. Antiretroviral prophylaxis for HIV prevention in heterosexual men and women. N Engl J Med 2012;367(5):399–410.
35. Choopanya K, Martin M, Suntharasamai P, et al. Antiretroviral prophylaxis for HIV infection in injecting drug users in Bangkok, Thailand (the Bangkok Tenofovir Study): a randomised, double-blind, placebo-controlled phase 3 trial. Lancet 2013;381(9883):2083–90.
36. Grant RM, Lama JR, Anderson PL, et al. Preexposure chemoprophylaxis for HIV prevention in men who have sex with men. N Engl J Med 2010;363(27):2587–99.

37. Marrazzo JM, del Rio C, Holtgrave DR, et al. HIV prevention in clinical care settings: 2014 recommendations of the International Antiviral Society-USA Panel. JAMA 2014;312(4):390–409.
38. Marrazzo JM, Ramjee G, Richardson BA, et al. Tenofovir-based preexposure prophylaxis for HIV infection among African women. N Engl J Med 2015;372(6):509–18.
39. Thigpen MC, Kebaabetswe PM, Paxton LA, et al. Antiretroviral preexposure prophylaxis for heterosexual HIV transmission in Botswana. N Engl J Med 2012; 367(5):423–34.
40. Van Damme L, Corneli A, Ahmed K, et al. Preexposure prophylaxis for HIV infection among African women. N Engl J Med 2012;367(5):411–22.
41. Corneli A, Wang M, Agot K, et al. Perception of HIV risk and adherence to a daily, investigational pill for HIV prevention in FEM-PrEP. J Acquir Immune Defic Syndr 2014;67(5):555–63.
42. Corneli AL, Deese J, Wang M, et al. FEM-PrEP: adherence patterns and factors associated with adherence to a daily oral study product for pre-exposure prophylaxis. J Acquir Immune Defic Syndr 2014;66(3):324–31.
43. McCormack S, Dunn DT, Desai M, et al. Pre-exposure prophylaxis to prevent the acquisition of HIV-1 infection (PROUD): effectiveness results from the pilot phase of a pragmatic open-label randomised trial. Lancet 2015;387(10013):53–60.
44. Patterson KB, Prince HA, Kraft E, et al. Penetration of tenofovir and emtricitabine in mucosal tissues: implications for prevention of HIV-1 transmission. Sci Transl Med 2011;3(112):112re14.
45. Desai K, Sansom SL, Ackers ML, et al. Modeling the impact of HIV chemoprophylaxis strategies among men who have sex with men in the United States: HIV infections prevented and cost-effectiveness. AIDS 2008;22(14):1829–39.
46. Paltiel AD, Freedberg KA, Scott CA, et al. HIV preexposure prophylaxis in the United States: impact on lifetime infection risk, clinical outcomes, and cost-effectiveness. Clin Infect Dis 2009;48(6):806–15.
47. Muessig KE, Cohen MS. Advances in HIV prevention for serodiscordant couples. Curr HIV/AIDS Rep 2014;11(4):434–46.
48. Volk JE, Marcus JL, Phengrasamy T, et al. No New HIV Infections With Increasing Use of HIV Preexposure Prophylaxis in a Clinical Practice Setting. Clin Infect Dis 2015;61(10):1601–3.
49. Grant RM, Liegler T, Defechereux P, et al. Drug resistance and plasma viral RNA level after ineffective use of oral pre-exposure prophylaxis in women. AIDS 2015; 29(3):331–7.
50. Lehman DA, Baeten JM, McCoy CO, et al. Risk of drug resistance among persons acquiring HIV within a randomized clinical trial of single- or dual-agent preexposure prophylaxis. J Infect Dis 2015;211(8):1211–8.
51. Liegler T, Abdel-Mohsen M, Bentley LG, et al. HIV-1 drug resistance in the iPrEx preexposure prophylaxis trial. J Infect Dis 2014;210(8):1217–27.
52. Glidden DV, Buchbinder S, Anderson PL, et al. PrEP Engagement for HIV Prevention: Results From the iPrEx Open Label Extension (OLE). Conference on Retroviruses and Opportunistic Infections (CROI 2015). Seattle, WA, USA, February 23–26, 2015. [Abstract: 970].
53. Molina JM, Capitant C, Spire B, et al. On Demand PrEP With Oral TDF-FTC in MSM: Results of the ANRS IPERGAY Trial. Conference on Retroviruses and Opportunistic Infections (CROI 2015). Seattle, WA, USA, February 23–26, 2015. [Abstract: 23LB].
54. Johnson JA, Sax PE. Beginning antiretroviral therapy for patients with HIV. Infect Dis Clin North Am 2014;28(3):421–38.

55. Gallant JE, Staszewski S, Pozniak AL, et al. Efficacy and safety of tenofovir DF vs stavudine in combination therapy in antiretroviral-naive patients: a 3-year randomized trial. JAMA 2004;292(2):191–201.
56. Martin A, Bloch M, Amin J, et al. Simplification of antiretroviral therapy with tenofovir-emtricitabine or abacavir-Lamivudine: a randomized, 96-week trial. Clin Infect Dis 2009;49(10):1591–601.
57. Taiwo BO, Chan ES, Fichtenbaum CJ, et al. Less Bone Loss With Maraviroc-Versus Tenofovir-Containing Antiretroviral Therapy in the AIDS Clinical Trials Group A5303 Study. Clin Infect Dis 2015;61(7):1179–88.
58. Brown TT, Moser C, Currier JS, et al. Changes in Bone Mineral Density After Initiation of Antiretroviral Treatment With Tenofovir Disoproxil Fumarate/Emtricitabine Plus Atazanavir/Ritonavir, Darunavir/Ritonavir, or Raltegravir. J Infect Dis 2015; 212(8):1241–9.
59. Duvivier C, Kolta S, Assoumou L, et al. Greater decrease in bone mineral density with protease inhibitor regimens compared with nonnucleoside reverse transcriptase inhibitor regimens in HIV-1 infected naive patients. AIDS 2009;23(7):817–24.
60. McComsey GA, Kitch D, Daar ES, et al. Bone mineral density and fractures in antiretroviral-naive persons randomized to receive abacavir-lamivudine or tenofovir disoproxil fumarate-emtricitabine along with efavirenz or atazanavir-ritonavir: Aids Clinical Trials Group A5224s, a substudy of ACTG A5202. J Infect Dis 2011;203(12):1791–801.
61. Tebas P, Powderly WG, Claxton S, et al. Accelerated bone mineral loss in HIV-infected patients receiving potent antiretroviral therapy. AIDS 2000;14(4):F63–7.
62. Brown TT, Qaqish RB. Antiretroviral therapy and the prevalence of osteopenia and osteoporosis: a meta-analytic review. AIDS 2006;20(17):2165–74.
63. Lo Re V 3rd, Volk J, Newcomb CW, et al. Risk of hip fracture associated with hepatitis C virus infection and hepatitis C/human immunodeficiency virus coinfection. Hepatology 2012;56(5):1688–98.
64. Yin MT, Shi Q, Hoover DR, et al. Fracture incidence in HIV-infected women: results from the Women's Interagency HIV Study. AIDS 2010;24(17):2679–86.
65. Young B, Dao CN, Buchacz K, et al, Investigators HIVOS. Increased rates of bone fracture among HIV-infected persons in the HIV Outpatient Study (HOPS) compared with the US general population, 2000-2006. Clin Infect Dis 2011; 52(8):1061–8.
66. McComsey GA, Tebas P, Shane E, et al. Bone disease in HIV infection: a practical review and recommendations for HIV care providers. Clin Infect Dis 2010;51(8): 937–46.
67. Pozniak A, Arribas JR, Gathe J, et al. Switching to tenofovir alafenamide, coformulated with elvitegravir, cobicistat, and emtricitabine, in HIV-infected patients with renal impairment: 48 week results from a single-arm, multi-center, open-label, Phase 3 study. J Acquir Immune Defic Syndr 2016;71(5):530–7.
68. Wohl D, Oka S, Clumeck N, et al. A Randomized, Double-Blind comparison of Tenofovir Alafenamide (TAF) vs. Tenofovir Disoproxil fumarate (TDF), each coformulated with Elvitegravir, Cobicistat, and Emtricitabine (E/C/F) for initial HIV-1 Treatment: Week 96 results. J Acquir Immune Defic Syndr 2016. [Epub ahead of print].
69. Foy M, Sperati CJ, Lucas GM, et al. Drug interactions and antiretroviral drug monitoring. Curr HIV/AIDS Rep 2014;11(3):212–22.
70. Vieira CS, Bahamondes MV, de Souza RM, et al. Effect of antiretroviral therapy including lopinavir/ritonavir or efavirenz on etonogestrel-releasing implant pharmacokinetics in HIV-positive women. J Acquir Immune Defic Syndr 2014;66(4): 378–85.

Index

Note: Page numbers of article titles are in **boldface** type.

Moving?

Make sure your subscription moves with you!

To notify us of your new address, find your **Clinics Account Number** (located on your mailing label above your name), and contact customer service at:

Email: **journalscustomerservice-usa@elsevier.com**

800-654-2452 (subscribers in the U.S. & Canada)
314-447-8871 (subscribers outside of the U.S. & Canada)

Fax number: **314-447-8029**

Elsevier Health Sciences Division
Subscription Customer Service
3251 Riverport Lane
Maryland Heights, MO 63043

*To ensure uninterrupted delivery of your subscription, please notify us at least 4 weeks in advance of move.

Printed and bound by CPI Group (UK) Ltd, Croydon, CR0 4YY

07/10/2024

01040506-0007